A PRIMER OF WATER, ELECTROLYTE, AND ACID-BASE SYNDROMES

A Primer of Water, Electrolyte, and Acid-Base Syndromes
Eighth Edition

Jeffrey M. Brensilver, MD, DIM (Nephrology)
Professor of Clinical Medicine
New York Medical College
Valhalla, New York
Chief of Medicine
New Rochelle Hospital Medical Center
New Rochelle, New York

Emanuel Goldberger, MD, FACP *(deceased)*
Clinical Associate Professor of Medicine
New York Medical College
Valhalla, New York
Attending Cardiologist
New Rochelle Hospital Medical Center
New Rochelle, New York

 F. A. Davis Company ● Philadelphia

F. A. Davis Company
1915 Arch Street
Philadelphia, PA 19103

Previous editions published by Lea & Febiger, Philadelphia, PA.

Printed in the United States of America

Last digit indicates print number: 10 9 8 7 6 5 4 3 2 1

Medical Editor: Robert W. Reinhardt
Medical Developmental Editor: Bernice M. Wissler
Production Editor: Glenn L. Fechner
Cover Designer: Louis J. Forgione

As new scientific information becomes available through basic and clinical research, recommended treatments and drug therapies undergo changes. The author(s) and publisher have done everything possible to make this book accurate, up to date, and in accord with accepted standards at the time of publication. The authors, editors, and publisher are not responsible for errors or omissions or for consequences from application of the book, and make no warranty, expressed or implied, in regard to the contents of the book. Any practice described in this book should be applied by the reader in accordance with professional standards of care used in regard to the unique circumstances that may apply in each situation. The reader is advised always to check product information (package inserts) for changes and new information regarding dose and contraindications before administering any drug. Caution is especially urged when using new or infrequently ordered drugs.

Library of Congress Cataloging in Publication Data

Brensilver, Jeffrey M.
    A primer of water, electrolyte, and acid-base syndromes / Jeffrey M. Brensilver, Emanuel Goldberger. — 8th ed.
        p.   cm.
    Goldberger's name appears first on previous edition.
    Includes bibliographical references and index.
    ISBN 0-8036-0054-2
    1. Water-electrolyte imbalances.   2. Acid-base imbalances.   3. Fluid therapy.
I. Goldberger, Emanuel, 1913–1994.   II. Title.
    [DNLM: 1. Water-Electrolyte Imbalance.   2. Acid-Base Imbalance.   3. Fluid Therapy.   WD 220 B838p 1995]
    RC630.G6   1996
    616.3'99—dc20
    DNLM/DLC
    for Library of Congress   95-11650

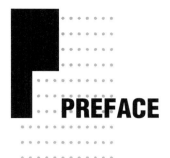

PREFACE

In the first edition of this Primer, Emanuel Goldberger, an innovative cardiologist known for his work in electrocardiography, organized material from the clinical disciplines that would later become the core of the nascent subspecialty of nephrology. The basic organization of the book, which is still retained into this eighth edition—35 years after the first edition—provides an introduction to the commonly encountered clinical syndromes and therapeutic dilemmas of electrolyte and acid-base medicine.

Numerous chapters have been completely revised and others have been added to update the Primer. But the focus remains consistent with the previous seven editions—to provide easily accessible, case-based discussions of electrolyte and acid-base disorders, organized in a fashion consistent with the practice of clinical medicine.

Emanuel Goldberger died at age 81, shortly before the final prepublication revisions of this eighth edition. The author of innumerable textbooks and articles, he had remained active in clinical cardiology and in scholarly medical endeavors until the last weeks of his life.

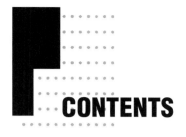

CONTENTS

THE EXTRACELLULAR WATER

1

THE BODY WATER

About a billion years ago, life began—in the sea. The sea possessed unique properties for the maintenance of life. For example, the water of the sea is a solvent for the electrolytes and the oxygen that are necessary for life. The sea is also a solvent for the carbon dioxide that accumulates during life's processes. Since the carbon dioxide is volatile, it can be easily dissipated from the surface of the sea. In addition, the volume of the sea is so great that it can absorb large amounts of heat, or lose large amounts of heat, with only relatively small changes in temperature. The volume of the sea is also so great that significant changes in its composition occur only over a period of hundreds of thousands of years. Finally, its dielectric constant, its surface tension, and other physical properties are all important in maintaining and protecting life.

As a result, the water that surrounds the cells of vertebrates and of humans, namely, the extracellular water, still has an electrolyte composition similar to what the sea had in prerecorded times, in spite of all the countless changes in evolution that have occurred. Over the eons, the rivers of the world have eroded land and have washed elements into the sea. This has caused the electrolytes of the sea to become more concentrated. In spite of this, there is still a remarkable similarity between the proportional composition of electrolytes in seawater and in extracellular water.

TOTAL BODY WATER

The total amount of water in the body can be determined by introducing into the body a known quantity of a substance that diffuses evenly throughout the extracellular water and the cells, and then determining its concentration. Antipyrine, urea, thiourea, and more recently "heavy water" (deuterium oxide or tritium oxide) have been used for this purpose.

THE EXTRACELLULAR WATER

The body water is usually divided into two main compartments: the *extracellular water* (extracellular fluid) and the *intracellular water* (intracellular fluid). The extracellular water includes the plasma water and the *interstitial water* (the fluid in the tissue spaces, lying between the cells). Gastrointestinal secretions, urine, sweat, exudates, and transudates can also be considered as specialized portions of the extracellular water, because when these are lost a severe loss of extracellular water occurs.

The relations of the body water to the body weight are as follows:

Water Compartment	Percentage of Body Weight	Volume in Liters (man, 70 kg)
Plasma water	4	2.8
(plus)		
Interstitial water	16	11.2
Total extracellular water	= 20	= 14
(plus)		
Intracellular water	40	28
Total average body water in a man	= 60	= 42
Total average body water in a 70-kg woman	50	35

These figures represent average values that we shall use in calculating water and electrolyte requirements in this book.

The total body water varies. It is related principally to the fat content of the body, and to sex. Fat has relatively little water associated with it. Therefore, a fat person will have relatively less water than a thin person. In addition, a woman has a lower content of body water than a man. The water content of the body also decreases with age.

The average water content of a man is approximately 60%. The average water content of a woman is approximately 50%.

Body water is also composed of inaccessible bone water and transcellular fluids.

Transcellular fluids include the fluids of organs such as the kidneys, liver, pancreas, skin, and the mucous membranes of the gastrointestinal and respiratory tracts; cerebrospinal fluid; the intraluminal fluid of the gastrointestinal tract; and so on. It is difficult to measure the volume of the fluid in these compartments.

Body water, including percentage of fat and of lean body tissue, can now be measured using a bioelectrical impedance analyzer.

The Electrolytes in the Extracellular Water

Chemists are able to determine the nature and the concentration of the electrolytes in both the extracellular water and the cells. However, the determination of electrolyte concentration in the cells requires special research techniques. Therefore, physicians must rely on the changes in electrolyte concentration in the extracellular water, particularly in the plasma or serum, in treating patients.

The relative concentration of electrolytes in the extracellular water and in the cells is shown in Table 1–1. Notice that sodium (Na) and chloride (Cl) are the principal electrolytes in the extracellular water. However, potassium (K) and phosphates (PO_4) are the principal electrolytes in the cells.

The extracellular preponderance of sodium and the intracellular preponderance of potassium are not due to the impermeability of the cell membrane to sodium, because recent studies with isotopic sodium have shown that the sodium passes rapidly across cell membranes. In other words, some mechanism exists by which sodium is actively extruded from the cells. The extracellular preponderance of sodium ions and the intracellular preponderance of potassium ions are maintained by an energy (ATP) dependent cell membrane "pump" that exchanges sodium and potassium ions.

It should be noted that the electrolyte concentration of the plasma (or serum) is slightly different from the electrolyte concentration in the interstitial portion of the extracellular water. The major difference is that the protein concentration of the plasma is greater than that of the interstitial portion of the extracellular water. This is due to the fact that the capillary walls prevent the outward movement of most of the protein from the plasma. As a result, the sodium concentration in plasma is slightly greater

TABLE 1–1
THE ELECTROLYTE CONCENTRATION OF BODY FLUIDS (mEq/L)*

Solution	Extracellular Fluid	Intracellular Fluid
Cations		
Sodium	142	10
Potassium	4.5	150
Magnesium	2	40
Calcium	4.5	
Total	153	200
Anions		
Chloride	102	
Phosphates	2	120
Sulfates	1	30
Bicarbonate	27	10
Protein	16	40
Organic Acids	5	
Total	153	200

*Adapted from Wilson, RF: Critial Care Manual: Applied Physiology and Principles of Therapy, ed 2. F.A. Davis, Philadelphia, 1992, p 656, with permission.

than the sodium concentration in the interstitial water. Conversely, the chloride concentration in the plasma is slightly less than the chloride concentration in the interstitial water. These differences can be explained by the Donnan equilibrium.

The Donnan Equilibrium

Let us place water on one side of a membrane, and a solution of sodium chloride (NaCl) on the other (Fig. 1–1A). If the membrane is permeable to sodium and chloride ions, the sodium and chloride will pass through the membrane until their concentrations on both sides are equal (Fig. 1–1B).

Now, let us place a sodium chloride solution, NaCl, on one side of the membrane, and a sodium salt of a protein, NaR, on the other side (the symbol R represents the protein ion) (Fig. 1–2A). Let us further suppose that the membrane is impermeable to the protein ion, R, but is permeable to all other ions.

The British physicist Donnan showed that, even in such a case, the sodium chloride on the right side of the membrane will diffuse across the membrane into the left side of the solution (Fig. 1–2B). Furthermore, at equilibrium, the product of the concentrations of the sodium ions and of the chloride ions on one side of the membrane will be the same as the product of the concentrations of the same ions on the other side of the membrane. In other words,

$$Na_1 \times Cl_1 = Na_2 \times Cl_2 \text{ (Fig. 1–2B)}.$$

In compartment (1), the concentration of sodium must be equal to the sum of the other ions, namely, R plus Cl. In compartment (2), on the other side of the membrane, the concentration of sodium (Na) must be the same as that of chloride (Cl). Since the products of sodium times chloride on both sides of the membrane are equal, it follows that the concentration of sodium ions in compartment (1) must be greater than in compartment (2), on the right. The reverse must be true for the chloride ions.

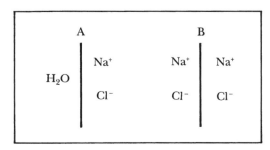

FIGURE 1–1. The Donnan equilibrium. See text.

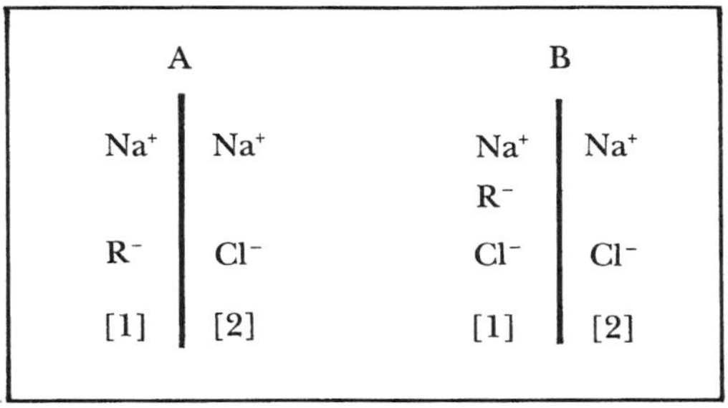

FIGURE 1–2. The Donnan equilibrium. See text.

The Concentration of Electrolytes in the Extracellular Water

Table 1–1 gives the values of the cations and the anions of the extracellular water. An *ion* is an atom or group of atoms with an electrical charge. When it has a positive electrical charge, it is called a *cation*. When it has a negative electrical charge, it is called an *anion*.

The terms "cation" and "anion" can be remembered by the following mnemonic device. A cation has a positive charge. It also has the letter T in it; the T resembles the (+) symbol for a positive charge.

The electrolyte concentrations are given in terms of milliequivalents per liter of serum or plasma (mEq/L).

Milliequivalents

Over 200 years ago, when modern chemistry began, it was noted that the weights of two given elements that could combine chemically with each other always had a fixed ratio or set of ratios. For example, 1 g of hydrogen would combine with 7.937 g of oxygen to form water, or with 35.5 g of chlorine to form hydrochloric acid. Chemists later determined that actually two *atoms* of hydrogen combined with one *atom* of oxygen. In other words, oxygen had a valence of 2, compared with hydrogen. In addition, weights of the hydrogen and oxygen atoms had a ratio of $1:(2 \times 7.937)$, or $1:15.873$.

For convenience, chemists later decided to set the atomic weight of oxygen arbitrarily at 16. The combining or equivalent weight of oxygen therefore became $\frac{16}{2}$ or 8; and hydrogen had both an atomic and a combining or equivalent weight of $\frac{1}{15.873} \times 16$, or 1.008.

This concept of combining or *equivalent weights* is useful. It enables the chemist to predict that 1 g of hydrogen (at. wt. 1; valence 1) will combine with 35.5 g of chlorine (at. wt. 35.5; valence 1), and that 2 g of hydrogen will combine with 16 g of oxygen (at. wt. 16; valence 2). Similarly, 23 g of sodium (at. wt. 23; valence 1) or 39 g of potassium (at. wt. 39; valence 1) will combine with 35.5 g of chlorine.

An equivalent weight or *equivalent* can therefore be described as the atomic weight of an atom (or a group of atoms, such as NH_4, which reacts chemically as a unit, or of a molecule) divided by its valence. Just as a millimeter is $1/1000$ of a meter, a milliequivalent weight or *milliequivalent* is $1/1000$ of an equivalent.

The electrolytes of the body are in solution, mostly in the form of ions. Their concentration can be described in terms of weight, such as milligrams (mg) per deciliter (dL) of blood (mg/dL: a deciliter, or one tenth of a liter, is the same as 100 mL). Since the concentrations of the various electrolytes are small, they are expressed as milliequivalents per liter, mEq/L.

These values are shown in Table 1–1. Notice that the concentration of the cations is the same as the concentration of the anions in blood serum or plasma when expressed in terms of milliequivalents. In other words, each liter of blood has 153 mEq of cations (Na, K, Ca, Mg) and 153 mEq of anions (bicarbonate, chloride, sulfate, phosphate, organic acid anions, and protein anions).

The Relationship Between Milliequivalents and Milligrams

The relationship between milliequivalents and milligrams can be expressed as follows: The weight of a salt in milligrams can be converted into milliequivalents by dividing its weight in milligrams by its molecular weight, and multiplying by the valence.

Example
1 g (1000 mg) NaCl = 17.1 mEq
Proof:
Na (at. wt. 23; valence 1) Cl (at. wt. 35.5; valence 1) Na + Cl = 58.5
$\dfrac{1000}{58.5} = 17.1$ mEq

Since the electrolyte concentrations in blood serum are usually expressed in mEq/L, the following formulas can be used to convert mg/dL into mEq/L, or vice versa:

$$mEq/L = \frac{mg/dL \times 10 \times valence}{atomic\ weight}.$$

$$mg/dL = \frac{mEq/L \times atomic\ weight}{10 \times valence}.$$

Table 1–2 gives conversion factors that enable these values to be obtained more easily.

Moles and Millimoles

There is another way of expressing the weight of chemical substances. A *mole* of a substance is the molecular weight of that substance in grams. For example, the chemical formula of the glucose molecule is $C_6H_{12}O_6$. Since

TABLE 1–2

TABLE FOR CONVERTING SERUM OR PLASMA ELECTROLYTE CONCENTRATIONS IN mEq/L, OR mg/100 mL*

Electrolyte	Calculated as	Atomic weight	Valence	Equivalent weight	Conversion Factors mEq/L from mg/dL—DIVIDE; mg/dL from mEq/L —MULTIPLY	NORMAL RANGES (SERUM OR PLASMA) mg/dL	NORMAL RANGES (SERUM OR PLASMA) mEq/L
Cations							
Sodium	Sodium	23	1	23	2.3	310–335	136–145
Potassium	Potassium	39	1	39	3.9	13.7–19.5	3.5–5.0
Calcium	Total calcium	40	2	20	2	9.0–11	4.5–5.5
Magnesium	Magnesium	24	2	12	1.2	1.8–3.0	1.5–2.5
Anions							
Bicarbonate	CO_2 content			22.26	2.2	53–75 (avg. 62) vol. %	24–33 (avg. 28)
Chloride	Chloride	35.5	1	35.5	3.5	350–375	98–106
Phosphate†	Phosphorus	31	1.8	17.2	1.7	2–4.5	1.2–3.0
Sulfate	Sulfur	32	2	16.	1.6	0.5–2.5	0.3–1.5
Protein	Protein				.41	6–8 g	14.6–19.4

*After Weisberg, and others.

†The phosphate is calculated as phosphorus, with a valence of 1.8. The reason for this is that at the normal pH of the extracellular water, 20% of the phosphate ions are in a form with one sodium equivalent (NaH_2PO_4), and 80% are in a form with two sodium equivalents (Na_2HPO_4). The total valence is therefore $(0.2 \times 1) + (0.8 \times 2) = 1.8$.

carbon has an atomic weight of 12, hydrogen, 1 and oxygen, 16, the molecular weight of glucose is 12×6 (carbon) plus 1×12 (hydrogen) plus 16×6 (oxygen) or 180. Therefore, 1 mole of glucose = 180 g.

A *millimole* (mM) is 1/1000 of a mole. Therefore, 1 millimole of glucose is 1/1000 of 180 g, or 180 mg.

Similarly, the molecular weight of NaCl is: sodium (at. wt. 23) plus chlorine (at. wt. 35.5) or 58.5 g. Therefore, 1 mole NaCl = 58.5 g, and 1 millimole (mM) = 58.5 mg.

The weight of a salt in milligrams can be converted into moles or millimoles by dividing the weight in milligrams by the molecular weight, in a way similar to that used to convert milligrams into equivalents and milliequivalents.

Example

1 g (1000 mg) NaCl = 17.1 millimoles.
1000 divided by the molecular weight of NaCl, which is 58.5 = 17.1.

The concept of moles and millimoles can also be applied to ions, such as Na, K, and HCO_3. A mole of any ion is its atomic weight (or the sum of the atomic weights of its elements) expressed in grams.

Example

1 mole Na (at. wt. 23 = 23 g)
1 mM Na = 23 mg
1 mole HCO_3, (sum of the atomic weights, H, C, and $3-0 = 61$)
  = 61 g

The concentration of gases can also be expressed in terms of milliequivalents. One mole of an ideal gas at a standard temperature of $0°C$, and 760 mm Hg pressure, occupies 22.4 liters. Therefore, 1 millimole occupies 22.4 mL. However, 1 mole of CO_2 occupies a slightly smaller volume of 22.26 liters, and a millimole of CO_2 occupies 22.26 mL.

The concentration of a gas dissolved in a fluid such as water can be expressed in terms of the milliliters of the gas dissolved in 100 mL of the fluid, or in terms of millimoles per liter.

The following formulas can be used to convert volumes percent of CO_2 (or bicarbonate) to millimoles per liter, (or milliequivalents per liter) and vice versa.

$$\text{mM } CO_2/L = \frac{\text{Vol \%* } CO_2}{22.2} \times 10.$$

$$\text{vol \% } CO_2 = \frac{\text{mM } CO_2/L^*}{10} \times 22.2.$$

---

*at $0°C$ and 760 mm Hg

The Relationship Between Milliequivalents and Millimoles

A *mole* is the atomic weight of a substance in grams. An *equivalent* is the atomic weight in grams, divided by the valence. Therefore, if an ion is univalent, an equivalent or a milliequivalent is the same as a mole or a millimole. However, if an ion is bivalent, such as calcium or sulfate, 1 mole equals 2 equivalents, and 1 millimole equals 2 milliequivalents. The reason for this is that 1 millimole of calcium (2 mEq) will react with 2 millimoles of chlorine (2 mEq) to form $CaCl_2$, for example.

THE ACTIVITY CONSTANT OF IONS

Measurement of the concentration of an ion or electrolyte in the blood does not necessarily indicate that this quantity is completely available for chemical reactions, because a portion may be bound to proteins, water, or other ions. A familiar example is the serum calcium concentration, which is partly bound to serum albumin, and is partly ionized. A similar situation exists with other ions, such as sodium and particularly chloride ions, as Dahms and others have shown. The ionized and nonionized percentages of these ions in the blood can both be measured. However, the clinical importance of this information is still not known.

Cation-Anion Balance

Table 1–1 shows that the sum of the cations in serum or plasma equals 153 mEq/L and the sum of the anions also equals 153 mEq/L.

This electrical equivalence of cations and anions in serum or plasma is maintained regardless of whether the sum of the cations (and anions) is greater or less than 153 mEq/L. It may be greater, for example, when water loss occurs. It is often less than 153 mEq/L when electrolytes are lost from the body, as in vomiting or diarrhea.

All the cations can be determined clinically, although it is usual to determine only sodium, potassium, and calcium routinely. Chloride is the only anion that is routinely determined in studying electrolyte disturbances. The bicarbonate concentration can be calculated from the CO_2 content. Under ordinary conditions it is usually between 0.6 and 1.8 mEq/L less than the CO_2 content. However, for purposes of simplicity, one can calculate all the bicarbonate concentrations by subtracting 1 mEq/L from the CO_2 content.

The sum of phosphates, sulfates, organic acid anions, and proteins is described by the symbol R, which is calculated as follows:

The Significance of Anions Labeled R

In previous editions of the book, the term R (residual ions) was used to describe unmeasured ions, such as plasma proteins and inorganic and organic acid anions in the plasma, which may be present normally or may accumulate in some patients with metabolic acidosis.

R is calculated as follows:

$$R = Na + K + 6.5 \text{ (the sum of Ca and Mg)} - (HCO_3 + Cl).$$
$$\text{Normally, the value of R is 22 mEq/L or less.}$$

However, measurement of the anion gap (see below) is a simpler way of describing an accumulation of abnormal anions.

The Anion Gap

The *anion* gap (or *delta*) also describes the residual or unmeasured anions.

Since the concentration of anions such as phosphates, sulfates, and organic acid and protein anions is not ordinarily measured, the sum of the *measured cations* (Na, K, Ca) will be greater than the sum of the *measured anions* (HCO_3 and Cl). This difference is known as the *anion gap* (or *delta*).

The following simple formula can be used to determine if an abnormal gap is present:

$$\text{Anion gap} = (Na + K) - (HCO_3 + Cl).$$

Normally, the anion gap is 16 mEq/L or less. (An anion gap of less than 9 mEq/L is extremely unlikely, and is probably the result of a laboratory error.)

An alternate formula for measuring the anion gap is:

$$Na - (HCO_3 + Cl).$$

When this formula is used, the average normal value for the anion gap is 12 mEq/L, with a range of 8 to 16 mEq/L.

Example
Na 142   K 4   HCO$_3$ 27   Cl 103 mEq/L
Anion Gap $= (Na + K) - (HCO_3 + Cl)$.
$(142 + 4) - (27 + 103)$.
$146 - 130 = 16$ mEq/L.
This is normal.

When metabolic acidosis is present with an *abnormal* anion gap, the value of the anion gap is usually more than 22 mEq/L.

INCREASED ANION GAP. This can occur in the following ways:

1. Increased unmeasured anions, such as the accumulation of lactic acid in lactic acidosis; aceto-acetic acid, in diabetic ketoacidosis; organic or keto acids caused by the ingestion of salicylates, paraldehyde, ethylene glycol, organic acids in hyperosmolal hyperglycemic nonketoacidotic

diabetic coma; phosphoric, sulfuric, and organic acids in azotemia; formic acid in methanol (methyl alcohol) poisoning: ketoglutaric acid in hepatic failure; other anions, including high doses of (sodium) penicillin, and (sodium) carbenicillin.

2. Decreased unmeasured cations, for example, potassium, in hypokalemia (if the alternate formula above is used); calcium in hypocalcemia; magnesium in hypomagnesemia.

3. Water loss.

   If water loss occurs in the patient described above and the serum concentrations rise 10%, the following concentrations would be present:

$$Na\ 156.2 \quad K\ 4.4 \quad HCO_3\ 29.7 \quad Cl\ 113.3\ mEq/L$$

$$
\begin{aligned}
\text{Anion gap} &= (Na + K) = (HCO_3 + Cl) \\
&= (156.2 + 4.4) - (29.7 + 113.3) \\
&= 160.6 - 143.0 \\
&= 17.6\ mEq/L. \text{ This is } 10\% \text{ greater than the} \\
&\quad \text{original ion gap.}
\end{aligned}
$$

4. Metabolic alkalosis. The plasma proteins give up H ions and increase their net negative charge. As a result, the measured anion concentration of the plasma is apparently low. In addition, alkalosis is associated with a decreased extracellular volume (water loss—see above).

   (The total anion value must equal the total cation value of the plasma. When alkalosis develops, the anion value of the proteins increases. However, the anion value of the proteins is not measured. Therefore, there is a spurious decrease of the measured anions, and an apparent increase in the anion gap.)

5. Increased unmeasured anions, such as increased phosphate, or sulfate ions, or due to treatment with intravenous solutions containing lactate, citrate or acetate ions.

6. Laboratory errors, with falsely high serum Na or falsely low serum Cl or HCO_3 values.

THE SIGNIFICANCE OF AN INCREASED ANION GAP IN METABOLIC ACIDOSIS. When a metabolic acidosis is present with an increased anion gap, the value of the anion gap is usually more than 22 mEq/L. Clinically, the anion gap is important, because, when a metabolic acidosis occurs, it may or may not be associated with an accumulation of abnormal unmeasured anions (and with an increased anion gap). For example, the anion gap is increased in metabolic acidosis patients described under category 1 above. However, other patients with metabolic acidosis do not have an accumulation of unmeasured anions and do not show an increased anion gap. Instead, they show an increased concentration of chloride ions (hyperchloremic metabolic acidosis). The separation of patients with a hyperchloremic metabolic acidosis from those with an increased anion gap is clinically useful and is described in Chapter 17.

DECREASED ANION GAP. This can occur in the following ways:

1. Decreased unmeasured anions, as in hypoalbuminemia. This is probably the most common cause of a decreased anion gap. A normal value of 4 g/dL of serum albumin provides 11 mEq/L of anions. Therefore, when the serum albumin content decreases from 4 to 3 g/dL, for example, the anion gap should decrease by 2.75 mEq/L.
2. Increased unmeasured cations; for example, increased serum calcium in hypercalcemia, increased serum magnesium in hypermagnesemia or increased serum potassium in hyperkalemia (if the alternate formula above has been used). Other abnormal cations include IgG globulin in multiple myeloma or other paraproteinemias, tromethamine (TRIS buffer), polymyxin B, lithium, or bromine. Bromide intoxication may give falsely low serum chloride levels, unless the Cl is measured by means of a potentiometer technique.
3. Water excess.

   If water excess occurs and the serum electrolyte concentrations decrease by 10% in the patient described above, the following concentrations would be present:

$$Na\ 127.8 \qquad K\ 3.6 \qquad HCO_3\ 24.3 \qquad Cl\ 92.7\ mEq/L$$
$$\begin{aligned} \text{Anion gap} &= (Na + K) - (HCO_3 + Cl) \\ &= (127.8 + 3.6) - (24.3 + 92.7) \\ &= 131.4 - 117.0 \\ &= 14.4\ mEq/L. \text{ This is } 10\% \text{ less than the} \\ &\quad \text{original anion gap of } 16\ mEq/L. \end{aligned}$$

4. Laboratory errors giving a falsely low serum Na or a falsely high serum Cl or HCO_3. A falsely low serum Na may also occur if the serum is viscous. As a result, the blood sample has a smaller volume than usual.

A simultaneous increase in both the anion gap and the gap between calculated and measured osmolality (see Chapter 11) suggests diabetic acidosis, alcoholic acidosis, or methanol or ethylene glycol poisoning. Methanol and ethylene glycol are metabolized to organic acids that cause a metabolic acidosis with an elevated anion gap. They also cause an osmolal gap (see Chapter 11).

The Relation of Serum Sodium to Bicarbonate and Chloride Concentrations

There is another relation between the cations and anions that can be used, namely, the relation between serum sodium concentration and the sum of the serum bicarbonate and chloride ions. In Table 1–1, it will be noted that the most important cation is sodium, and that the most important anions are bicarbonate and chloride. In most cases, the following relations between these three ions exist:

$$Na = HCO_3 + Cl + 12\ mEq/L$$

Example

Na 142 HCO_3 27   Cl 103 mEq/L

142 = 27 + 103 + 12.

In other words, if the bicarbonate and chloride ion concentrations in serum or plasma are known, the concentration of sodium can be determined from these values, using the above rule.

The major exceptions to this rule occur in patients with a metabolic acidosis who show an abnormal anion gap, because the abnormal anions are not ordinarily measured (see above). This increased anion concentration in the plasma causes the bicarbonate concentration to be reduced without necessarily affecting the sodium or chloride concentrations. The reason for this is discussed in the chapters on metabolic acidosis.

The calculated serum sodium concentration may also be incorrectly high if hyperchloremia is present.

The calculated serum sodium concentration may also be incorrectly low if the bicarbonate concentration is high due to a respiratory acidosis.

Bibliography

Blume, RS, MacLowry, JD, and Wolff, SM: Limitations of chloride determination in the diagnosis of bromism. N Engl J Med 279:593, 1968.

Brozek, J: Body composition. Ann New York Acad Sci 110:425, 1963.

Dahms, H, Rock, R, and Seligson, D: Ionic activities of sodium, potassium, and chloride in human serum. Clin Chem 14:859, 1968.

Edelman, IS, and Leibman, J: Anatomy of body water and electrolytes. Am J Med 27:256, 1959.

Gamble, JL: Chemical Anatomy: Physiology and Pathology of Extracellular Fluid, 6th ed. Cambridge, Harvard University Press, 1954.

Hald, PM, Heinsen, AJ, and Peters, JP: Estimation of serum sodium from bicarbonate plus chloride. J Clin Invest 26:983, 1947.

Hays, RM: Dynamics of body water and electrolytes. In Maxwell, MH and Kleeman, CR (eds): Clinical Disorders of Fluid and Electrolyte Metabolism. New York, McGraw-Hill Book Co., 1980.

Henderson, LJ: The Fitness of the Environment. New York, Macmillan, 1913.

Leaf, A, and Newburgh, LH: Significance of Body Fluids in Clinical Medicine, 2nd ed. Springfield, Ill.,Charles C Thomas, 1955.

Maccallum, AB: The paleochemistry of the body fluids and tissues. Physiol Rev 6:316, 1926.

Moore, FD, Haley, HB, Bering, EA, Brooks, L, and Edelman, IS: Further observations on total body water. Surg Gynec Obstet 95:155, 1952.

Moore, FD, Olesen, KH, McMurrey, JD, Parker, HV, Ball, MR, and Boyden, CM: The Body Cell Mass and Its Supporting Environment. Philadelphia, W.B. Saunders, 1963.

Olmstead, EG: Mammalian Cell Water. Physiologic and Clinical Aspects. Philadelphia, Lea & Febiger, 1966.

Robin, ED, and Bromberg, PA: Claude Bernard's milieu interieur extended: Intracellular acid-base relationships. Am J Med 27:689, 1959.

Ross, EJ, ed: Clinical Effects of Electrolyte Disturbances. Philadelphia, J.B. Lippincott, 1959.

Snively, WD, Jr: An example of atavistic physiology? JAMA 204:392, 1968.

Steele, JM, et al: Total body water in man. Am J Physiol 162:313, 1950.

Strauss, MB: Body Water in Man. Boston, Little, Brown & Co., 1957.

Ussing, HH: Ion transport across biological membranes. In Ion Transport Across Membranes (Clarke, HT, ed). New York, Academic Press, 1954.

Williams, RJP, and Wacker, WEC: Cation balance in biological systems. JAMA 201:18, 1967.

Anion Gaps

Askenazi, J, et al: Spurious increases in the anion gap due to exposure of serum to air. Letter. N Engl J Med 307:190, 1982.

Cole, DEC, and Scriver, CR: Unexplained serum anion gap. Letter. N Engl J Med 304:542, 1981.

de Troyer, A, et al: Value of anion gap determination in multiple myeloma. N Engl J Med 296:858, 1977.

Emmett, M, and Narins, RG: Clinical use of the anion gap. Medicine (Baltimore), 56:38, 1977.

Gabow, PA, and Kaehny, WD: The anion gap. Its meaning and clinical utility. The Kidney 12:(2), March 1979.

Graber, ML, et al: Spurious hyperchloremia and decreased anion gap in hyperlipidemia. Ann Intern Med 98:607, 1983.

Gabow, PA, et al: Diagnostic importance of an increased serum anion gap. N Engl J Med 303:854, 1980.

Goldstein, RJ, et al: The myth of the low anion gap. JAMA 253:1737, 1980.

Jacobsen, D, et al: Anion and osmolal gaps in the diagnosis of methanol and ethylene glycol poisoning. Acta Med Scandinav 212:17, 1982.

Keshgegian, AA: Hypoalbuminemia and decreased anion gap. Letter. JAMA 247:1697, 1982.

Madrias, NE, Ayus, CJ, and Adrogue, HJ: Increased anion gap in metabolic alkalosis. The role of plasma-protein equivalency. N Engl J Med 300:1421, 1979.

Oh, MS, and Carroll, HJ: Current Concepts. The anion gap. N Engl J Med 297:814, 1977.

Smithline, N, and Gardner, KD, Jr: Gaps—anionic and osmolal. JAMA 236:1594, 1976.

Weisberg, H: Water, Electrolyte and Acid-Base Balance, Baltimore, Williams & Wilkins, 1953.

2

THE OSMOTIC PRESSURE
AND THE VOLUME OF THE
EXTRACELLULAR WATER

OSMOTIC PRESSURE

A *solute* is a substance, such as sodium chloride, potassium phosphate, glucose, or protein, which can dissolve in a *solvent*, such as water, to make a *solution*.

If we take a solution of sodium chloride in water, for example, and place it on one side of a membrane that is permeable to both the sodium and chloride ions and to the water molecules, and if we place water on the other side of the membrane, the sodium and chloride ions and the water molecules will pass freely through both sides of the membrane until the concentration of sodium and chloride on both sides is equal.

However, we can prepare a membrane that will allow a solvent such as water to pass freely, but that will not allow a substance such as sodium chloride or glucose or protein to pass. If we place such a sodium chloride solution in a funnel, the mouth of which is sealed by such a semipermeable membrane, and then place the mouth of the funnel in a container of water, the sodium and the chloride ions will not be able to pass through the membrane. However, the water molecules will be able to pass through in either direction and they will enter the funnel and the level of the solution in the funnel will rise (Fig. 2–1). The rise continues until the hydrostatic pressure exerted by the column of fluid in the funnel is equal to the pressure exerted by the water molecules as they pass through the membrane into the funnel. When this occurs, the hydrostatic pressure prevents any further increase of volume in the salt solution. The height of the fluid in the funnel tube is therefore a measure of the osmotic pressure of the salt solution, and is dependent upon the

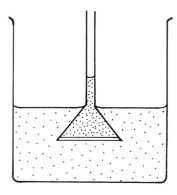

FIGURE 2–1. Diagram showing the effect of osmotic pressure. See text.

number of particles or ions of the salt in a given volume of solution. In other words, a more concentrated salt solution would have a greater osmotic pressure, and a less concentrated salt solution would have a lesser osmotic pressure.

Osmotic pressure is measured in terms of osmoles (Osm) or *milliosmoles* (mOsm). An osmole (or a milliosmole) of a substance such as glucose, which does not dissociate into ions, is the same as a mole (or a millimole). However, a mole of a salt such as sodium chloride, which dissociates almost completely into sodium and chloride ions, equals 2 osmoles.

A mole of a salt such as sodium bicarbonate, which dissociates into sodium, Na, and bicarbonate (HCO_3) ions, also equals 2 osmoles. A mole of a more complex salt such as Na_2HPO_4, which dissociates into 2 Na and 1 HPO_4 ions, equals 3 osmoles. The total osmotic pressure of a solution therefore is calculated from the sum of all the ions in solution.

We can now perform another experiment. For example, in Figure 2–2 a sodium chloride solution and a potassium phosphate solution are separated by a membrane that is impermeable to all these ions, but that is freely permeable to the water in which the ions are dissolved.

Let us assume that the concentration of sodium chloride is 310 mOsm/L, and that the potassium phosphate solution has equal osmolal concentration. Since the osmotic *pressure* is the same on both sides of the membrane, there will not be any movement of water, regardless of the volume on either side of the membrane (Fig. 2–2).

However, if we place a solution of sodium chloride with a lower osmotic concentration, for example, 290 mOsm/L, on one side of the membrane, and a solution of potassium phosphate with a higher osmotic concentration of 310 mOsm/L on the other side, the osmotic pressure of the sodium chloride solution will be less than that of the potassium phosphate solution. Be-

NaCl	K_2HPO_4
14 L	28 L
310 mOsm/L	310 mOsm/L
4340 mOsm	8680 mOsm

FIGURE 2–2. Diagram showing osmotic equilibrium. See text.

cause of this, water will flow from the sodium chloride solution to the potassium phosphate solution in order to equalize the osmotic pressures. As a result of this, the volume of the sodium chloride solution will decrease, and the concentration of the sodium chloride will rise toward normal (Fig. 2–3). (The method of calculating the shift in water is described in Appendix 1.)

These experiments demonstrate a fundamental rule of osmotic pressure, namely: *water will flow from a region of low to a region of higher osmotic pressure.*

In the human and in animals, it is assumed that the osmotic pressures of the extracellular water and of the cells are the same. However, there are

Before osmotic equilibrium

14 L	28 L
290 mOsm/L	310 mOsm/L
4060 mOsm	8680 mOsm
NaCl	K_2HPO_4

After osmotic equilibrium

13.4 L	28.6 L
303 mOsm/L	303 mOsm/L
4060 mOsm	8680 mOsm
NaCl	K_2HPO_4

FIGURE 2–3. Diagram showing the shift of water due to a disturbance in osmotic equilibrium. See text.

observations that this may not be correct. The osmotic pressure of the cells may be higher than that of the extracellular water and a constant gradient may normally be maintained between them by a constant active extrusion of water by the cells. However, even if this is so, it does not invalidate the concept that the osmotic pressures of the extracellular water and of the cells are in equilibrium, and that a change in the osmotic pressure of either the extracellular water or the cells will cause a flow of water either into or out of the cells.

In the human, the osmotic pressure of the extracellular water and of the cells is 310 mOsm/L. The significance of this is the following: In the plasma (or serum) and in the extracellular water, the sodium concentration is 142 mEq/L and the total cation concentration is 155 mEq/L. Practically all the osmotic pressure of the extracellular water is a result of monovalent salts, which ionize into two ions each. Therefore, the osmotic pressure of the extracellular water is twice the cation (or anion) concentration, or $2 \times 155 = 310$ mOsm/L. We can make the following assumption: Sodium is the chief cation of the extracellular water. Therefore, the osmotic pressure of the extracellular water should vary proportionately with the sodium concentration of the serum or plasma. In other words, we should be able to use the serum sodium concentration as a measure of the osmotic pressure of the extracellular water. Unfortunately, this relationship is valid only in normal subjects. This is discussed further in Chapter 6.

THE DIFFERENCE BETWEEN OSMOTIC PRESSURE AND ONCOTIC PRESSURE

The term "osmotic pressure" should be differentiated from the term "oncotic pressure," or "colloid osmotic pressure." The osmotic pressure of a solution varies with the number of molecules in a solution, as was pointed out above. When the molecular weight of a substance is low, there will be more molecules of the substance per unit weight, and the osmotic pressure will be greater. For example, a substance such as mannitol, which has a low molecular weight, will increase the osmotic pressure when given intravenously. However, a substance such as human albumin, or dextran, which has a high molecular weight around 80,000, will not increase the osmotic pressure greatly. However, such a substance exerts an oncotic pressure (colloid osmotic pressure) because it is confined by a membrane (the vascular system) to which it is relatively impermeable. Therefore, an infusion of albumin or dextran will greatly increase the oncotic pressure of the blood and will prevent the loss of excessive fluid from the capillaries. However, it will have an almost negligible effect on the osmotic pressure of the blood. Oncotic pressure is measured in terms of pressure units (mm Hg).

FACTORS REGULATING THE OSMOTIC PRESSURE AND THE VOLUME OF THE EXTRACELLULAR WATER

We have just pointed out that a primary change of osmotic pressure, either in the extracellular water or in the cells, is associated with a shift of water into or out of the extracellular water, and consequently is associated with a change in the volume of the extracellular water.

In the maintenance of life, the body has homeostatic or regulatory mechanisms that help to maintain the osmotic pressure and the volume of the extracellular water within physiological limits. The osmotic pressure of the extracellular water is controlled by the posterior pituitary antidiuretic hormone (ADH). The volume of the extracellular water is controlled partly by the adrenal cortical hormone aldosterone. We can now consider the action of these two hormones.

ADH, the Antidiuretic Hormone of the Posterior Pituitary Gland

Some authors use the abbreviation AVP (arginine vasopressin), the chemical name of the antidiuretic hormone, instead of ADH. However, the abbreviation ADH is so well known that we shall continue to use it.

ADH, the antidiuretic hormone of the posterior pituitary gland, is an octapeptide (arginine vasopressin). It is produced by neurons of the supraoptic nuclei of the hypothalamus, and is stored in axon endplates that terminate in the posterior pituitary gland.

The site of action of ADH is probably the distal tubules and collecting ducts of the kidneys. ADH increases the permeability of these structures to water. When this occurs, an increased amount of water is reabsorbed, the volume of urine decreases, and the osmolality of the urine increases.

ADH secretion can be stimulated in three ways:

1. Osmotic stimulation of ADH secretion—hyperosmolality. The most important action of ADH is to maintain the osmotic pressure of the extracellular water in relation to the osmotic pressure of the cells. The stimulus for the secretion of ADH is the *relative* osmotic pressure of the neurons (cells) of the supraoptic nuclei of the hypothalamus, that is, the osmotic pressure of these neurons in relation to the osmotic pressure of the extracellular water. When the osmotic pressure of the extracellular water becomes relatively greater than the osmotic pressure of these neurons, ADH secretion increases. For example, if a large amount of glucose is infused into the body, it will raise the osmotic pressure of the extracellular water. Therefore the osmotic pressure of the extracellular water will rise above that of the neurons. As a result, ADH secretion will occur and water excretion by the kidneys will decrease.

2. Nonosmotic stimulation of ADH secretion. ADH secretion can also be stimulated by way of central neural pathways, from the midbrain reticular formation to the supraoptic area. These neural receptors respond to emotional stress, fever, trauma, infections, major operations, most anesthetics, and most analgesics, anticholinergic drugs, barbiturates, morphine, meperidine (Demerol), cytoxan, carbamazine, vincristine, and others.

3. ADH secretion is also partly controlled by changes in blood volume. There are volume receptors in the left atrial wall that are stimulated when the left atrial pressure falls. Therefore, procedures that promote pooling of blood in peripheral vessels, such as warm ambient temperature or quiet standing, tend to decrease left atrial filling and stimulate ADH secretion. Similarly, intermittent or continuous positive pressure respiration also decreases left atrial filling pressure and stimulates ADH secretion. A decreased arterial blood pressure resulting from contraction of the vascular or extracellular volume or from a decreased cardiac output also stimulates ADH secretion.

Inhibition of ADH secretion can also occur from osmotic or nonosmotic causes.

1. Osmotic inhibition of ADH secretion—hypo-osmolality. When the osmotic pressure of the neurons of the supraoptic nuclei of the hypothalamus show an increased osmotic pressure *relative* to the osmotic pressure of the extracellular water, ADH secretion is inhibited. For example, if a person drinks plain water, the immediate effect of the imbibed water is to dilute the extracellular water. This causes the osmotic pressure of the extracellular water to become lower (at least temporarily) than the osmotic pressure of the neurons. As a result, ADH secretion decreases or stops and a water diuresis occurs.

2. Nonosmotic inhibition of ADH secretion. Increased arterial blood pressure, increased tension in the left atrial wall and great pulmonary veins secondary to expansion of the vascular or extracellular volume with a rise in cardiac output, quiet resting in a supine position, exposure to cool ambient temperature, or negative-pressure breathing will increase left atrial filling and decrease ADH secretion. Drugs such as alcohol and phenytoin will also inhibit ADH secretion.

The usual stimulus for the secretion of ADH is water loss. This causes the osmotic pressure of the extracellular water to become greater than that of the cells. ADH secretion occurs in an attempt to decrease water loss through the kidneys. In addition, ADH secretion often occurs as a result of other factors, as mentioned above.

The regulation of osmotic pressure is more important than the regulation of blood and extracellular water volume. Therefore, when the osmotic pressure of the blood and extracellular water (in relation to the osmotic pressure of the cells) decreases, and the blood and extracellular volume also decrease, *the osmotic pressure should be corrected first.*

If the volume deficit is corrected with a solution of 5% dextrose in water, for example, which does not significantly raise the plasma osmolality, the blood and extracellular water will be further diluted, their osmotic pressures will decrease further, and more water will pass into the cells, again decreasing the blood volume, after the initial temporary increase in blood volume resulting from the dextrose and water infusion. However, if a solution of isotonic saline (sodium chloride solution), or dextrose in isotonic saline, or plasma, or dextran, etc., which has a significant osmolality, is infused, the increased osmolality will draw water from the cells into the extracellular water and blood, thereby increasing the blood volume as well as restoring plasma osmolality.

Haberich and others have shown that the liver also acts as an osmoreceptor to regulate the intake of water from the gastrointestinal tract. When water is imbibed, it is absorbed into the splanchnic circulation and is brought to the liver by way of the portal vein. This causes the osmolality of the portal vein to decrease rapidly. This stimulates the liver, and afferent stimuli are sent to the hypothalamus by way of the vagus nerve. The hypothalamus then stimulates the kidneys to excrete water.

Aldosterone and the Volume of the Extracellular Water

Aldosterone is secreted by the cells of the glomerulosa zone of the adrenal cortex. Its secretion can be stimulated in several ways:

1. It responds to factors (sodium depletion, hemorrhage, diuretic therapy, and so on) that decrease the effective circulating blood volume and reduce renal perfusion. Apparently, the renal afferent arterioles act as volume receptors, which respond to decreased renal arterial pressure and decreased renal blood flow by increasing the release of renin from the juxtaglomerular cells. Renin causes the formation of angiotensin II in the blood. This directly stimulates aldosterone secretion. As a result, sodium ions (and water) are retained and the circulating blood volume rises. When this occurs, the juxtaglomerular cell secretion of renin is inhibited and aldosterone secretion stops.
2. Aldosterone secretion is also influenced by serum potassium concentration. Any factor that raises the serum potassium concentration stimulates aldosterone secretion. As a result, a diuresis of potassium ions occurs. Conversely, hypokalemia is associated with a reduced aldosterone secretion and a retention of potassium ions.
3. ACTH can also cause a transient increase in aldosterone secretion.

A deficiency of aldosterone secretion occurs usually in Addison's disease, although it may be present as an isolated abnormality (hypoaldosteronism). It is associated with a loss of sodium ions (and water), hypotension or shock, and hyperkalemia.

Patients with increased aldosterone secretion may show various syndromes. Patients with primary aldosteronism show hypokalemia but usually no edema. Patients with secondary aldosteronism caused by congestive heart failure, cirrhosis of the liver, the nephrotic syndrome, or malignant hypertension may show extensive edema.

Natriuretic Hormone (Atrial Natriuretic Factor [ANF])

It has been known for many years that dogs respond to saline infusions with a prompt increase both in sodium excretion and in glomerular filtration rate. Originally, this increased excretion of sodium was attributed to the increased filtration of sodium through the glomeruli. Studies by deWardener and many others have indicated that the increased excretion of sodium is related to a *decreased* tubular reabsorption of sodium from the proximal tubules of the kidneys. A similar loss or "escape" of sodium from the kidneys occurs when salt-retaining hormones, such as aldosterone and 11-desoxycorticosterone, are administered over a prolonged period of time to normal human subjects. This is an explanation for the observation that patients with primary hyperaldosteronism do not develop marked edema.

The cardiac atria are the site of ANF. Specific receptors occur throughout the arterial vasculature and in the tubules.

SIMULTANEOUS CHANGES IN OSMOTIC PRESSURE AND IN THE VOLUME OF EXTRACELLULAR WATER

Isolated changes in osmotic pressure and in the volume of extracellular water can occur. Under most conditions, there are simultaneous changes in osmotic pressure and volume. It is preferable to consider these changes from the broad clinical point of view of the patient rather than from a limited physiological point of view. Therefore, in the chapters that follow, these disturbances in volume and osmotic pressure are described in terms of the clinical syndromes with which they are associated.

Bibliography

Barron, WM, et al.: Transient vasopressin—resistant diabetes insipidus of pregnancy. N Engl J Med 310:442, 1984.
Burg, MB, and Orloff, J: Control of fluid absorption in the renal proximal tubules. J Clin Invest 47:2016, 1968.
deWardener, HE, and Clarkson, EM: The natriuretic hormone. Recent developments. Clin Sci 63:415, 1982.
Davis, JO: Aldosterone and angiotensin. Interrelationship in normal and diseased states. JAMA 188:1062, 1964.

Davis, JO, Urquhart, J, and Higgins, JT, Jr: Effects of alterations of plasma sodium and potassium concentration on aldosterone secretion. J Clin Invest 42:597, 1963.

de Zeeuw D, Janssen WMT, de Jong PE: Atrial natriuretic factor: Its (patho) physiological significance in humans. Kidney Int 41:1115, 1992.

Fauchald PF: Transcapillary colloid osmotic pressure gradient and body fluid volumes in renal failure. Kidney Int 29:895, 1986.

Galambos, JT, Herndon, EG, Jr., and Reynolds, GH: Specific-gravity determination. Fact or fancy? N Engl J Med 270:506, 1964.

Gann, DS, Delea, CS, Gill, JR, Jr., Thomas, JP, and Bartter, FC: Control of aldosterone secretion by change in body potassium in normal man. Am J Physiol 207:104, 1964.

Gauer, OH: Osmocontrol versus volume control. Fed Proc 27:1132, 1968.

Gross, F: The regulation of aldosterone secretion by the renin-angiotensin system under various conditions. Acta Endocr Suppl. 124, 41, 1967.

Haberich, FJ: Osmoreception in the portal circulation. Fed Proc 27:1137, 1968.

Hays, RM: Antidiuretic hormone. N Engl J Med 295:659, 1976.

Jacobson, MH, Levy, SE, Kaufman, RM, Gallinek, WE, and Donnelly, OW. Urine osmolality. Arch Intern Med 110:121, 1962.

Kiil F: Molecular mechanisms of osmosis. Am J Physiol 256:R801, 1989.

Laragh, JH: Potassium, angiotensin and the dual control of aldosterone secretion. N Engl J Med 289:745, 1973.

Lichardus, B, and Pearce, JW: Evidence for a humoral natriuretic factor released by blood volume expansion. Nature 209:407, 1966.

Maffly, LH, and Leaf, A: The intracellular osmolality of the mammalian tissues. J Clin Invest 37:916, 1958.

Mills, IH: Atrial natriuretic factor. A new hormone? Editorial BMJ 289:210, 1984.

Rector, FC, et al: Demonstration of a hormonal inhibitor of proximal tubular reabsorption during expansion of extracellular volume with isotonic saline. J Clin Invest 47:761, 1968.

Robinson, JR: Osmoregulation in surviving slices from the kidneys of adult rats. Proc Roy Soc London, Series B, 137:378, 1950.

Share, L: Effects of carotid occlusion and left atrial distention on plasma vasopressin titer. Am J Physiol 203:219, 1965.

Sonnenberg, H, et al: A humoral component of the natriuretic mechanism in sustained blood volume expansion. J Clin Invest 51:2631, 1972.

Verney, EB: Absorption and excretion of water: The antidiuretic hormone. Lancet 2:739, 781, 1946. Also Surg Gynecol Obstet 106:441, 1958.

Zehr, JE, Johnson, JA, and Moore, WE: Left atrial pressure, plasma osmolality and ADH levels in the unanesthetized ewe. Am J Physiol 217:1672, 1969.

Zerbe, RL, and Robertson, GL: A comparison of plasma vasopressin measurements with a standard indirect test in the differential diagnosis of polyuria. N Engl J Med 305:1540, 1981.

SYNDROMES ASSOCIATED WITH WATER DISTURBANCES

3

WATER LOSS SYNDROMES

Desiccation occurs as a result of a loss of water from the body, which can be caused by either a decreased intake of water or an excessive loss of water through the lungs, skin, kidneys, or gastrointestinal tract. In most patients, it is a result of a decreased intake of water.

Synonyms for desiccation are pure dehydration, dehydration hypertonicity, water deficit, water deficiency, pure water depletion.

The term "dehydration" has been used to describe not only the syndromes associated with a loss of water but also the completely different syndromes associated with a loss of salt (sodium ions), with or without a concomitant loss of water. Therefore, we shall not use it in this book.

ETIOLOGY

Water loss can occur in the following ways:

1. Water loss secondary to inadequate water intake. This can occur in several ways:
   a. In shipwrecked sailors, people lost in the desert, or those who have been injured and are immobilized. Water loss will occur more rapidly if a castaway tries to drink seawater, because the kidneys have to excrete the extra salt with a large amount of water. Similarly, those stranded on land will become desiccated more quickly if they are directly exposed to the sun.
   b. When swallowing is difficult or impossible. This occurs in debilitated patients, comatose patients, or in patients with dysphagia.
   c. When the sense of thirst is impaired, as in elderly patients with cerebral atherosclerosis, patients with cerebral tumors, poliomyelitis of the bulbar type, meningitis, or cerebral injury. (Cerebral injury can also cause diabetes insipidus and water loss in this way.)

2. Water loss secondary to loss through the kidneys. This can occur in patients with normal or with impaired renal function.
   a. Water loss in patients with normal kidneys can occur with:
      i. Central (neurogenic, vasopressin-sensitive) diabetes insipidus. Here, the kidneys are unable to concentrate water normally, because of a lack of the posterior pituitary antidiuretic hormone ADH. Alcoholics may lose water in a similar way, because the alcohol inhibits the secretion of ADH.
      ii. Solute excess (Chapter 4) or hyperosmolality (Chapter 5).
   b. Water loss in patients with impaired kidney function can occur when the kidneys show a decreased ability to conserve water because of renal tubular dysfunction (*nephrogenic diabetes insipidus*). As a result, the kidneys do not respond normally to ADH.

      This can occur in chronic pyelonephritis, glomerulonephritis, polycystic kidneys, during the diuretic phase of acute renal failure, partial urinary tract obstruction, hypokalemia, hypercalcemia, primary aldosteronism, amyloidosis, gout, multiple myeloma, Sjögren's syndrome, sickle-cell anemia affecting the kidneys, after transplantation of a kidney, as a result of high-dose lithium carbonate intake, demeclocycline (declomycin), ethanol, opium antagonists, or as a toxic effect of penthrane (methoxyflurane) anesthesia. It can also occur as a congenital anomaly.
3. Water loss arising from other causes, for example,
   a. Excessive loss of water from the lungs. Prolonged exposure to the sun's heat without water intake, hyperventilation, and fever can cause a large loss in water volume this way. A tracheotomy accelerates the pulmonary water loss, because it reduces the dead air fraction of the tidal volume. A cerebral injury may cause hyperventilation and an increased water loss.
   b. Excessive loss of water through the skin. This occurs in burns, especially with open treatment.

PATHOPHYSIOLOGY

Water loss causes physiological changes in the following ways:

1. **Changes due to osmolality.** We know that the osmotic pressure of the extracellular water tends to remain equal to the osmotic pressure of the cells at all times. Following a loss of water, the osmotic pressure of the extracellular water becomes higher than that of the cells. Since water passes from a region of lower to a region of higher osmolality according to the osmotic rule, water will flow out of the cells into the extracellular water. This tends to lower the osmotic pressure of the extracellular water toward normal and to increase its volume toward normal.

2. **Changes due to hormonal effects.** Because of the loss of water and resultant hypertonicity the posterior pituitary gland secretes ADH. This in turn causes the kidney tubules to reabsorb more water, which helps minimize the water loss. In addition, the water loss has caused a decrease in the volume of extracellular water. This causes the adrenal glands to secrete aldosterone. This in turn causes a retention of sodium, which tends to raise the osmotic pressure of the extracellular water still further and tends to negate the effect of the secretion of ADH.

3. **Potassium loss in the urine.** The increased serum aldosterone level results in substantial urinary potassium loss. The potassium that is excreted comes mostly from the cells, because potassium is found in greatest concentration in the cells. Therefore, when this loss of cellular potassium occurs, the osmotic pressure of the cells falls and becomes relatively less than that of the extracellular water. As a result, more cellular water will flow from the cells into the extracellular water to equalize the osmotic pressure.

4. **Changes in the brain cells.** The brain cells respond to water loss in a different way from all other cells in the body, because the brain cells are able to synthesize new substances (solute) called *osmolytes*. In this way, the osmolality of the brain cells is increased, less water is withdrawn from the brain cells, and less injury to the brain cells occurs. These osmolytes, which appear within 1 hour after experimental water loss is produced, are protein and carbohydrate molecules.

Starvation, or partial starvation, may have a sparing effect upon water loss; however, ketonemia may eventually obligate excess water loss in the urine. In contrast, a high-protein diet increases urea output, which results in an increased excretion of water.

SYMPTOMS

Thirst is the earliest symptom of water loss. It occurs when the water loss is equal to about 2% of the body weight (about 3 lb, or 1.4 liters in a 70-kg [154-lb] patient). As extracellular water is lost and its osmotic pressure increases, water passes from the cells to the extracellular water, decreasing the volume of the cells. A center in the brain, probably in the hypothalamus, is sensitive to this decreased cell volume and causes the sensation of thirst. Later, the tongue sticks and there is an inability to swallow dry food. However, thirst may not be present, even with severe water loss, in patients with cerebral lesions, for reasons already mentioned.

Thirst can also develop when the extracellular fluid volume decreases. This occurs in the following way: when the extracellular and the circulating blood volumes decrease, the juxtaglomerular cells of the kidneys are stimulated to secrete renin. This in turn causes an increase of angiotensin II, which stimulates thirst receptors in the hypothalamus. It also stimulates the posterior pituitary gland to secrete vasopressin, which in turn causes the kidneys to retain water. Angiotensin II also stimulates the secretion of aldosterone, which causes the kidneys to retain sodium ions.

Thirst and polyuria have also been described in patients with chronic potassium loss, and in patients with hypercalcemia. The potassium loss causes injury to the kidney tubules. This prevents them from concentrating water and causes a condition similar to diabetes insipidus (water-losing nephritis, nephrogenic diabetes insipidus). Persistent hypercalcemia causes similar changes in the kidney tubules.

SIGNS

The clinical signs depend on the extent of the desiccation. The patient appears weak and ill. Weight loss is proportional to the degree of desiccation. A fever may be present. The temperature may reach 105°F or more when the desiccation is marked.

Skin and Mucous Membranes

The following signs are present:

1. The skin may be flushed. Sweating is decreased. The axilla and groin are dry.
2. There is little saliva or tears.
3. The tongue is dry and fissured and may be red and swollen. Phonation may be difficult and words may be poorly pronounced. These signs can also occur in patients who are not desiccated, but who are mouth-breathers, or have been receiving oxygen by mask. In desiccation, examination of the mucous membranes will reveal dryness. When you place a finger in the patient's mouth and palpate the mucous membranes where the gums and cheek meet, you will find that your finger does not glide easily because of the dryness of the mucous membranes.
4. Skin turgor remains normal. However, the skin may have a thick, "doughy" or "rubbery" feeling. (Loss of skin turgor occurs characteristically with sodium loss [Chapter 8].)

Cardiovascular System

Since water is drawn from the cells into the extracellular fluid, as a result of the water loss, the circulating blood volume and the efficiency of the cardiovascular system remain relatively unchanged and signs of shock do *not* usually appear. However, a tachycardia may develop when fever is present.

Central Nervous System

Generalized muscle weakness, muscle rigidity, or muscle tremors may develop. Epileptiform convulsions may appear (particularly if the water loss is treated too energetically with an infusion of dextrose and water). Occasionally a patient develops muscle weakness instead of muscle rigidity. Hallucinations, delirium, and manic behavior may also develop. Death usually occurs from respiratory arrest. Before this, the patient may develop hyperpnea.

These central nervous system changes may be functional. However, the water loss can also cause subdural or intracranial hemorrhage, particularly in children.

LABORATORY FINDINGS

Blood

In the early stages of water loss, the blood findings may be within the normal range because some cellular water passes to the extracellular fluid in response to osmotic pressure changes. However, as water continues to be lost, hemoconcentration occurs, and the hematocrit, the serum sodium, and other blood values begin to rise proportionately.

A rise in the hematocrit is a good sign of either water loss or sodium loss (unless red blood cells are also being lost by way of hemorrhage or hemolysis). The normal range of the hematocrit is 47% ± 5% for men, and 42% ± 5% for women.

A hematocrit of 55% in a patient with water loss is a much more serious sign than a hematocrit of 55% in a patient with sodium loss. The reason is that, in water loss, the extracellular fluid is diluted with water from the cells as a result of osmotic pressure changes. This tends to lower the hematocrit. Therefore, the water loss is actually greater than the rise in hematocrit would indicate.

However, when sodium loss occurs, as in vomiting, diarrhea, burns, and other conditions, water flows from the extracellular fluid into the cells because of osmotic pressure differences. This also causes the hematocrit to rise. Here, however, the water loss is actually less than the hematocrit would indicate, because it represents (in part) a shift of water into the cells rather than a true loss of water from the body. (This is described in detail in Chapter 9. [It should also be pointed out that a high hematocrit can also occur with overtransfusion.])

Other serum electrolyte and protein values are also elevated because of the water loss. An elevated blood urea nitrogen may be present. This may indicate inadequate kidney function arising from a decreased renal blood flow. The plasma osmolality is high, because of the water loss.

If the patient has abnormal quantities of nonelectrolyte substances in the blood, such as glucose in a diabetic patient, the serum sodium concentration may rise only slightly, or may be low, even though the water loss is marked. However, the plasma osmolality will be high in such patients (Chapter 11). (The effects of an increased blood sugar concentration on the serum sodium concentration are described in Appendix IV.)

Cation-Anion Balance

The normal values of the serum electrolytes and of the anion gap are given on pages 164 and 165. The anion gap normally has a value of 16 mEq/L or less. When water loss occurs, the serum electrolytes become more concentrated and the value of the anion gap becomes proportionately higher than 16 mEq/L (Chapter 1).

Urine

Because the renal blood flow is decreased, the urinary volume is small. However, it cannot fall below a minimum of 250 to 350 mL a day (unless the patient develops shock and renal shutdown). The specific gravity of the urine increases as the desiccation becomes aggravated and may reach 1.030. However, if the patient previously was unable to concentrate urine normally, the specific gravity may not rise greatly even if severe water loss is present. Albumin, casts, and even acetone may be present. An interesting urinary finding is the continued presence of sodium and chloride. However, with severe water loss, sodium and chloride may virtually disappear from the urine.

(In diabetes insipidus, the urine specific gravity remains below 1.010 and usually below 1.005. The urine osmolality is below 280 mOsm/kg and may decrease to 40 mOsm/kg when the polyuria is extreme. Also see page 38.)

Hypernatremia (a serum sodium concentration greater than 145 mEq/L) almost always indicates that there is too little water for the amount of sodium ions and other solutes in the body. Clinically, it is important to determine whether this relative water deficit has occurred in spite of normal kidney tubular function to conserve water, or because the kidney tubules have lost their ability to conserve the excretion of water.

If hypernatremia is present with a small amount of maximally concentrated urine (that is, with a high osmolality or specific gravity), this indicates that there is adequate ADH (the antidiuretic hormone of the posterior pituitary gland) and that the kidney tubules are functioning normally. Therefore, there is an external cause for the water loss, or the patient has "essential hypernatremia."

In *essential hypernatremia,* a rare syndrome associated with cerebral disease, the serum sodium concentration is continually higher than normal, but the patient does not show any apparent loss of water. Many of these patients have no symptoms. However, there may be attacks of muscle weakness or muscle paralysis, possibly related to a reduced total body potassium content, although the serum potassium concentration in these patients may be normal. Alford and Scoggins have treated a symptomatic patient with a low-sodium, high-potassium diet.

If hypernatremia is present with a dilute urine, this indicates that there is either a lack of ADH or the kidney tubules are not responsive to ADH and nephrogenic diabetes insipidus (see above) is present.

Mild hypernatremia also occurs in primary aldosteronism and in Cushing's syndrome.

DIAGNOSIS

Water loss should also be differentiated from three other clinical syndromes associated with exposure to high environmental temperatures:

HEAT CRAMPS

Years ago, miners and steel factory workers who worked day after day in a hot environment developed heat cramps (miner's cramps, stoker's cramps) caused by a loss of sodium and other electrolytes. However, the heat cramps that occur in athletes during hot weather, particularly early in the season, are caused by a loss of water. The cramps usually affect the gastrocnemius muscles or thigh muscles, but can affect other muscles. Spasm of the abdominal muscles may simulate an acute abdomen.

Treatment consists of removal from direct sunlight, rest, ice packs to the affected muscles, and replacement of water orally.

Prevention includes adequate water during strenuous exercises or sports.

Athletes should not use so-called athletic drinks and sport beverages to replace losses of sweat. These beverages contain electrolytes and large concentrations of sweeteners to mask the bitter taste of the electrolytes. This makes the beverages hypertonic. Because they are hypertonic, they leave the stomach slowly. This produces a sensation of satiety that discourages the athlete from ingesting much-needed water (Smith).

HEAT EXHAUSTION (HEAT PROSTRATION, HEAT SYNCOPE)

Heat exhaustion is caused by a loss of water, which results in reduced extracellular fluid and blood volume. As a result, circulation to the brain decreases. Symptoms include weakness, visual disturbances, vertigo, pounding headache, and syncope. The skin is warm and moist. The pulse is weak and rapid, the blood pressure is decreased. The body temperature may be normal or slightly elevated.

Treatment includes removal from direct sunlight, rest, oral fluids (1 to 2 L in 2 to 4 hours). If the patient is unconscious, it may be necessary to give fluids intravenously. It is rarely necessary to give sodium chloride intravenously.

Prevention is the same as that used to prevent heat cramps (see above).

HEAT STROKE (HEAT PYREXIA)

Heat stroke can be (1) induced by excessive physical exertion, in a hot environment, when it is not possible to dissipate the heat produced. This usually occurs in young healthy persons. Obesity, inadequate acclimatization to physical exertion, or potassium or salt depletion are contributing factors. (2) In the absence of physical exertion, heat stroke can occur in older persons, particularly with congestive heart failure, malnutrition, or alcoholism, who are exposed to a high environmental temperature and are also deprived of an adequate amount of salt and water. It can also occur in patients who have dysfunction of the sweat glands, as in scleroderma or cystic fibrosis.

The following factors can aggravate or precipitate either type of heat stroke: drugs that *decrease thirst,* such as haloperidol; drugs that *decrease sweating,* such as anticholinergics, antihistamines, antiparkinsonism drugs, propranolol; drugs that *increase heat production,* such as amphetamines, tricyclic antidepressants, MAO inhibitors, LSD (lysergic acid diethylamide), thyroid extract.

The patient may at first complain of weakness, headache, dizziness, mental confusion, muscle cramps, a feeling of impending doom, or conversely, euphoria, as sweating decreases markedly or stops. In other patients, coma may occur abruptly. Delirium, generalized convulsions, abnormal Babinski reflexes, cerebellar disturbances, or hemiplegia may also develop.

The rectal temperature rises rapidly to 41°C (106°F) or higher and may reach 43° to 45°C (110° to 113°F). The skin is hot and dry and may show a pink or ashen color. Tachycardia is present and the heart rate may exceed 200 beats per minute. Respirations are rapid. The electrocardiogram may show nonspecific ST and T changes.

Complications of heat stroke include acute renal failure, particularly in the exertional type; rhabdomyolysis (skeletal muscle necrosis), only in the exertional type; disseminated intravascular coagulation; necrosis of liver cells with abnormal liver function test values and an elevated blood bilirubin (and jaundice); necrosis of heart muscle cells; electrolyte and acid-base disturbances, including hypernatremia, hypokalemia and hyperkalemia, hypocalcemia, hyperphosphatemia, hyperuricemia, respiratory alkalosis (in the nonexertional type) or lactic acidosis (in the exertional type of heat stroke).

Death usually occurs in the first 3 days, particularly with coma lasting more than 8 hours, shock, or a rectal temperature higher than 42°C (108°F). A patient who survives may develop delirium or aggressive behavior (which may last for several days after consciousness returns) and may require restraints. Abnormal neurological findings may persist indefinitely.

The usual recommended treatment when the rectal temperature is 41.1°C (106°F) or higher is to place the patient in an ice water tub bath until the temperature falls to 38.8°C (102°F). An equally effective treatment is to place the patient on a bed with a large, high-powered fan blowing over him or her, and give vigorous massage with ice (Knochel). The rectal temperature should be taken every 10 minutes, because once it falls below 39.4°C (103°F) it may drop precipitously and shock may develop. Therefore, active cooling should be stopped when the temperature reaches 38.8°C (102°F).

The use of IV fluids or electrolytes will be determined by serum sodium and other electrolyte determinations.

When the temperature has fallen, the patient should be kept in a cool ventilated room with an electric fan facing the bed. If the temperature rises again, active cooling with ice should be resumed. The patient should be kept in bed for at least several days until the temperature control becomes stable again.

If shock occurs, IV full-strength saline or lactated Ringer's solution may be of value. The patient may need 1200 to 1400 mL or more IV during the first 4 hours. The saline solution should not be used until the temperature has been lowered. (During the hyperpyrexia, particularly when the temperature is 39.4°C [103°F] or higher, there is marked vasodilatation. Vasoconstriction occurs as the temperature falls. If the saline solution is given when the patient shows vasodilatation, the circulating blood volume may become excessive when vasoconstriction occurs.)

Intravenous isoproterenol or dobutamine may be helpful if shock occurs. An alpha-adrenergic vasoconstrictor should not be infused when the temperature is still high, because it decreases the dissipation of heat.

Auxiliary treatment with chlorpromazine (Thorazine) in a dose of 50 mg intravenously at 4- to 6-hour intervals has also been used as the temperature is being lowered. It prevents shivering or convulsions, which would cause the temperature to rise. It probably also lowers body temperature by means of a direct action on the central nervous system.

Acute renal failure is an indication for early hemodialysis, and a severe acidosis may require intravenous sodium bicarbonate (Barcenas, Hoeffler, and Lie).

Prevention of heat stroke is the same as for heat exhaustion or heat cramps.

THE DIFFERENTIAL DIAGNOSIS OF CENTRAL DIABETES INSIPIDUS

The polyuria of central neurogenic (vasopressin-sensitive) diabetes insipidus should be differentiated from that caused by diabetes mellitus, chronic renal disease (nephrogenic diabetes insipidus), and by compulsive water drinking. The diagnosis of diabetes mellitus or chronic renal disease is usually simple. However, the patient with compulsive water drinking may be difficult to distinguish from the patient with diabetes insipidus.

In diabetes insipidus, the initial disturbance is water loss resulting from polyuria. The excessive drinking is an attempt to overcome the loss of water. In compulsive water drinking, the initial disturbance is water excess, due to the excessive water drinking. The polyuria is an attempt to overcome the water excess. Therefore, the serum sodium concentration tends to be higher than normal in diabetes insipidus patients, and lower than normal in compulsive water drinkers.

Diabetes insipidus occurs equally in both sexes and may occur at any age. In approximately one half the patients, no causative factor is found. In other patients, it occurs after hypophysectomy, from basilar skull fractures, primary or metastatic brain tumors (particularly after breast carcinoma), or with cerebral histiocytosis (eosinophilic granuloma, Hand-Schüller-Christian disease), granulomatous infections (tuberculosis or sarcoidosis), other infections, or cerebral vascular insufficiency.

Patients who have had intracranial surgery may develop acute diabetes insipidus for a few days after surgery. This may then be followed by a period of severe water retention for 2 to 6 days. Then the patient may develop normal water metabolism, or permanent diabetes insipidus.

Compulsive water drinking (psychogenic polydipsia) occurs most commonly in psychotic women over 40 years. The patient with diabetes insipidus shows a rather constant intake of water from day to day. The compulsive water drinker shows a marked fluctuation in the daily volume of water imbibed, depending on the emotional state. Nocturia is common in diabetes insipidus, rare in compulsive water drinking.

A simple test for the diagnosis of diabetes insipidus is the water deprivation test. Water is withheld for 6 to 8 hours. Plasma and urine osmolality are measured at the beginning and end of the test. Normal persons will show little or no change in plasma osmolality, which remains below 300 mOsm/kg even at the end of the test. The urine osmolality is usually higher than the serum osmolality at the beginning of the test. Its osmolality becomes even higher at the end of the test so that urine-plasma osmolality ratio will always exceed 1, and even 2.

If diabetes insipidus is present, the plasma osmolality at the beginning of the test is usually higher than normal, and will rise above 300 mOsm/kg at the end of the test. The urine osmolality will be less than the plasma osmolality at the beginning of the test and will not change significantly.

Therefore, the urine-plasma osmolality ratio will either remain unchanged or may even fall.

In a compulsive water drinker, the initial plasma osmolality is usually low (because of water dilution). The initial urine osmolality is also low. Both the plasma and urine osmolalities rise at the end of the test so that the urine-plasma osmolality ratio is approximately 1. However, the plasma osmolality remains below 300 mOsm/kg.

In doing the water deprivation test, it is necessary to monitor the patient's weight carefully because a patient with severe diabetes insipidus may lose as much as 0.5 kg of body water per hour. The test should be stopped if the patient loses 3% or more of body weight.

Concomitant measurement of plasma ADH levels during the water deprivation test adds diagnostic precision in subtle cases.

COURSE AND PROGNOSIS

This depends on the extent of the water loss, on the presence of associated losses of sodium and other electrolytes, on the physical condition of the patient, on the presence of central nervous system injury, and on the rapidity with which water is replaced.

When 12% of the body weight is lost, the patient loses the ability to swallow. Death usually occurs when 15% to 25% of the body weight is lost.

PROPHYLAXIS

Water loss can be avoided if one remembers the daily water requirements. For example, Table 3–1 shows the average daily water balance in an adult.

When a patient is not eating because of starvation, a surgical operation, or any other cause, water is formed in the body as a result of three other mechanisms, namely, the lysis of muscle (lean) tissue,* the oxidation of muscle protein, and the oxidation of body fat.

The oxidation of body fat is the most important source of calories in a patient who is not eating, because each gram of fat provides 9 calories. Approximately 250 g or more of fat and 250 g of muscle tissue are catabolized daily under these circumstances.

The oxidation of 250 g of fat produces about 250 mL of water of oxi-

---

*Muscle tissue consists of approximately 73% water and 27% protein. Therefore, when 1 g of muscle tissue is lysed, 0.73 mL water is released from the cells. This is known as *preformed water, bound water, water of solution.* In addition, the oxidation of the 0.27 g of protein produces 0.11 mL of water. (1 g protein produces 0.41 mL of water of oxidation.) The total amount of water made available by the lysis and oxidation of 250 g of muscle tissue is therefore $250 \times (0.73 \text{ mL} + 0.11 \text{ mL}) = 210$ mL of water.

TABLE 3–1
DAILY WATER BALANCE

Water Intake		Water Excretion	
In fluids	1500 mL approx.	Urine	1500 mL
In solid food	800 mL	Insensible perspiration	600 mL
In a mixed		Vaporization from lungs	400 mL
2500-calorie diet		In feces	100 mL
(from oxidation of			
hydrogen)	300 mL approx.	Total	2600 mL
in 100 g protein	41 mL		
in 110 g fat	118 mL		
in 244 g carbohydrate	135 mL		
	294 mL		
Total	2600 mL approx.		

dation (1 g fat produces 1.07 mL water). The lysis of 250 g of muscle tissue and the oxidation of the protein that is present in this tissue produce another 210 mL of water daily under these circumstances.

The minimal volume of water needed by the kidneys to excrete waste materials is dependent on the presence or absence of kidney disease. Urinary solutes consist largely of urea and electrolytes. When kidney function is normal, 50 g of solute can be excreted in about 800 mL of urine. When renal disease is present and the kidneys are able to concentrate urine only to 1.010, for example, approximately 3500 mL of urine would be required to excrete 50 g of solute. A smaller urinary volume will be required with the ingestion of glucose (dextrose), which has a protein-sparing effect. The urinary volume will also be affected by changes in the relative amounts of urea and electrolytes affecting the specific gravity of the urine. Such changes might result from a high-protein or low-sodium diet, for instance.

Approximately 12 mL of water per kg body weight is lost by way of insensible perspiration and vaporization from the lungs daily. However, high ambient temperature, humidity, fever, and active sweating can greatly increase this loss. For example, a patient with a temperature of 104°F, breathing at a rate of 30 to 40 respirations per minute, can lose as much as 2500 mL of water through the lungs daily.

As a general rule, an average adult requires approximately 1500 to 2000 mL of pure water a day. If the patient has a high fever, an additional 500 to 1500 mL of water daily is necessary. If the patient is sweating moderately, an additional 500 mL of water daily is also needed, and if there is profuse perspiration, 1000 mL of water will be needed to compensate for the loss of water in the sweat. If renal disease is present, the patient may require 3000 mL of water a day. People engaged in strenuous exercise in hot weather should drink water more frequently than thirst dictates. Runners should drink up to 100 to 300 mL of water or a hypotonic glucose solution (Gatorade and others) 15 to 20 minutes before beginning a race and should drink about 250 mL every 3 to 4 km.

TREATMENT

In water loss and desiccation, water, and water alone, is needed. However, the patient may have lost sodium and other ions as well as water. In such a case, these ions must be replaced. The loss of sodium in addition to water can be suspected if the patient has had a high fever and has sweated profusely, or if there has been vomiting, diarrhea, gastrointestinal drainage, and other findings. (The subject of sodium loss is discussed in detail in Chapter 8.)

Treatment of moderate hyperthermia includes taking the patient's clothes off, sprinkling water over the patient, and fanning. Ice packs can be applied to the head, neck, abdomen, axillae, and groin.

Type of Fluid Needed

Pure water is needed. Water alone can be given orally or rectally. However, pure water cannot be infused because it causes the red blood cells to swell and hemolyze. It must be given in an isotonic (isosmotic) solution. An isotonic solution is one which will cause neither an increase nor a decrease in the size of the red blood cells when given intravenously. A 5% dextrose (glucose) solution in water is approximately isotonic.

Volume of Fluid Needed

There are several methods of calculating the volume of water needed to treat water loss. However, one should remember that, regardless of the method of calculating water loss, additional water must be given to supply the daily water needs. For example, suppose that you calculate that a water loss of 4000 mL is present. The patient needs not only the 4000 mL, but an additional 1500 mL or more water daily to cover the daily water losses due to insensible perspiration, urinary output, and other causes.

Method 1

A simple way to calculate the water deficit is the following:

1. If thirst is present, but other clinical signs are minimal, one can assume that the water deficit is about 2% of the body weight. Thus, in a 70-kg (154-lb) patient, the water deficit would be approximately 1400 mL.
2. If the patient has gone 3 to 4 days without water, and if there is marked thirst, a dry mouth, and oliguria, the water deficit is approximately 6%

of the body weight. In a 70-kg patient, the water deficit would be approximately 4200 mL.

3. The above signs are present. In addition, if there are marked physical weakness and severe mental changes, such as confusion or delirium, the water deficit is 7 to 14% of the body weight. In a 70-kg patient, this would be approximately 5 to 10 liters.

Method 2

If the patient has been weighed daily, and it is known, for example, that he or she has lost 4 kg weight during an *acute* period of desiccation, the water deficit is approximately 4000 mL, or 4 liters.

Method 3

This method is based on the fact that the plasma sodium concentration varies inversely with the volume of extracellular water. It assumes, however, that only water has been lost and that the sodium content of the body has remained unchanged.

The following formula is used:

$$Na_2 \times BW_2 = Na_1 \times BW_1.$$

Na_2 represents the present serum sodium concentration. BW_2 represents the present body water volume. Na_1 represents the original, or normal, serum sodium concentration of 142 mEq/L. BW_1 represents the original volume of body water. This is 60% of the body weight of a man (50% in a woman).

The loss of body water therefore equals $BW_1 - BW_2$.

Example

Man, weighing approximately 70 kg. Present serum sodium concentration, 162 mEq/L.

$$Na_2 \times BW_2 = Na_1 \times BW_1$$
$$162 \times X = 142 \times 42$$
$$X = \frac{142 \times 42}{162} = 37 \text{ liters.}$$

The water loss is therefore $42 - 37 = 5$ liters.

Route of Fluid Administration

If the patient can drink water, the water should be given orally, unless vomiting is present. Water can also be given by means of an intranasal gastric tube, or rectally by means of a Murphy drip. If enteral administration is impossible, an intravenous solution of dextrose in water is required. However, hyperglycemia may occur (even in the nondiabetic patient) when infusion rates exceed 300 mL/hr with 5% dextrose.

Rate of Administration

Ordinarily the water loss can be corrected in a period of 2 days. One half the necessary volume of water is given the first day. This can be done either orally or by means of an infusion of 5% dextrose in water. A rate of administration of 120 to 1000 mL/hr can be used. (The relation between the number of drops per minute and the total volume per hour is described in Chapter 36.)

(Water must never be given by nasogastric tube to a comatose patient unless a cuffed endotracheal tube is in place.)

If severe water loss is present and water is infused too rapidly, it may cause transient water intoxication and convulsions, because the brain cells have a higher osmolality than the other cells of the body, because of organic osmolytes that have been synthesized (see above). If water is given too rapidly, the brain cells will swell excessively. This can be avoided by giving the infusion slowly and by determining the serum sodium concentration after one-half the calculated volume of dextrose in water has been infused. As a general rule, the serum sodium should be decreased at a rate less than 0.5 mEq/hr.

Patients with neurogenic diabetes insipidus usually respond to IM vasopressin tannate in oil (Pitressin), to aqueous Pitressin, or to a nasal spray of synthetic lysine-8-vasopressin (lypressin, Dyapid-Sandoz). Desmopressin (DDAVP-Ferring), a synthetic analog of argenine vasopressin, the natural human antidiuretic hormone (ADH), is now available for intranasal use.

Such patients also respond to the thiazides and to the antidiabetic chlorpropamide. The thiazides probably act by decreasing the amount of sodium ions that reach the distal tubules of the kidneys. This is secondary to the sodium deficit induced by the thiazides. The thiazides are particularly effective in patients with nephrogenic diabetes insipidus.

Chlorpropamide and other sulfonylureas probably potentiate the action of ADH on the kidney tubules. (They can also cause hypoglycemia as a side effect, particularly if the patient fasts.)

The thiazides and chlorpropamide have additive effects and can be used simultaneously. Small doses, such as 125 to 375 mg chlorpropamide and 50 mg hydrochlorothiazide daily, are effective.

Bibliography

Alford, FP, and Scoggins, BA: Symptomatic normovolemic essential hypernatremia. Am J Med 54:359, 1973.

Arieff, AI, Guisado, R, and Lazarowitz, VC: Pathophysiology of hyperosmolar states. I. TE Andreoli, JJ Grantham, SC Rector, Jr., (eds) Disturbances in Body Fluids. American Physiology Society, Bethesda, Maryland, 1977.

Barlow, ED, and deWardner, HE: Compulsive water drinking. Quart J Med 28:235, 1959.

Barcenas, C, Hoeffler, HP, and Lie, JT: Obesity, football, dog days and siriasis. A deadly combination. Am Heart J 92:237, 1976.

Barron, WM, et al.: Transient vasopressin-resistant diabetes insipidus of pregnancy. N Engl J Med 310:442, 1984.

Belding, HS: Hazards to health. Work in hot weather. N Engl J Med 266:1052, 1962.

Beyer, CB: Heat stress and the young athlete. Recognizing and reducing the risks. Postgrad Med 76:109, 1984.

Black, DAK, McCance, RA, and Young WF: A study of dehydration by means of balance experiments. J Physiol 102:406, 1944.

Boyd, AE, and Beller, GA: Heat exhaustion and respiratory alkalosis, letter. Ann Intern Med 83:835, 1975.

Bricker, NS, and Klahi, S: Obstructive uropathy. In Diseases of the Kidney, 2nd ed. (Strauss, MB, and Welt, LG, eds.) Boston, Little, Brown & Co., 1971.

Costrini, AM, et al.: Cardiovascular and metabolic manifestations of heat stroke and severe heat exhaustion. Am J Med 66:296, 1979.

Clowes, GHA, and O'Donnell, TF, Jr: Heat stroke. N Engl J Med 291:564, 1974.

Coburn, JW, and Reba, RC: Potassium depletion in heatstroke. Milit Med 131:678, 1966.

Cushard, WG, Jr., et al: Oral therapy of diabetes insipidus with chlorpropamide. Calif Med 115:1, 1971.

Dashe, AM, Cramm, RF, Crist, CA, Habener, JF, and Solomon, DH: A water deprivation test for the differential diagnosis of polyuria. JAMA 185:699, 1963.

Daugirdas, JT, Kronfol, NO, Tzamaloukas, AH, Ing, TS: Hyperosmolar coma: Cellular dehydration and the serum sodium concentration. Ann Intern Med 110:855–857, 1989.

DeRubertis, FR, Michelis, MF, and Davis, BB: "Essential" hypernatremia. Arch Intern Med 134:889, 1974.

Dies, F., Rangel, S, and Rivera, A: Differential diagnosis between diabetes insipidus and compulsive polydipsia. Ann Intern Med 54:710, 1961.

England, AC, et al: Preventing severe heat injury in runners. Ann Intern Med 97:196, 1982.

Feig, PU, and McCurdy, DK: The hypertonic state. N Engl J Med 297:1444, 1977.

Fine, J: Disseminated intravascular coagulation in heat stroke, letter. JAMA 233:1164, 1975.

Fitzsimons, JT: The physiological basis of thirst. Kidney Int 10:3, 1976.

Gamble, JL: Chemical Anatomy, Physiology and Pathology of Extracellular Fluid, 6th ed. Cambridge, Harvard University Press, 1954.

Gordon, GL, and Goldner, F: Hypernatremia, azotemia and acidosis after cerebral injury. Am J Med 23:543, 1957.

Hariprasad, MK, et al: Hyponatremia in psychogenic polydipsia. Arch Intern Med 140:1639, 1980.

Hayek, A, and Ramirez, I: Demeclocycline-induced diabetes insipidus. JAMA 229:676, 1974.

Hays, RM: Antidiuretic hormone. N Engl J Med 295:659, 1976.

Hoagland, RJ, and Bishop, RJ, Jr: A physiologic treatment of heat stroke. Am J Med Sci 241:415, 1961.

Hockaday, TDR: Diabetes insipidus. BMJ 1:210, 1972.

Kaplan, SA, Yuceoglu, AM, and Strauss, J: Vasopressin-resistant diabetes insipidus. J Dis Child 97:308, 1959.

Knochel, JP: Environmental heat illness. Arch Intern Med 133:841, 1974.

Knochel, JP: Dog days and siriasis. How to kill a football player. JAMA 233:513, 1975.

Knochel, JP: Clinical physiology of heat exposure. In Maxwell, MH, and Kleeman, CR, (ed). Clinical Disorders of Fluid and Electrolyte Metabolism, 3rd ed. New York, McGraw-Hill, 1980.

Knochel, JP, and Caskey, JH: The mechanism of hypophosphatemia in acute heat stroke. JAMA 238:425, 1977.

Leaf, FA: Dehydration in the elderly. Editorial. N Engl J Med 311:791, 1984.

Marsden, PA, and Halperin, ML: Pathophysiological approach to patients presenting with hypernatremia. Am J Nephrol 5:229–235, 1985.

Massry, SG, and Coburn, JW: Clinical physiology of heat exposure. In Maxwell, MH, and Kleeman, CR, (eds): Clinical Disorders of Fluid and Electrolyte Metabolism. 2nd ed. New York, McGraw-Hill, 1972.

The Medical Letter on Drugs and Therapeutics: Treatment of Heat Injury. Abramowicz, M (ed). New Rochelle, NY, 32:66–68, July 13, 1990.

Mellinger, RC, and Zafar, S: Primary polydipsia syndrome of inappropriate thirst. Arch Intern Med 143:1249, 1983.

Middleton, DB: Treatment of hypernatremic dehydration. N Engl J Med 291:683, 1974.

Morris-Jones, PH, and Houston, IB: Prognosis of the neurological complications of acute hypernatremia. Lancet 2:1385, 1967.

Murphy, RJ: Heat illness in the athlete. Am J Sports Med 12:258, 1984.

Nelson, DC, et al: Hypernatremia and lactulose therapy. JAMA 249:1295, 1983.

O'Donnell, TF, and Clowes, GHA: The circulatory abnormalities of heat stroke. N Engl J Med 287:734, 1972.

Phillips, PA, et al: Reduced thirst after water deprivation in healthy elderly men. N Engl J Med 311:753, 1984.

Raff, SB, and Gershberg, H: Night sweats. A dominant symptom in diabetes insipidus. JAMA 234:1252, 1975.

Robinson, AG: DDAVP in the treatment of central diabetes insipidus. N Engl J Med 294:507, 1976.

Sandifer, M: Hyponatremia due to psychotropic drugs. J Clin Psychiatry 44:301, 1983.

Shibolet, S, et al: Heatstroke. Its clinical picture and mechanism in 36 cases. Quart J Med 36:525, 1967.

Smith, NJ: The prevention of heat disorders in sports. Am J Dis Child 138:786, 1984.

Statland, H: Fluid and Electrolytes in Practice, 3rd ed. Philadelphia. JB Lippincott, 1963.

Sturtz, GS, and Burke, EC: Obstructive water losing uropathy. JAMA 166:45, 1958.

The Medical Letter: Demopressin for diabetes insipidus, 20: no. 5, March 10, 1978.

Weitzman, R, and Kleeman, CR: Water metabolism and the neurohypophyseal hormones. In Maxwell, MH, and Kleeman, CR, (ed): Clinical Disorders of Fluid and Electrolyte Metabolism. 3rd ed., New York, McGraw-Hill, 1980.

Zelman, S, and Guillan, R: Heat stroke in phenothiazine-treated patients. A report of three fatalities. Am J Psychiatr 126:1787, 1970.

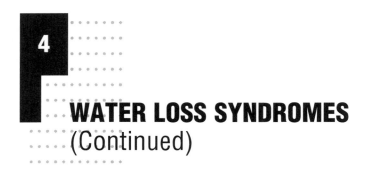

WATER LOSS SYNDROMES
(Continued)

WATER LOSS DUE TO SOLUTE EXCESS

This type of water loss is caused by the urinary excretion of an excessive amount of solutes such as sodium, chloride, potassium, and other anions and cations, or nonionic solutes such as dextrose, fructose, or other sugars, or urea, amino acids, or other nitrogenous products, that act as osmotic diuretics and cause an obligatory loss of water.

Synonym: Solute loading hypertonicity.

ETIOLOGY

Water loss due to solute excess can occur:

1. When an unconscious patient is given nasogastric feedings that supply a large amount of solutes, such as salt, dextrose, proteins, and other substances, with an inadequate volume of water. When a patient is given nasogastric feeding with a high-protein mixture, particularly if the daily protein intake is more than 150 g, much of the protein is not utilized and is converted to urea, which is excreted in the urine along with water.
2. When a patient with a bleeding peptic ulcer is given frequent feedings of milk and cream without water. Here, the absorption of partially digested blood, as well as the milk and cream, causes a great increase in the solute concentration of the blood.
3. When a patient convalescing from a severe burn is given a high-carbohydrate diet, particularly more than 300 g of carbohydrate a day. The patient may not be able to metabolize such a large amount of carbohy-

drate and the excessive glucose is excreted in the urine along with water (burn stress pseudodiabetes).

4. With many conditions associated with hyperosmolality particularly during parenteral hyperalimentation (Chapter 5).

PATHOPHYSIOLOGY

Substances such as dextrose and amino acids that are used for nasogastric feedings act as osmotic diuretics. In other words, when they reach the kidneys in excessive concentrations, they are automatically excreted along with a large amount of water. This can cause a large water loss. The kidneys may also excrete sodium with the water. This can cause a sodium loss in addition to a water loss. Excessive gastrointestinal water loss due to osmotic diarrhea may contribute to the syndrome in patients receiving nasogastric feeding formulas.

When the water loss occurs, the compensatory mechanisms described in Chapter 3 occur.

SYMPTOMS, SIGNS, AND LABORATORY FINDINGS

These are similar to those that occur in ordinary water loss due to a decreased water intake or the inability of the kidney tubules to conserve water. However, the following differences are present:

1. In water loss due to solute excess, the patient may gain weight, instead of losing, as the syndrome develops.
2. In water loss due to solute excess, the patient passes large amounts of urine as the water loss develops, whereas in water loss due to decreased water intake, or defective renal tubular function, the patient becomes oliguric as the water loss develops.
3. In water loss due to solute excess, the plasma osmolality can rise to very high levels, due to the excessive amounts of solutes in the blood, but the hematocrit remains essentially normal. For example, a plasma osmolality of 340 mOsm/kg can be present with a hematocrit of 45%. In ordinary water loss, the plasma osmolality and the hematocrit will rise proportionately. For example, a plasma osmolality of 340 mOsm/kg with a hematocrit of 55 to 66% or higher is not uncommon.
4. The polyuria associated with solute excess can be differentiated from the polyuria due to water excess, as occurs in diabetes insipidus, for example, in the following ways: When solute excess is present, the urine specific gravity tends to be higher (1.009 to 1.035 or higher) than when the polyuria is due to water diuresis (1.001 to 1.005). Similarly, when solute excess is present, the urine osmolality is higher (250 to 320

mOsm/kg) than when the polyuria is due to water diuresis (50 to 150 mOsm/kg) (Berman).

DIAGNOSIS

Water loss due to solute excess should be suspected in patients who are receiving nasogastric tube feedings or parenteral hyperalimentation or in diabetic or other patients who are receiving large amounts of saline but who show clinical signs of desiccation. A serum sodium concentration of 150 mEq/L or more indicates the presence of water loss (unless the patient has been receiving large volumes of saline solution intravenously).

When water loss is present with hyperglycemia, the serum sodium concentration in relation to the glucose concentration may be of value in differential diagnosis. In water loss due to solute excess, the increased serum sodium is unmasked as the blood sugar falls, as in a patient with diabetic acidosis who is being treated with insulin and saline solution. Marked elevation of blood urea nitrogen (BUN) is characteristic, reflecting the administered protein load and reduced renal blood flow.

COURSE AND PROGNOSIS

Water loss due to solute excess is even more serious than water loss due to decreased water intake, because nasogastric tube feedings are usually used for seriously ill patients. Death will occur unless the condition is recognized early.

PROPHYLAXIS

When a patient is being given nasogastric tube feedings, particularly if the daily protein intake is 150 g or more, he or she should be observed carefully for clinical signs of desiccation. If such signs develop, the concentration of the tube feedings should be decreased, and more water should be given.

TREATMENT

The treatment is the same as that for water loss caused by a decreased water intake. The volume of water lost can be calculated from the increased serum sodium concentration, and the water can be given orally or intravenously. In addition, if the patient has been receiving nasogastric tube feedings, these should be stopped temporarily. During treatment with water, the patient will continue to pass large volumes of urine.

Bibliography

Berman, LB: An abundance of urine. JAMA 229:203, 1974.

Daugirdas, JT, Kronfol, NO, Tzalaloukas, AH, Ing, TS: Hyperosmolar coma: Cellular dehydration and the serum sodium concentration. Ann Intern Med 110:855, 1989.

Engel, FL, and Jaeger, C: Dehydration with hypernatremia, hyperchloremia and azotemia complicating nasogastric tube feeding. Am J Med 17:196, 1954.

Fonkalsrud, EW, and Keen, J: Hypernatremic dehydration from hypertonic enemas in congenital megacolon. JAMA 199:584, 1967.

Gault, MH, et al: Hypernatremia, azotemia, and dehydration due to high-protein tube feeding. Ann Intern Med 68:778, 1968.

Kleeman CR: Metabolic coma. Kidney Int 36:1142, 1989.

Moder, KG, and Hurley, DL: Fatal hypernatremia from exogenous salt intake: Report of a case and review of the literature. Mayo Clin Proc 65:1587, 1990.

Moore, FD: Metabolic Care of the Surgical Patient. Philadelphia, W.B. Saunders, 1959.

Wilson, WS, and Meinert, JK: Extracellular hyperosmolarity secondary to high-protein nasogastric tube feeding. Ann Intern Med 47:585, 1957.

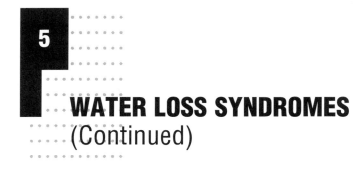

WATER LOSS SYNDROMES
(Continued)

WATER LOSS DUE TO HYPEROSMOLALITY

Water loss due to hyperosmolality can occur whenever the extracellular water becomes hyperosmal for any reason. The hyperosmolality due to the administration of food in excess of water has been described in Chapter 4. In this chapter, hyperosmolality that may occur in diabetic patients (hyperosmolal, hyperglycemia, nonketoacidotic diabetic coma) and the hyperosmolality associated with the parenteral or rectal administration of substances that increase the osmolality of the blood will be described.

HYPEROSMOLAL, HYPERGLYCEMIC, NONKETOACIDOTIC DIABETIC COMA

Hyperosmolal, hyperglycemic, nonketoacidotic diabetic coma may occur in middle-aged or elderly diabetic patients whose diabetes is not severe. Most patients are over 60 years old. Rarely, the condition occurs in young patients.

Precipitating factors include treatment with corticosteroids, chlorpromazine, antimetabolites, or phenytoin (Dilantin), thiazide diuretics, furosemide or ethacrynic acid, propranolol, cimetidine, diazoxide, mannitol, mafenide burn ointment, peritoneal dialysis with a high-glucose solution, or diseases such as pancreatitis or carcinoma of the pancreas, acute pyelonephritis, acute myocardial infarction, subdural hematoma, hemorrhage from the gastrointestinal tract, burns, systemic lupus erythematosus, pemphigus, and hypothermia. Frequently, a serious infection or a cerebrovascular accident can precipitate hyperosmolal diabetic coma. Neurological impairment limiting access to water may accelerate the process.

Pathophysiology

The precipitating factor is reduced insulin activity. This may be due to a decreased insulin reserve or to insulin resistance. The decreased insulin activity is adequate to prevent acidosis, but is not adequate to control the hyperglycemia.

The condition slowly develops over many days. The hyperglycemia increases and the osmotic pressure of the extracellular water rises much higher than that of the cells. As a result, water flows from the cells to the extracellular water. This decreases the water content of the cells and temporarily increases the water content of the extracellular water. However, the large amount of glucose that is brought to the kidneys acts as an osmotic diuretic. When the glucose is filtered through the glomeruli and enters the kidney tubules, it has to be excreted with water. The large amount of glucose excreted produces a large water loss. The increased serum sodium concentration that results from the water loss also contributes to the hyperosmolality.

Cerebral symptoms and signs occur as a consequence of severe dehydration of the brain cells. Intracerebral or subarachnoid hemorrhages may also develop.

Renal tubular dysfunction may also be present and may be one of the factors that cause a loss of water (Chapter 3).

Symptoms and Signs

During this time, the patient continues to eat, but becomes thirsty from the water loss. He or she often drinks a large amount of juice or carbonated beverage that contains carbohydrate to slake the unquenchable thirst. This aggravates the condition. (Many patients are not aware that they are diabetic.)

When the water loss becomes excessive, the patient becomes less aware that he or she is thirsty and drinks less. Therefore, the hyperglycemia and the hyperosmolality increase.

At this time, abnormal neurological signs may develop. These include stiffness of the neck, extensor plantar responses, focal or generalized convulsive seizures, and coma. In addition, the patient shows the characteristic physical signs of water loss (Chapter 3) and may show signs of shock, arterial or venous thrombosis, or acute renal failure. A high fever may develop because of the water loss.

Laboratory Findings

The serum glucose concentration is usually above 1000 mg/dL. The serum osmolality is greatly increased. The serum sodium concentration may or may not be increased (see Appendix IV). The serum potassium concentration may be normal or decreased. The plasma shows no acetone or only a trace. The pH is within normal or may show a slight acidosis. The BUN concentration is elevated because of decreased renal blood flow. Therefore, the serum creatinine concentration remains essentially normal and the BUN:creatinine ratio becomes much higher than the normal 10:1 ratio.

The urine characteristically shows a 4 plus glucose reaction, but no ketonuria. (Occasionally, the urine may show a small or moderate amount of ketones.)

The white blood count may rise even to 50,000/mL^3.

The patient continues to have a seemingly adequate urine output. This may be misleading because the physician may misinterpret this as a sign of adequate water intake.

Treatment

Relatively small amounts of regular insulin are needed. Initially, 10 to 20 units of regular insulin can be given intramuscularly, or a slow intravenous insulin drip may be started. This can be followed by 5 units of regular insulin intramuscularly every hour until the blood glucose level falls to 300 mg/dL. When this occurs, the insulin can be stopped. (Some patients may show insulin resistance.)

The insulin therapy can result in severe hypokalemia, particularly if the serum potassium level was low before treatment. In such cases, potassium chloride, in a dose of 20 to 40 mEq, can be added to each liter of intravenous fluid. However, no parenteral potassium chloride should be given until the patient shows an adequate urinary output.

If the patient is able to drink, water should be given orally. Water can also be given by way of a nasogastric tube.

There are differences of opinion about the best fluid to give intravenously. Most physicians prefer to start with a hypotonic saline solution (half strength), and agree that dextrose solutions should *not* be used at the beginning of treatment. Dextrose solutions can be given when the blood glucose concentration has fallen to 250 mg/dL.

A variable amount of intravenous fluid is needed. It has been calculated that as much as 6 to 16 liters of fluid may be needed the first 24 hours. If hypotonic solutions are continually used, there is a danger that water excess will develop. Therefore, isotonic saline can be used when the serum sodium concentration (corrected for the hyperglycemia [Appendix IV]) begins to fall. Replacement of potassium ions may also be necessary.

Prognosis

In spite of treatment, the mortality of hyperosmolal, hyperglycemic, nonketoacidotic diabetic coma patients is high, often reflecting the serious nature of concomitant conditions.

HYPEROSMOLALITY DUE TO OTHER CONDITIONS

Water loss due to hyperosmolality can also occur in diabetic patients who do not have nonketoacidotic diabetic coma, for example, in untreated diabetic acidosis, a large amount of glucose is excreted by the kidneys. This is associated with polyuria and water loss.

A similar clinical picture of water loss due to hyperosmolality can occur in another way when diabetic acidosis is present. When the blood glucose concentration is high, the osmotic pressure of the extracellular water becomes greater than that of the cells, and water will flow from the cells into the extracellular water, diluting it. When the serum sodium concentration is measured in such a patient, it may be low. However, this is more apparent than real, since it is produced by the dilution of the extracellular water (Appendix IV).

When the patient is given insulin, the blood glucose concentration falls; the osmotic pressure of the extracellular water also falls and becomes lower than that of the cells. Water therefore flows from the extracellular water into the cells, and the concentration of the extracellular electrolytes, including the serum sodium concentration, becomes elevated. If a large amount of sodium chloride and other sodium salts, such as bicarbonate or lactate, and other substances have been used in the treatment of the diabetic acidosis, the total electrolyte concentration may rise steeply and a serious water loss due to the excretion of these substances may develop, even though the diabetic acidosis is controlled.

Hyperosmolality can also occur after repeated angiocardiography with contrast material, after the intravenous use of sodium bicarbonate for lactic acidosis or the use of sodium sulfate for hypercalcemia, after repeated hypertonic enemas for congenital megacolon and after sodium phosphate administration for constipation in the elderly. It can occur as a complication of therapeutic abortion, when hypertonic sodium chloride solution is inadvertently injected intraperitoneally or intravascularly instead of into the amniotic cavity.

Hyperosmolality is also often present in patients with chronic renal disease, due to the marked increase in nitrogenous substances in the extracellular water and blood. In many of these patients, the hyperosmolality may be overlooked because the serum sodium concentration is low (for reasons discussed in Appendix IV). However, the serum osmolality is high.

A similar syndrome may occur in patients convalescing from severe burns. These patients may be unable to metabolize diets high in carbohydrate, particularly over 300 g of carbohydrate a day. This syndrome can be prevented by avoiding a high carbohydrate intake.

Bibliography

Arieff, AI, and Carroll, HJ: Nonketotic hyperosmolar coma with hyperglycemia. Medicine 51:73, 1972.
Arieff, AI., et al.: Pathophysiology of hyperosmolar states, in TE Andreoli, JJ Grantham, and

FC Rector, Jr., (eds.) Disturbances in Body Fluid Osmolality. Chap. 11, Bethesda, Maryland, American Physiology Society, 1977.

Boyer, J, Gill, GN, and Epstein, FH: Hyperglycemia and hyperosmolality complicating peritoneal dialysis. Ann Intern Med 67:568, 1967.

Boyer, MH: Hyperosmolar anacidotic coma in association with glucocorticoid therapy. JAMA 202:1007, 1967.

Fulop, M, Tannenbaum, H, and Dreyer, N: Ketotic hyperosmolar coma. Lancet 2:635, 1973.

Gerich, JE, Martin, MM, and Recant, L: Clinical and metabolic characteristics of hyperosmolar nonketotic coma. Diabetes 20:228, 1971.

Giammona, ST, Lurie, PR, and Segar, WE: Hypertonicity following selective angiocardiography. Circulation 28:1096, 1963.

Lindsey, CA, et al.: Plasma glucagon in nonketotic hyperosmolar coma. JAMA 229:1771, 1974.

McCurdy, DK: Hyperosmolar hyperglycemic nonketotic diabetic coma. Med Clin North Am 54:683, 1970.

Perry, TL: et al.: Nonketotic hyperglycemia. N Engl J Med 292:1269, 1975.

Phillips, PA, Bretherton, B, Johnston, CI, and Gray, L: Reduced osmotic thirst in healthy elderly men. Am J Physiol 261:R166, 1991.

Podolsky, S: Nonketotic diabetic coma in the cardiac patient. Cardiovasc Reviews & Reports 4:201, 1983.

Questions and Answers: Hypernatremia from intravascular saline infusion during therapeutic abortion. JAMA 220:1749, 1972.

Rosenberg, SA, et al.: The syndrome of dehydration, coma, and severe hyperglycemia without ketosis in patients convalescing from burns. N Engl J Med 272:931, 1965.

Ross, EJ, and Christie, SBM: Hypernatremia. Medicine 48:441, 1969.

Sament, S: Hyperosmolar coma in diabetes. Lancet 1:1153, 1966. Also N Engl J Med 276:1385, 1967.

Sherwood, LM: Hypernatremia during sodium sulfate therapy. N Engl J Med 277:314, 1967.

Whelton, MJ, Walde, D, and Harvard, CWH: Hyperosmolar non-ketotic diabetic coma, with particular reference to vascular complications. BMJ 1:85, 1971.

Woods, JE, et al.: Hyperosmolar non-ketotic diabetic coma, with particular reference to vascular complications. BMJ 1:85, 1971.

Woods, JE, et al.: Hyperosmolar nonketotic syndrome and steroid diabetes. Occurrence after renal transplantation. JAMA 232:1261, 1975.

Zileli, MS, et al.: Oxazepam intoxication simulating non-ketoacidotic coma. JAMA 215:1986, 1971.

6

WATER EXCESS SYNDROMES

Water excess occurs when a patient receives more water than the kidneys can excrete.

Synonyms: Water intoxication, overhydration, dilution syndrome.

ETIOLOGY

When the posterior pituitary gland, the kidneys, and the adrenal glands are normal, it is almost impossible for a person to take enough water by mouth to produce water excess (except in the case of a psychotic patient). However, water excess can be experimentally produced by infusing water at a rate faster than the kidneys can excrete it (about 13 mL/min).

Water excess is likely to occur when the following groups of patients are given excessive water or hypotonic (hyposmotic) solutions either orally, subcutaneously, intravenously, or rectally:

1. When ADH secretion is excessive. This can occur as a result of fear, pain, analgesics or anesthetics, an acute infection such as pneumonia, an acute medical stressful situation such as an acute myocardial infarction, an acute surgical stressful situation, such as trauma or a major operation, or even being hospitalized. Excessive ADH secretion can also occur in many other clinical conditions (see Chapter 7).
2. When the renal blood flow is low and the kidneys are not able to excrete water normally. This is seen in:
   a. Addison's disease, and other conditions of adrenocortical insufficiency. Water excess can also occur and produce stupor and coma in patients with hypopituitarism (pituitary coma). Deficient ACTH results in deficient secretion of adrenal cortical steroids that normally enable the kidneys to excrete water when necessary.
   b. Acute renal insufficiency. Water excess occurs when the physician

attempts to increase the urinary volume by giving large infusions of dextrose in water.

   c. Severe congestive heart failure or cirrhosis of the liver with low renal blood flows.

3. From absorption of the irrigating fluid during transurethral electroresection of the prostate or during hysteroscopic uterine fibroid resection.

4. Sodium loss from any reason (vomiting, diuretics, low sodium intake, and so on). The reason for this is that when sodium is lost, the osmotic pressure of the blood and the extracellular water is lower than that of the cells. Therefore, water flows from the blood and extracellular water into the cells, which swell. Sodium depletion reduces tubular urine flow, thereby substantially limiting the renal capacity to excrete ingested water.

5. Water excess may occur in compulsive water drinkers, who usually show symptoms suggestive of diabetes insipidus, but who may present clinically with delirium or seizures due to acute hyponatremia.

6. Habitual excessive beer drinking (exceeding 4 liters daily) may also cause water excess with severe neurological signs. Here again, other factors, such as sodium loss, are probably also present. The term "beer potomania" is used to describe this unusual condition.

7. When a continual intravenous infusion (usually of 5% dextrose in water) is administered to a hospitalized patient to keep a vein open (KVO). If a microdrip bulb is not attached to the IV tubing, and if the rate of flow is not kept minimal, as much as a liter or more of fluid will be infused in each 24-hour period.

8. In hospitalized patients as a result of fluids taken with medication, little sips of water, or mouth washing. It has been calculated that as much as 500 to 1000 mL of water can be imbibed daily in this way. In addition, chronically or seriously ill patients are usually anorexic and prefer liquids to solids. If they imbibe sodium-free liquids such as ginger ale, water, or fruit juices rather than eating solid food, this can also result in water excess.

9. From absorption of the irrigating fluid during transurethral electroresection of the prostate or during hysteroscopic uterine fibroid resection.

PATHOPHYSIOLOGY

When a normal person is given an excess of water, the water will dilute the extracellular water, and its osmotic pressure will become less than that of the cells. As a result, water will flow into the cells. This will cause the posterior pituitary gland to stop secreting ADH, and a water diuresis will occur. However, if the patient is in an antidiuretic state due to excessive secretion of ADH, the water will be retained. This causes a further decrease in the osmotic pressure of the extracellular water, and a further flow of water into the cells.

The retention of water causes an increased volume of the extracellular water. Normally, when the volume of the extracellular water rises, aldosterone secretion stops and the kidneys stop retaining sodium, which is then excreted along with water (Chapter 2). Here, the increased volume of the extracellular water also causes aldosterone secretion to stop. Therefore, the kidneys excrete sodium, but a free water diuresis does not occur because of the presence of excessive ADH. This loss of sodium ions by the kidneys merely aggravates the water excess, because it causes the osmotic pressure of the extracellular fluid to fall still further. Thus, a vicious cycle is created. A patient with latent epilepsy may develop a convulsive seizure when only minimal water excess is present.

The mechanism causing convulsions is not known. One explanation is that the convulsions are due to the entrance of water into the cells of the central nervous system.

SYMPTOMS

Wynn has pointed out that in acute water excess, the symptoms start dramatically and suddenly. The patient develops strange behavior, loss of attention, confusion, staring, aphasia, incoordination, sleepiness interposed with periods of violent behavior, shouting, delirium, and extreme muscle weakness. This may be followed by convulsive seizures, coma, and overbreathing.

If the water excess occurs slowly, the patient may complain of weakness, apathy, sleepiness, and may have anorexia, nausea, and vomiting. Headache and muscle cramps are rare. Later, personality changes occur, with disorientation or psychotic behavior, convulsive seizures, or coma.

Salivation and lacrimation may be marked, and a watery diarrhea may occur because of the water excess. However, there is no unusual sweating. The patient may complain of thirst, though it is difficult to explain this symptom. When water excess develops slowly, the patient may have minimal symptoms.

SIGNS

There is a history of an acute gain of weight.

Skin

The skin is warm, moist and may be flushed. It may become edematous and show "fingerprinting," which is elicited in the following way: If you roll your finger over a bony prominence such as the patient's sternum or tibia, your fingerprint will become visible on the patient's skin.

Central Nervous System

There is gross muscle weakness, and isolated muscle twitching may occur. The tendon reflexes are usually diminished or absent. However, when convulsions or coma occur, a positive Babinski reflex may appear. The patient may also develop a hemiplegia. Papilledema may occur in association with an increased pressure of the cerebrospinal fluid.

The electroencephalogram may show abnormalities such as theta and delta waves.

Cardiovascular System

The cardiovascular system remains normal. Subcutaneous edema or pulmonary edema may occur, or become aggravated, particularly if the patient has congestive heart failure.

LABORATORY FINDINGS

Blood

Hemoglobin and mean corpuscular hemoglobin concentration (MCHC) are decreased because of the water dilution. The mean corpuscular volume (MCV) of the red blood cells is increased because the osmotic pressure of the plasma (and the extracellular water) is lower than that of the cells. This causes water to enter the cells, including the red blood cells, making them swell. The hematocrit remains relatively unchanged because the swelling of the red cells is proportional to the increased plasma volume.

Serum Electrolyte Concentrations

The serum sodium and other electrolyte concentrations may be low as a result of the water dilution. The blood urea nitrogen is normal or low, unless it was previously high. Potassium concentration is either normal or low.

The serum sodium concentration is below 130 mEq/L. It may fall to 115 mEq/L, or even lower. However, the rate of lowering is more important than the absolute concentration reached, and convulsions may occur when the serum sodium concentration falls rapidly, even to 120 mEq/L.

A marked lowering of the bicarbonate level may occur in acute water excess. This is due to overbreathing and the development of an acute respiratory alkalosis.

Urine

The urinary volume may be low or high. The specific gravity is usually low, especially if the urinary volume is high. Sodium and chloride may be present in the urine, in spite of the low sodium and chloride concentrations in the serum. In some patients, however, the urinary sodium and chloride content becomes low.

DIAGNOSIS

Water excess should be suspected when a postoperative patient develops strange behavior, a convulsive seizure or hemiplegia, or becomes comatose. A sudden lowering of the serum sodium concentration is also a good sign of water excess, unless sodium has been lost by some extrarenal route, such as vomiting, diarrhea, or paracentesis.

The presence of a low serum sodium concentration by itself is not pathognomonic of water excess. It can occur also in patients with a true sodium loss, or in diabetic or uremic patients when the serum glucose or BUN concentration is high (see Appendix IV). However, in water excess, the serum osmolality is characteristically low, whereas in diabetic patients with low serum sodium concentrations, the serum osmolality may be high or normal, and will be low only when water excess is also present.

A low serum sodium concentration can also occur in the syndrome of inappropriate secretion of ADH (the antidiuretic hormone) (Chapter 7).

COURSE AND PROGNOSIS

If moderate water excess is present and no further water is given, the patient will usually recover spontaneously. However, if the patient has developed a convulsive seizure, or has become comatose, or has developed a hemiplegia, death may occur even when the patient is treated vigorously.

The water excess syndrome that occurs after trauma and postoperatively is usually self-limited. However, if it occurs in a severe form, the serum potassium concentration may rise to very high levels. This may be dangerous to life, particularly since the toxic effects of potassium ions on the heart are aggravated by hyponatremia, which is present, and by hypocalcemia, which may also be present.

The exact cause of the marked increase in serum potassium concentration that may occur is not known. The elevated serum potassium and the low serum sodium concentrations resemble the electrolyte patterns of acute adrenal cortical insufficiency. However, it has been shown that the concentration of free blood corticosteroids is high (40 to 80 mg/dL) in these patients after extensive surgery. This indicates that the adrenal cortex is functioning normally.

PROPHYLAXIS

There is a tendency to give postoperative patients and patients with acute renal shutdown too much water. Methods of avoiding this are described in Chapters 36 and 37. Similarly, the physician should remember that water excess can occur if too much water is given, regardless of the route of administration.

TREATMENT

Type of Fluid Needed

Water excess is treated in two ways:

1. Fluids should be withheld for 24 hours. In this way at least 1000 mL will be lost through the skin and lungs, and a large volume will be excreted in the urine. This alone will correct a moderate water excess.
2. If convulsions or hemiplegia have occurred, or if the patient is comatose, fluids must be withheld. In addition, hypertonic sodium chloride solution (3% to 5%) should be given.

If the patient is acidotic and chloride ions are contraindicated, a one third or one half molar lactate solution can be used instead of the hypertonic sodium chloride solution.

Volume of Fluid Needed

It is not necessary to calculate the exact volume of water excess that is present in order to determine the volume of 5% sodium chloride solution needed. The reason for this is that the body is not a closed system, and a relatively small volume of hypertonic sodium chloride solution will prevent death and enable the kidneys to respond by the excretion of large volumes of water.

A simple rule to use is to give the patient 6 mL hypertonic (5%) sodium chloride solution per kg of body weight.

Example: Patient weighing 70 kg.
$6 \times 70 = 420$ mL 5% sodium chloride solution needed.
This will raise the serum sodium concentration approximately 10 mEq/L.

The derivation of this rule is given in Appendix III.

If there is doubt whether water excess is present, one fourth to one half of the calculated hypertonic sodium chloride solution can be given and the patient can be checked by noting signs of clinical improvement, or a rise in serum sodium concentration.

Route of Fluid Administration

Hypertonic sodium chloride solution can be given only intravenously.

Rate of Fluid Administration

The rate of administration must be adjusted to the severity of the clinical syndrome. In patients having serious cerebral symptoms, the goal should be to raise serum sodium by 1 to 2 mEq/hr. Accordingly, in a 70-kg adult, 100 mL of hypertonic sodium chloride solution should be given at a rate of 100 mL/hr. The patient should then be observed for a half hour. At this time, another 100 mL can be infused. Not more than 400 mL of 5% sodium chloride solution should be infused in 1 day.

Bibliography

Beresford, HR: Polydipsia, hydrochlorothiazide, and water intoxication. JAMA 214:879, 1970.
Berl, T: Treating hyponatremia: Damned if we do and damned if we don't. Kidney Int 37:1006, 1990.
Bewley, TH: Acute water intoxication from compulsive water drinking. BMJ 2:861, 1964.
Cheng, JC, Zikos D, Skopicki, HA, and Peterson, DR: Long term neurologic outcome in psychogenic water drinkers with severe symptomatic hyponatremia: the effect of rapid correction. Am J Med 88:561–566, 1990.
Cluitmanns, FHM, and Meinders, AE: Management of hyponatremia: Rapid or slow correction? Am J Med 88:161, 1990.
Demanet, JC, et al: Coma due to water intoxication in beer drinkers. Lancet, 2:1115, 1971.
Desmond, J: Serum osmolality and plasma electrolytes in patients who develop dilutional hyponatremia during transurethral resection. Can J Surg 13:116, 1970.
Editorial: The hazard of water enemas. Lancet, 1:559, 1959.
Friedman, E, Shadel, M, Halkin, H, and Farfel, Z: Thiazide-induced hyponatremia. Reproducibility by single-dose challenge and an analysis of pathogenesis. Ann Intern Med 110:24, 1989.
Goldman, MB, Luchins, DJ, and Robertson, GL: Mechanisms of altered water metabolism in psychotic patients with polyuria and hyponatremia. N Engl J Med 318:397, 1988.
Gupta, DR, and Cohen, NH: Oxytocin, "salting out" and water intoxication. JAMA 220:681, 1972.
Halma, C, et al: Life threatening water intoxication during somatostatin therapy. Ann Int Med 107:518, 1987.
Klonoff, DC, and Jurow, AH: Acute water intoxication as a complication of urine testing in the work-place. JAMA 265:84, 1991.
Marx, GF: Koenig, JW, and Orkin, LR: Dilutional hypervolemia during transurethral resection of the prostate. JAMA 174:1834, 1960.
Papadakis, MA, Fraser, CL, and Arieff, AL: Hyponatremia in patients with cirrhosis. Q J Med 76:675, 1990.
Richards, MR, and Hiatt, RB: Untoward effects of enemata in congenital megacolon. Pediatrics 12:253, 1953.
Rose BD: New approach to disturbances in the plasma sodium concentration. Am J Med 81:1033, 1986.

Shalhoub, RJ, and Antoniou, LD: The mechanism of hyponatremia in pulmonary tuberculosis. Ann Intern Med 70:943, 1969.

Sterns RH: The treatment of hyponatremia: First, do no harm. Am Med 88:557, 1990.

Van Buren, MJ, Singelyn, F, Donnez, J, and Bribomont B: Dilutional hyponatremia associated with intrauterine endoscopic laser surgery. Anes 71:449–450, 1989.

White, JC: The risks of excessive water drinking in epileptic patients, letter. N Engl J Med 312:246, 1985.

Wynn, V, and Rob, CG: Water intoxication: differential diagnosis of hypotonic syndromes. Lancet 1:587, 1954. Also Metabolism 5:490, 1956.

7

WATER EXCESS SYNDROMES
(Continued)

INAPPROPRIATE ADH SECRETION SYNDROMES (SIADH)

The syndrome of inappropriate ADH (antidiuretic hormone) secretion (SIADH) is a form of dilutional hyponatremia and low serum osmolality due to the retention of water, produced by an inappropriate or an excessive secretion of ADH. In addition, there is failure to excrete a dilute urine in the presence of the low serum osmolality, and excessive loss of sodium ions in the urine in the absence of renal or adrenal disease. The syndrome is not caused by excessive water intake.

In 1953, Leaf and associates showed that when long-acting pitressin was given to humans, water retention, hyponatremia, a decreased serum osmolality, and an increased urine osmolality due to increased sodium excretion (*renal sodium wasting*) developed.

In 1957, Schwartz and associates described two patients with bronchogenic carcinoma who showed similar signs. They postulated that the syndrome was due to an "inappropriate" secretion of ADH. (Ordinarily, when hyponatremia and a decreased serum osmolality occur, urine with a low sodium concentration and a low osmolality is formed because of an increased urinary excretion of free water, in an attempt to restore the serum osmolality to normal.) Since then, the syndrome has been described in many other groups of patients.

PATHOPHYSIOLOGY

The physiological mechanisms for the secretion of ADH have been described in Chapter 2.

The basic physiological disturbance in this syndrome is an inappropriate or an excessive secretion of ADH. The secretion of ADH results in water retention and an expansion of the blood and extracellular volume. This causes a suppression of aldosterone secretion and the release of atrial natriuretic factor. As a result, sodium ions are lost through the kidneys into the urine. The serum osmolality falls because of the increased retention of water and a modest loss of sodium ions. The urine osmolality rises because of the decreased urinary excretion of water and the continued excretion of sodium ions. As a result, the osmolality of the urine becomes higher than the osmolality of the plasma.

The inappropriate ADH secretion can be due to many factors.

1. ADH secretion due to cerebral stimulation, as in:
    a. Central nervous system diseases such as brain abscess, hypopituitarism, encephalitis, Guillain-Barré syndrome, head injuries, meningitis, subarachnoid hemorrhage, concussion, electroconvulsive therapy.
    b. Stress reactions, including fear, pain, trauma, or major operations. The period of postoperative ADH secretion is usually 12 to 36 hours, but may last longer.
    c. Drugs, including hypoglycemic drugs such as chlorpropamide (Diabenese) and tolbutamide (Orinase); antineoplastic drugs, such as cyclophosphamide and vincristine; tricyclic drugs acting on the central nervous system, such as amitriptyline (Elavil), barbiturates, carbamazepine (Tegretol), fluphenazine (Permitil, Prolixin), haloperidol (Haldol), thioridazine (Mellaril), and thiothixene (Navane); and miscellaneous drugs including acetaminophen (Tylenol), tranylcypromine (Parnate), clofibrate (Atromid S), isoproterenol, morphine, meperidine (Demerol), oxytocin, and most anesthetics.

    Chlorpropamide probably produces the SIADH by potentiating the action of ADH on the kidneys, although it may also stimulate ADH secretion centrally.
2. Secretion of ADH-like peptides by tumor or inflammatory tissue such as tumors of the lung (particularly oat cell bronchogenic carcinoma), pancreas, thymus, duodenum, or other organs; Ewing's sarcoma; or inflammatory lung diseases such as pneumonia, tuberculosis, chronic pulmonary infections, status asthmaticus, and pulmonary aspergillosis with cavitation.
3. Excessive ADH secretion due to unknown factors, such as acute intermittent porphyria.

Also note the following:

1. Endocrine disturbances such as myxedema, Addison's disease, and hypopituitarism may simulate SIADH and must be excluded by specific testing.

2. Thiazide diuretics may produce an SIADH-like syndrome. However, serum potassium depletion is characteristic.

SYMPTOMS AND SIGNS

Symptoms and signs are related to the rapidity with which the water excess has developed and to the extent of the lowering of the serum sodium concentration.

The water excess usually develops slowly, so that symptoms and signs are rarely present when the serum sodium concentration is more than 125 mEq/L. However, when the serum sodium concentration falls to 115 mEq/L or less, serious neurological disturbances, including mental depression, convulsive seizures, or coma, commonly develop. In addition, symptoms and signs will be aggravated by any coincidental condition that produces water excess or sodium loss.

Many nonspecific symptoms related to the underlying disease rather than to the water excess may also be present.

LABORATORY FINDINGS

Blood

The serum sodium concentration and the serum osmolality are low.

The serum chloride concentration is also low. The serum potassium concentration may be normal or low. It is low, in association with a high serum bicarbonate concentration (metabolic alkalosis), when the syndrome has been produced by excessive diuretic therapy. Hypokalemia may also occur when the patient has a chronic wasting disease and does not eat adequately.

The BUN concentration is usually low, as is the serum uric acid level.

Bioassay of ADH in the plasma will show elevated levels.

Urine

The excretion of sodium ions in the urine continues despite the low serum sodium concentration. The sodium excretion will be equal to or greater than the sodium intake. (The sodium concentration in the urine is usually more than 20 mEq/L. However, if the patient is on a low-sodium diet, sodium excretion in the urine may be less than this.)

The urine is usually hypertonic to plasma because the plasma is diluted with water, and the urine contains an appreciable amount of sodium ions. Therefore, the urine osmolality is usually higher than the plasma osmolality. However, in mild cases of SIADH, the urine osmolality may be as low as 200 mOsm/kg.

Normal amounts of adrenocortical hormones are excreted in the urine.

DIAGNOSIS

An inappropriate ADH secretion syndrome can be suspected if the following conditions are present:

1. Hyponatremia and decreased osmolality of the serum.
2. Urine osmolality usually higher than serum osmolality.
3. Continued urinary excretion of sodium in spite of hyponatremia (unless the patient is on a low-sodium diet).
4. Normal renal function tests (BUN, serum creatinine, creatinine clearance).
5. Normal aldosterone blood levels and normal urinary excretion of aldosterone.
6. Absence of hypotension or dehydration.
7. Absence of clinical edema
8. Improvement in the clinical condition by fluid restriction.
9. Absence of endocrine disturbance.

Example: Oat cell carcinoma of the lung
Na 121   K 3.7 HCO_3 29   Cl 85
Serum osmolality: 240 mOsm/kg
Urine osmolality: 590 mOsm/kg
BUN 5 mg/dL
Serum creatinine 0.9 mg/dL

TREATMENT

There is no specific treatment. If convulsions or other serious neurological symptoms of water excess develop, hypertonic sodium chloride solution may be needed intravenously (Chapter 6). However, the goal of such therapy should be modest—with serum sodium rising by more than .5 mEq/hr. Hypertonic saline must be discontinued when the serum sodium reaches 125 mEq/L. Furosemide administration is useful to enhance water excretion and prevent iatrogenic salt overload when hypertonic saline is being given in extreme cases. If lesser symptoms are present, the intake of water should be restricted, even to 500 mL a day, for several days, and the amount of salt in the diet can be increased. Patients with bronchogenic carcinoma may improve when the tumor is removed surgically, or with appropriate chemotherapy. Phenytoin (Dilantin) has also been used to inhibit the excessive ADH secretion.

If the syndrome is due to thiazides, the diuretic should be stopped and potassium chloride should be given to correct the hypokalemia. Sodium chloride may also be helpful, although it is contraindicated when the syndrome is due to other causes.

Demeclocycline (Declomycin), a broad spectrum antibiotic has been used to treat the SIADH because it can interfere with the action of ADH on the kidneys and therefore can produce a diabetes insipidus-like effect (Cherrill et al.) A dose of 300 mg can be given three times a day. It may take several days before its effects are noted. Transient azotemia may occur as a side effect.

Lithium carbonate has also been recommended for the SIADH syndrome, because it interferes with the action of ADH on the distal tubules of the kidneys. However, it may cause toxicity, and it may interfere with the action of aldosterone, so that a loss of sodium ions may occur. It can also cause a nephrogenic type of diabetes insipidus.

Intravenous or oral urea has also been used (see Urea in Part 5).

The underlying condition producing the SIADH should be treated, if possible.

PROPHYLAXIS

The inappropriate ADH secretion syndrome is aggravated by any condition associated with a loss of sodium ions or an excess of water in the extracellular spaces. Therefore, diuretics should not be used unless necessary, and when used should be given in minimal doses. Similarly, intravenous fluids must be given very cautiously, to avoid water excess. Oral water intake should also be limited, depending on the serum sodium concentration.

Bibliography

Ajilouni, K, et al: Thiothixene-induced hyponatremia. Arch Intern Med 134:1103, 1974.
Ayus, JC, Wheeler, JM, Arieff, AL: Postoperative hyponatremic encephalopathy in menstruant women. Ann Intern Med 117:891, 1992.
Baker, JW, et al: Elevated plasma antidiuretic hormone levels in status asthmaticus. Mayo Clin Proc 51:31, 1976.
Baylis, PH, et al: Water disturbances in patients treated with oral lithium carbonate. Ann Intern Med 88:607, 1978.
Beresford, HR: Polydipsia, hydrochlorothiazide, and water intoxication. JAMA 214:879, 1970.
Berl, T: Treating hyponatremia: damned if we do and damned if we don't. Kidney International 37:1006–1018, 1990.
Cherrill, DA, Stote, RM, Birge, JR, and Singer, I: Demeclocycline treatment in the syndrome of inappropriate antidiuretic hormone secretion. Ann Intern Med 83:654, 1975.
Cusik, JF, et al: Inappropriate secretion of antidiuretic hormone after transsphenoidal surgery for pituitary tumors. N Engl J Med 311:38, 1984.
Decaux, G, et al: Hyponatremia in the syndrome of inappropriate secretion of antidiuretic hormone. Rapid correction with urea sodium chloride and water restriction therapy. JAMA 247:471, 1982.
Decaux, G, et al: Treatment of the syndrome of inappropriate secretion of antidiuretic hormone with furosemide. N Engl J Med 304:329, 1981.
Decaux, G, et al: Hyponatremia in the syndrome of inappropriate secretion of antidiuretic

hormone. Rapid correction with urea, sodium chloride, and water restriction therapy. JAMA 247:471, 1982.

DeFronzo, RA, et al: Water intoxication in man after cyclophosphamide therapy. Ann Intern Med 78:861, 1973.

Dempster, WJ: Syndrome of inappropriate secretion of antidiuretic hormone. Lancet 1:970, 1971.

DeRubertis, FR, et al: Complications of diuretic therapy. Severe alkalosis and syndrome resembling inappropriate secretion of antidiuretic hormone. Metabolism 19:709, 1970.

Dingman, JF: What is an 'inappropriate' ADH syndrome? Mod Med May, 36, 1973.

Fine, D, and Shedrovilzky, H: Hyponatremia due to chlorpropamide. A syndrome resembling inappropriate secretion of antidiuretic hormone. Ann Intern Med 72:83, 1970.

Fishman, MP, Kleeman, CR, and Bethune, JE: Inhibition of antidiuretic hormone secretion by diphenylhydantoin. Arch Neurol 22:45, 1970.

Fishman, MP, et al: Diuretic-induced hyponatremia. Ann Intern Med 75:853, 1971.

Glassock, RJ, Cohen, AH, Danovitch, G, Parsa, KP: Human immunodeficiency virus (HIV) and the kidney. Ann Intern Med 112:35, 1990.

Goldstein, CS, et al: Idiopathic syndrome in inappropriate antidiuretic hormone secretion possibly related to advanced age. Ann Intern Med 99:185, 1983.

Greenberg, SR, and Yudis, M: Rapid reversal of inappropriate antidiuretic-hormone syndrome. Lancet 1:547, 1971.

Gupta, DR, and Cohen, NK: Oxytocin, "salting out," and water intoxication. JAMA 220:681, 1972.

Hamburger, S, et al: Thiazide-induced syndrome of inappropriate secretion of antidiuretic hormone. JAMA 246:1235, 1981.

Hantman, D, et al: Rapid correction of hyponatremia in the syndrome of inappropriate secretion of antidiuretic hormone. An alternative to hypertonic saline. Ann Intern Med 78:870, 1973.

Hendler, N, et al: Problems with lithium as treatment of inappropriate ADH secretion, letter. N Engl J Med 294:446, 1976.

Hill, AR, Uribarri, J, Mann, J, and Berl, T: Altered water metabolism in tuberculosis: Role of vasopressin. Am J Med 88:357, 1990.

Kaplowitz, LG, and Robertson, GL: Hyponatremia in rocky mountain spotted fever. Role of antidiuretic hormone. Ann Intern Med 98:334, 1983.

Khokhar, N: Inappropriate secretion of antidiuretic hormone. Postgrad Med 62:73, 1977.

Lauersen, NH, and Birnbaum, SJ: Water intoxication associated with oxytocin administration during saline-induced abortion. Am J Obstet Gynecol 121:2, 1975.

Marcaron, C, and Olufunsho, F: Hyponatremia of hypothyroidism. Arch Intern Med 138:820, 1978.

Miller, M, and Moses, AM: Urinary antidiuretic hormone in polyuric disorders and in inappropriate ADH syndrome. Ann Intern Med 77:715, 1972.

Novik, RK: Drug-induced dilutional hyponatremia. N Engl J Med 292:810, 1975.

Raskind, MA, et al: Acute psychosis, increased water ingestion and inappropriate antidiuretic hormone secretion. Am J Psychiatry 132:407, 1975.

Robertson, GL: Physiology of ADH secretion. Kidney Int 32 (suppl 21): S–20, 1987.

Rosenow, EC, II, Segar, WE, and Zehr, JE: Inappropriate antidiuretic hormone secretion in pneumonia. Mayo Clin Proc 47:169, 1972.

Sandifer, M: Hyponatremia due to psychotropic drugs. J Clin Psychiatry 44:301, 1983.

Schwartz, WB, Bennet, W, Curelop, S, and Bartter, FC: A syndrome of renal sodium loss and hyponatremia probably resulting from inappropriate secretion of antidiuretic hormone. Am J Med 23:529, 1957.

Sexton, DJ, and Clapp J: Inappropriate and antidiuretic hormone secretion. Occurrence in a patient with Rocky Mountain Spotted Fever. Arch Intern Med 137:362, 1977.

Sterns, RH: The treatment of hyponatremia: first, do no harm. Am J Med 88:557–560, 1990.

Tanay, A, et al: Long-term treatment of the syndrome of inappropriate antidiuretic hormone secretion with phenytoin. Ann Intern Med 90:50, 1979.

Weissman, PN, Shenkman, L, and Gregerman, RI: Chlorpropamide hyponatremia. Drug-induced inappropriate antidiuretic-hormone activity. N Engl J Med 284:65, 1971.

White, MG, and Fetner, CD: Treatment of the syndrome of inappropriate secretion of antidiuretic hormone with lithium carbonate. N Engl J Med 292:390, 1975.

SYNDROMES ASSOCIATED WITH SODIUM DISTURBANCES

8

SODIUM LOSS SYNDROMES

The sodium loss syndrome is due to a loss or depletion of sodium from the extracellular water. There may be no accompanying water loss; if water loss is present, it is proportionately less than the loss of sodium ions.

Synonyms: Sodium depletion, pure salt depletion, desalting water loss, sodium deficiency, low sodium syndrome, dehydration.

PATHOPHYSIOLOGY

The sodium loss that occurs in the sodium loss syndrome is not related to a decrease in total exchangeable body sodium. The sodium loss that causes the physiological disturbances, symptoms, and signs is localized to the extracellular water. The total exchangeable body sodium may be low or normal, and may often be high. As a matter of fact, an internal shift of sodium and water to a localized area, such as in severe burns, or in peritonitis, or in an accumulation of pleural or ascitic fluid, can cause a severe and fatal sodium loss syndrome without any sodium having been lost from the body. In addition, a severe and even fatal sodium loss syndrome can occur in a patient with congestive heart failure who shows marked edema (which indicates that there is an excess of total exchangeable body sodium).

We know that the concentration in the extracellular water is relatively so great that the loss of sodium (with a loss of chloride or other anions) can cause a marked decrease in the osmotic pressure of the extracellular water. When this occurs, water will flow from the extracellular water into the cells, because of the lowered osmotic pressure of the extracellular water. As a result, the volume of the extracellular water, including the volume of the blood plasma, will fall and produce a decreased circulating blood volume and shock. The shock that occurs as a result of sodium loss is characterized by a lack of response to pressor substances, such as norepinephrine

(Levophed), dopamine (Intropin), and other similar drugs; the shock responds only to solutions containing isotonic, hypotonic, or concentrated sodium salts.

In addition, the loss of sodium is associated with a loss of circulating plasma proteins, particularly albumin, from the bloodstream. This causes the osmotic pressure of the blood to become lower than that of the extravascular portion of the extracellular water. As a result, water flows out of the plasma and the circulating blood volume falls still further. The reason for the loss of plasma albumin is not clear. It may be that as the cardiac output falls there is a decreased return of the extracellular and lymphatic fluid (which is rich in albumin) to the heart.

ETIOLOGY

Sodium loss can occur in the following situations:

1. Loss of sodium in gastrointestinal secretions. The electrolyte concentrations of the various gastrointestinal secretions are shown in Table 8–1. Notice that when these secretions are lost, a marked loss of sodium as well as other electrolytes occurs. The sodium can be lost as a result of:
   a. Vomiting.
   b. Dysentery, cholera, diarrhea, ulcerative colitis, pseudomembranous colitis.

      A patient with a mucus-secreting villous adenoma of the rectum or sigmoid may excrete several liters of mucus a day, and as a result may develop shock from the loss of sodium ions and water (in the mucus). In addition, a large amount of potassium ions may also be lost in this way, and symptomatic hypokalemia may also develop.
   c. Gastric, biliary, pancreatic, or intestinal lavage by means of a Levin or Abbott-Miller tube.
   d. Gastrointestinal or biliary fistulas.
   e. Cation exchange resins. These absorb sodium from food in the stomach and cause its excretion in the stool. (Cations, such as potassium and magnesium, are also lost in addition to the sodium.)
2. Loss of sodium through the skin. This can occur in
   a. Excessive sweating, particularly if a large amount of water is imbibed to quench thirst.
   b. Extensive, exudative skin lesions or burns.
   c. Fibrocystic disease of the pancreas (mucoviscidosis).

      The diagnosis of cystic fibrosis of the pancreas is based on four criteria: increase in the concentration of sodium or chloride in sweat; absence of the pancreatic enzyme trypsin, obtained by duodenal drainage; signs of chronic pulmonary involvement (obstructive emphysema and history of bilateral bronchopneumonia); and a family history of this disorder. All these criteria need not be present.

TABLE 8–1
WATER AND ELECTROLYTE LOSSES IN GASTROINTESTINAL SECRETIONS, AND IN SWEAT

Fluid	Average Volume (mL/24 hr)	ELECTROLYTE CONCENTRATIONS (mEq/L)			
		Na+	K+	Cl	HCO$_3$
Blood plasma		136–145	3.5–5.0	98–106	23–28
Gastric juice*	2500				
achlorhydric		8–120	1–30	100	20
containing HCl		10–110	1–32	8–55	0
Bile	700–1000	134–156	3.9–6.3	83–110	38
Pancreatic juice	>1000	113–153	2.6–7.4	54–95	110
Small bowel					
(Miller-Abbott suction)	3000	72–120	3.5–6.8	69–127	30
Ileostomy					
(a) recent	100–4000	112–142	4.5–14	93–122	30
(b) adapted	100–500	50	3	20	15–30
Cecostomy	100–3000	48–116	11.1–28.3	35–70	15
Feces	100	<10	<10	<15	<15
Sweat	500–4000	30–70	0–5	30–70	0

*The electrolyte concentrations in gastric juice vary widely—the higher the acidity, the lower the sodium concentration. Thus, when normal gastric acidity is present, the average sodium concentration of gastric juice is approximately 45 mEq/L. When hypoacidity or anacidity is present (as in elderly patients or those with carcinoma of the stomach), the average sodium concentration of gastric juice is approximately 100 mEq/L.

3. Loss of sodium in bronchial secretions. This is a relatively rare cause of sodium loss. It occurs, for example, in patients with bronchorrhea due to pulmonary adenomatosis. Some patients can expectorate 500 mL or more of bronchial secretions daily for weeks or months.

4. Sequestration of sodium within the body. This can occur in several ways:

    a. In small bowel obstruction, where large volumes of intestinal fluid can exudate into the intestinal lumen. In these patients, little or no visible loss of fluids may be noted because the patient may not vomit.

    b. A sequestration of extracellular water in the abdomen in peritonitis patients, in acute spreading cellulitis, in acute venous obstruction, such as portal vein thrombosis, and in so-called tourniquet lesion, with "release edema."

    c. In severe burns, where the edema accumulates under the burn, withdrawing salt, water, and protein from the plasma and the extracellular water. This edema continues to accumulate for 48 to 72 hours after the burn, and may be complicated by an external loss of water and salt through the burned skin.

    The external loss of extracellular water and sodium into the burn area is maximal in wet burns and scalds and reaches 1000 to 2000 mL a day. In dry, charred burns, such a loss of sodium and water is minimal. However, in dry burns treated with the open method, there may be a considerable loss of water by evaporation, particularly as sloughing begins. This can cause a severe water loss syndrome. (Burns are discussed in detail in Chapter 9.)

    d. As a result of hypodermoclysis of dextrose in distilled water. When this is done, sodium, chloride, and other electrolytes diffuse into the subcutaneous pool of dextrose and water. (No solution should ever be given subcutaneously unless it contains electrolytes in either isotonic or half-isotonic strength (see Chapter 37).

5. Sodium loss through the kidneys. This can occur in the following ways:

    a. With intrinsic renal disease. The usual patient with chronic renal disease does not lose an excessive amount of sodium ions through the kidneys. However, many patients with chronic renal disease may lose a small but definite amount of sodium ions daily this way and can develop a sodium loss syndrome quickly if they are placed on a low-sodium diet, or if they lose sodium ions extrarenally in any other way. The terms *renal salt wasting* or *salt-losing nephritis* have been used to describe patients with chronic renal disease who lose so many sodium ions that they require massive amounts of sodium chloride daily to prevent a sodium loss syndrome. Although such patients are rare, certain chronic conditions have been associated with salt wasting (e.g., medullary cystic disease, sarcoidosis). Transient salt wasting can occur during the polyuric phase of acute renal failure, after relief of urinary obstruction, and rarely after transplantation of a kidney.

    b. In the syndrome of inappropriate secretion of antidiuretic hormone (ADH) (Chapter 7). These patients show a retention of water and an increased circulating blood volume due to the continuous secretion of ADH. However, aldosterone secretion decreases and atrial natriuretic factor secretion increases as a result of the increased circulating blood volume and the kidneys excrete a large amount of sodium ions. The low serum sodium concentration in these patients is therefore partly due to water excess and partly due to true sodium loss.

    c. In Addison's disease and other forms of adrenocortical insufficiency, as after the withdrawal of cortisone or other corticosteroids.

    d. In diabetic acidosis. Sodium loss may occur in patients with diabetic acidosis even if they have not vomited. Apparently, the diuresis of large quantities of glucose is associated with a large urinary loss of sodium. This is due to the fact that the glucose excreted by the kidneys acts as an osmotic diuretic and causes sodium and other electrolytes to be eliminated into the urine.

e. As a result of drugs:
    i. Carbonic anhydrase inhibitors, such as Diamox. These drugs inhibit the action of carbonic anhydrase in the kidney tubular cells Chapter 12). When this happens, hydrogen ions are retained, and sodium and potassium are excreted instead.
    ii. Excessive ammonium chloride administration. The ammonium ion is converted to urea by the liver. The chloride is excreted along with sodium and other cations.
    iii. Diuretics such as the thiazides, spironolactone, furosemide, and ethacrynic acid.
6. Loss of sodium from serous cavities, or the subcutaneous tissues. This can occur after abdominal paracentesis, when a large volume of ascitic fluid is removed, or after repeated thoracenteses, or with the use of Southey tubes to relieve severe edema of the lower extremities. In such cases, the fluid quickly reaccumulates, or the patient becomes thirsty and drinks a large amount of water. This further lowers the osmotic pressure of the extracellular water and causes more water to flow into the cells, thereby further decreasing the volume of the extracellular water.
7. Loss of sodium as a result of severe hemorrhage.

In all of the above patients, the sodium loss syndrome is aggravated by a low-sodium diet. In addition, just as sodium loss aggravates the water excess syndrome (Chapter 6), water excess will aggravate the sodium loss syndrome.

SYMPTOMS AND SIGNS

The clinical picture depends on the rapidity of the sodium loss. When it occurs acutely, the clinical picture is that of severe shock. When it occurs slowly, the following symptoms and signs may appear.

General Symptoms

These include weakness, apathy, and lassitude. McCance, in his classic studies of experimentally induced salt loss, described how he and the other subjects all suffered from excessive fatigue and a general sense of exhaustion. They were content to sit and do nothing for hours on end. Muscle weakness was also present, and McCance found that his arm became tired while shaving and his jaws became tired when he ate.

Headache is an early sign. It is dull and becomes more marked on standing. In addition, giddiness and a feeling of faintness on standing may occur because of the decreased circulating blood volume. Muscle cramps may also occur. These can be precipitated if the patient drinks water freely, because the water aggravates the sodium loss.

When the sodium loss is marked, mental confusion, delirium, delusions, stupor, or coma may develop.

Gastrointestinal symptoms such as anorexia, nausea, or vomiting may occur. Thirst is characteristically absent; however, cases of sodium loss have been reported where thirst has been present. This is due to the decreased extracellular and circulating blood volume (see Chapter 3).

The patient appears apathetic and acutely ill. The eyeballs may be sunken and soft on palpation. The eyes have a glassy stare. The tongue may appear softened and shrunk, and may show longitudinal wrinkling.

The Skin

Skin turgor and elasticity disappear. Normally, when the skin of the inner forearm or arm is picked up and released, it returns to its previous shape almost immediately. When sodium loss is present, the skin tends to remain folded for one-half minute or more. (This sign can occur in elderly or cachectic patients in the absence of sodium loss.)

Cardiovascular Signs

These depend on the extent to which the circulating blood volume has diminished. There may be orthostatic hypotension, tachycardia, a low blood pressure and small pulse pressure, and a collapsing pulse. The extremities may be cold and the body temperature subnormal. The peripheral pulses may be absent. In severe cases, the typical signs of shock with cold, clammy skin and sweating may be present.

The peripheral veins, such as the hand veins, may be collapsed and may fill slowly (in more than 5 seconds) when the hand is held dependent, or if an occlusive venous tourniquet is placed around the hand.

A patient with congestive heart failure who develops sodium loss may show an aggravation of the heart failure, such as increasing edema, the development of pulmonary edema, or pleural effusion. A patient with coronary artery disease may show increased coronary insufficiency, or may develop a myocardial infarct.

LABORATORY FINDINGS
Blood

Hemoconcentration is present, with an elevated hematocrit. However, the mean corpuscular volume of the red blood cells is high, due to the entrance of water into the cells. This occurs because the osmotic pressure of the extracellular water is lower than that of the cells, as a result of the loss of sodium. For this same reason, the mean corpuscular hemoglobin concentration is low. In spite of the hemoconcentration, the serum sodium concentration is low—135 mEq/L, or lower. This differentiates sodium loss from water loss, where a high hematocrit is associated with a high serum sodium concentration.

The concentration of chloride or bicarbonate is also low, depending on which ion has been lost in association with the sodium. The BUN concentration is high because of the decreased renal blood flow. The serum potassium concentration is often high. (There is a tendency for the serum potassium and sodium concentrations to vary in opposite directions, because salt depletion syndromes will cause diminished urinary potassium excretion.)

Urine

The specific gravity is usually normal. The urinary volume is low and anuria may occur as a result of shock. Sodium and chloride concentrations are characteristically low in the urine.

The concentration of sodium in the urine tends to be proportional to the serum sodium concentration. In the sodium loss syndrome, it is therefore low and is characteristically below 10 mEq/L. It may even fall below 1 mEq/L. The urinary sodium concentration should be measured at a time when a sodium salt is not being given intravenously, and when the patient is not receiving a diuretic. In addition, the sodium concentration in the urine should be determined from a 24-hour collection.

When hyponatremia is associated with low urinary excretion of sodium ions, regardless of the dietary intake of salt, this is a sign either that the extracellular and blood volume is low, or that a condition, such as congestive heart failure with edema, cirrhosis of the liver, or the nephrotic syndrome, associated with an increased retention of sodium ions by the kidneys, is present. (A patient with inappropriate secretion of ADH [SIADH] [Chapter 7] may also have a low urinary excretion of sodium ions, if the dietary salt intake is low.)

A urinary sodium concentration of more than 10 mEq/L can occur in the sodium loss syndrome in two different conditions:

1. When the kidneys are unable to conserve sodium ions, as in patients with renal salt wasting.
2. When the adrenal cortex is not secreting sufficient aldosterone, as in Addison's disease or transient adrenocortical insufficiency. This may occur postoperatively.

A high urinary sodium concentration also occurs in the syndrome of inappropriate secretion of ADH (SIADH) (Chapter 7), when the dietary intake of salt is adequate.

DIAGNOSIS

Hyponatremia without true sodium loss may also occur when marked hyperglycemia, hyperlipidemia, or hyperproteinemia is present (see Chapter 11). This type of hyponatremia is asymptomatic and the patient does not require treatment. However, one should be certain that the hyponatremia is caused by one of these conditions, because sodium loss or water excess may also be present.

The use of serum osmolality measurements to differentiate true sodium loss or water excess from other syndromes associated with a low serum sodium concentration is described in Chapter 11.

The sodium loss syndrome is also frequently confused with another condition in which a low serum sodium concentration is found, namely, water excess syndrome.

The laboratory findings in water excess and sodium loss are similar because in both conditions the osmotic pressure of the extracellular water is lower than that of the cells, and each condition aggravates the other. However, the clinical picture of the two conditions is different. Patients with water excess will give a history of weight gain. Central nervous system disturbances, particularly convulsions, dominate the clinical picture. In sodium loss, weight loss, loss of skin turgor, and shock are characteristic. Water excess is described in detail in Chapters 6 and 7.

Acute Adrenal Crisis

Adrenal crisis (acute adrenocortical insufficiency) can be suspected when a patient receiving long-term corticosteroid therapy, or one who has had bilateral adrenalectomy or hypophysectomy, for example, develops one or more of the following symptoms and signs: severe weakness or lethargy, nausea and vomiting and abdominal pain, hypotension or shock, hyponatremia and hyperkalemia, hyperthermia and hypoglycemia.

The decreased circulating blood volume that occurs as a result of the sodium loss is often associated with decreased renal blood flow and a high BUN concentration. A metabolic acidosis is also present. The plasma cortisol level will be low. Some patients may show an apparently normal plasma cortisol level, but this is really inappropriately low in the presence of the stress situation.

PROPHYLAXIS

In the absence of sweating, a normal person requires little salt. It has been shown that as little as 200 mg of sodium (approximately 0.5 g of salt) or less is needed daily.

When sweating is present, the patient will require salt as well as water. So-called *insensible* perspiration contains practically pure water. It occurs continually in cold as well as warm weather. *Sensible* or visible sweat, on the other hand, occurs with excessive heat production by the body as a result of fear, or other strong stimuli. It can be considered as a hypotonic (hyposmotic) solution with a sodium and chloride concentration ranging from about 30 to 70 mEq and a small amount of potassium (Table 8–1). When sensible perspiration is excessive, the patient will require supplemental salt. This can be given in the form of salt tablets (0.5 g). Water with one tablet per pint (0.5 g per 500 mL) (0.1% solution) can be imbibed freely. As a general rule, one 0.5-g salt tablet and 1 pint of water for each pound of weight lost should provide a satisfactory amount of salt and water.

A patient who is perspiring excessively and cannot take salt orally can be given an infusion composed of 1 part of isotonic saline (sodium chloride) solution and 2 parts of dextrose in water. (This contains approximately 50 mEq sodium per liter and is similar to the composition of sweat; Table 8–1.)

Sodium loss can be prevented if the physician is aware of the conditions in which it can occur and is alert to recognize premonitory symptoms and signs.

Several preventive measures can be taken. For example, if the patient has pyloric obstruction and is vomiting greatly, or if gastric suction is being used, a volume-for-volume replacement of the water and electrolytes (including potassium) should be done daily. The volume of gastric fluid in the suction bottle can be measured every 4, 6, or 12 hours, and an equivalent amount of fluid infused. In addition, since the patient is not taking fluids orally, enough water, sodium, potassium, and protein for ordinary daily needs (Chapter 37) must be given.

The type of fluid used for replacement of gastrointestinal losses depends on the type of fluid being lost.

If fluid is being lost by gastric suction, or from vomiting due to pyloric obstruction, an adequate gastric replacement solution can be prepared in the following way:

If the gastric juice is highly acid (pH 1.5 to 2.5) replace one third of the volume lost with isotonic saline solution and two thirds with dextrose in water, and add 20 mEq potassium chloride (1.5 g) per liter.

If the gastric juice has a low acidity (pH 5.0 to 5.5), give half-strength saline solution to which 20 mEq potassium chloride (1.5 g) per liter has been added. Such solutions can be given at a rate up to 500 mL/hr.

In acute gastric dilatation, the fluid may have a high chloride concentration of 150 mEq/L. In such a patient, isotonic saline solution should be used to replace the fluid lost.

If gastrointestinal fluids are being lost from a pancreatic or small intestinal fistula, or from intestinal obstruction, the electrolyte concentration of lactated Ringer's solution (Chapter 38) is similar to that of the duodenal and small intestinal secretions, and it can be used to replace duodenal or small intestinal losses. Additional KCl can be added if necessary.

In pancreatic fistulas, the fluid may have a high sodium concentration, even 185 mEq/L. Isotonic saline solution should be used to replace fluid losses. In addition, it may be necessary to use small amounts of hypertonic 5% sodium chloride to maintain a normal sodium concentration.

Ileostomy fluid may have a high potassium concentration, even 70 mEq/L. Sufficient potassium must be added to the lactated Ringer's solution to maintain the serum potassium concentration.

A volume-by-volume replacement of the intestinal fluid losses should be made, and the patient's daily needs for water, sodium, potassium, and protein (Chapter 36) should be maintained.

One should remember that patients with small-bowel obstruction may lose enormous volumes of fluid, as much as 5 to 10 liters, in the distended intestine, even though vomiting is not present. Similarly, patients with duodenal or jejunal fistulas can lose 3 to 6 liters daily through the fistula alone. Patients with pancreatic fistula usually lose less than 2 liters a day through the fistula. A patient with acute gastric dilatation who is being treated with nasogastric suction can lose 8000 mL or more fluid a day, which must be replaced (also see Chapter 37).

Bile secretion has a composition that is approximately similar to that of the plasma. Therefore, losses from biliary fistula can be replaced with lactated Ringer's solution (Chapter 38).

When gastrointestinal suction is being used, the tube should be irrigated with isotonic saline, or saline solution to which 1 g of potassium chloride per liter has been added, but not with water.

TREATMENT

In treating sodium loss, one should:

1. Treat shock. Large quantities of sodium chloride, water, and plasma may be needed (see below). In addition, we have already mentioned the fact that severe shock due to sodium loss will not respond to pressor amines, such as dopamine (Intropin), or norepinephrine (Levophed). However, pressor amines may become effective after an infusion of sodium chloride has been started. (The pressor amines can be used immediately if they are given in a solution that contains sodium chloride. Norepinephrine should be given in a solution that contains dextrose as well as sodium chloride when treating a patient with shock due to sodium loss. Otherwise it will oxidize and become ineffective.)

2. Stop further sodium loss from the body. This has already been discussed under Prophylaxis. In addition, if Addison's disease is present, hydrocortisone or large quantities of salt orally are indicated (also see below). If the patient is on a low-sodium diet, the sodium intake should be increased. In a patient with renal salt wasting as much as 15 to 20 g of salt orally may be needed daily.

3. Give sufficient sodium chloride, water, and plasma, if necessary, to compensate for the loss of sodium. In addition, other electrolytes such as potassium, chloride, or bicarbonate may have to be replaced.

Type of Solution Needed

Most patients with acute sodium loss and shock respond to isotonic 0.9% sodium chloride (saline). In addition, colloid solutions such as albumin or plasma expanders such as dextran may be helpful in treating the shock.

In patients with chronic sodium loss, hypertonic 5% sodium chloride solution can be given intravenously (see Chapter 6).

If the patient is acidotic, one-third molar sodium lactate (Chapter 38), or 3.75% sodium bicarbonate (Chapter 38) can be substituted for the 5% sodium chloride.

Potassium Solutions

When gastrointestinal secretions are lost, potassium as well as sodium is lost and must be replaced. Table 8–1 gives average values for the electrolyte concentrations in the various gastrointestinal secretions. The potassium can be given as potassium chloride in the infusion bottle. As much as 80 mEq/L potassium (6 g KCl) can be placed in the infusion bottle, but the potassium must be infused at a rate that does not exceed 20 mEq (rarely, 35 mEq) per hour. In addition, if the patient is oliguric, potassium should not be given until the urinary volume increases.

Even when sodium loss is not related to a loss of gastrointestinal secretions, potassium chloride orally may be helpful in raising the serum sodium concentration. It probably is effective by entering the cells and exchanging with intercellular sodium ions, which pass into the extracellular water and blood.

Volume of Solution to Be Used

There are several methods for calculating the volume of sodium chloride and colloid solution to be given. Any one of the following is satisfactory:

Method 1

If one knows the acute weight loss, the loss of sodium (in mEq) equals 142 times the loss of weight in kilograms (kg). This assumes that the normal sodium concentration of the extracellular water is 142 mEq/L and that the weight loss has been due entirely to a loss of extracellular water and its electrolytes.

Example: The patient has lost 2 kg weight in a period of one day. Therefore, the loss of sodium would be $142 \times 2 = 284$ mEq sodium.
1 mEq sodium = approximately 1 mL hypertonic 5% NaCl solution.
1 mEq sodium = approximately 6 mL isotonic 0.9% NaCl solution.
Therefore, the patient would receive $284 \times 6 = 1704$ mL, or approximately 2 liters of isotonic sodium chloride (saline) solution.

Method 2

If accurate weight loss is not available, the sodium loss can be calculated from the hematocrit. This method also assumes that only extracellular water and electrolytes have been lost, and that there has not been any hemorrhage.

Example: Woman weight 70 kg; hematocrit 55%.

We know that the normal extracellular water volume is approximately 20% of the body weight. (The plasma volume is about 4% of the body weight, or one-fifth the volume of the extracellular water.) The average normal hematocrit is 42% ± 5% in a woman and 47% ± 7% in a man.

Therefore, a rise in the hematocrit from 42 to 55% in a woman indicates that approximately 25% of the extracellular water has been lost (55 − 42 = 13%; 13/42 = 1/4, or 25% loss).

The extracellular water volume of this patient is 20% of 70 kg = 14 liters. The loss of sodium and water is 25% of 14 liters = 3.5 liters. Therefore, 3.5 liters of isotonic sodium chloride solution are urgently needed.

Method 3

The sodium loss can also be calculated from changes in the serum sodium concentration. Superficially, it might seem that the changes in serum sodium concentration in relation to the volume of extracellular water should be measured. However, when sodium salts are given, a similar rise must occur in the osmolality of both the extracellular water and of the cells. This is the reason that changes in the serum sodium concentration must be calculated in relation to the total body water volume (unit serum sodium deficit per mEq/L *times* volume of body water).

Example: Patient weight 70 kg; serum sodium 122 mEq/L.

We know that the total body water volume is 60% of the weight, $0.6 \times 70 = 42$ liters. The unit sodium deficit equals 142 mEq/L (the normal concentration) − 122 mEq/L = 20 mEq/L.

In other words, a deficit of 20 mEq sodium is present in each liter of body water. Since the total body water volume is 42 liters, the total sodium deficit is $20 \times 42 = 840$ mEq. However, it is neither necessary nor desirable to give such a large quantity of sodium chloride.

Not more than one-half this amount, or 840/2 = 420 mEq, should be given. One reason for this is that as the sodium and water are infused the circulation improves and the kidneys are able to excrete water. This increases the serum sodium concentration and helps decrease the need for further salt.

Method 4. Treatment of Sodium Loss Complicated by Water Excess

This usually occurs in patients with chronic sodium loss. It also is common in patients with congestive heart failure, who have lost sodium, and also occurs in patients with sodium loss who have been incorrectly treated with dextrose in water, or with pressor amines in dextrose and water.

These patients should be treated by withholding water and giving sodium chloride. The water intake can be kept below 1000 mL a day, and even withheld for the first 12 hours. Salt can be added to the diet. For example, if a cardiac patient who has been on a low-sodium diet complains of progressive weakness and shows other signs of sodium loss, 2 to 3 g of table salt can be added daily to the food. This can be done by using an ordinary No. 0 gelatin capsule. When the capsule is filled with salt, it holds almost 1 g (400 mg sodium). The salt is sprinkled on the food, because salt on the food tastes better than salt in the food. This can be done easily by puncturing an end of the capsule a few times with a pin, making the capsule a miniature salt shaker.

If a patient with congestive heart failure who shows sodium loss and water excess is given hypertonic sodium chloride intravenously, the heart failure may become aggravated. However, one may use hypertonic sodium chloride intravenously, even in congestive heart failure patients, if signs of acute water intoxication, such as the sudden development of delirium, are present. A small infusion of 50 to 100 mL 5% sodium chloride is usually adequate.

Patients with cardiac decompensation and a combination of sodium loss and water excess (as indicated by a low serum sodium concentration) can be treated with "loop" diuretics, such as furosemide (Lasix) or ethacrynic acid (Edecrin). Both of these diuretics are able to cause a diuresis of water in excess of sodium ions.

Rate of Administration of the Solution

When shock is present, isotonic sodium chloride can be given rapidly, at a rate of 1 to 2 L/hr. Marriott, for example, describes the following schedule in the treatment of shock due to severe acute sodium losses:

500 mL in 10 minutes. Then,
500 mL in 15 minutes. Then,
500 mL in 10 minutes. Then,
500 mL in 30 minutes. Then,
500 mL every 2 hours until the blood pressure is normal.

Such massive doses are rarely needed, because after the first 500 mL or 1 liter has been infused, the shock can be alleviated either with plasma or dextran.

When isotonic sodium chloride is given at a rate faster than 500 mL an hour, the patient should be watched constantly by the physician for the development of signs of congestive heart failure or metabolic acidosis.

The rate of administration of hypertonic sodium chloride solution is described in Chapter 6.

Route of Administration

Intravenous administration is advisable. However, large volumes of isotonic sodium chloride solution can be given by means of a nasogastric tube, or rectally by means of a Murphy drip apparatus, or by hypodermoclysis. Salt can also be given orally. Isotonic sodium chloride solution is irritating to the gastrointestinal tract of many patients, and may be deleterious in the treatment of patients with cholera. However, Moyer has found that large amounts of a salt solution having less than 0.6% salt can be imbibed without difficulty, especially if the solution also contains sodium bicarbonate. He recommends a mixture of 3 to 4 g (1 level teaspoonful) of sodium chloride and 1.5 to 2 g (1 level teaspoonful) of sodium bicarbonate or citrate per liter of water. Salt tablets can also be given orally in mild sodium loss.

Carpenter has made extensive studies in the treatment of patients with cholera. He has shown that cholera stool is approximately isotonic and has a bicarbonate concentration of 45 to 50 mEq/L.

WHO (World Health Organization) has recommended the use of the following oral replacement solution for severe diarrhea, including cholera:

	g/L		mmol/L
Sodium chloride	3.5	Na	90
Potassium chloride	1.5	K	20
Sodium bicarbonate	2.5	Cl	80
Glucose	20	HCO_3	30

Dextrose is used in the solution because it stimulates active transport of sodium ions and water from the intestines into the bloodstream.

The oral solution can be given on a basis of equal volumes for stool losses. If the stool volume exceeds oral intake in any 4-hour period, intravenous therapy should be given if possible.

Treatment of Renal Salt Wasting

When a patient with moderate renal salt wasting is placed on a low-sodium diet, a continued excretion of sodium ions in the urine occurs, so that a sodium loss syndrome may develop, often in a few days. This can be prevented by allowing a regular diet without added salt. (This contains about 7 g of salt a day.) When renal salt wasting is severe, as in a patient with medullary cystic disease of the kidneys, as much as 10 to 40 g of salt a day may be needed to maintain sodium balance.

Treatment of Acute Adrenocortical Insufficiency (Adrenal Crisis)

Acute adrenocortical insufficiency is associated with a deficiency of both the glucocorticoid and mineralocorticoid adrenal cortical hormones.

Emergency treatment includes the following (after Himathongkam et al.):

Treatment of Glucocorticoid Lack

A solution of 100 mg hydrocortisone succinate (Solu-Cortef) dissolved in 2 to 10 mL water is given as an intravenous bolus. Then 100 mg hydrocortisone succinate is given continuously in an intravenous infusion every 8 hours, for at least 36 or 48 hours. A total dose of 300 mg hydrocortisone over 24 hours is adequate to control the stressful situation that precipitated the crisis.

After this period, 5 mg hydrocortisone, or cortisone acetate, is given orally every 6 hours. In addition, 50 mg cortisone acetate can be given intramuscularly every 12 hours to maintain adequate cortisol blood levels until the acute crisis disappears. The glucocorticoid dosage can be decreased over a period of several days to a maintenance dose of approximately 10 mg hydrocortisone 2 or 3 times a day.

Treatment of Mineralocorticoid Lack

While the patient is receiving large doses of hydrocortisone, it is not necessary to use any supplementary adrenal mineralocorticoid hormones. However, when the daily hydrocortisone dosage decreases below 100 mg, it may be necessary to give the patient a mineralocorticoid such as fludrocortisone acetate (Florinef), 0.1 mg every 24 hours, or desoxycorticosterone acetate (DOCA), 2.5 to 5.0 mg intramuscularly every 24 hours, to prevent a loss of sodium ions in the urine.

Treatment of Hyponatremia and Hypotension

Intravenous saline solution is necessary to raise the serum sodium concentration, increase the circulating blood volume, and counteract the hypotension. One liter of 5% dextrose in isotonic saline is given intravenously in a period of 1 to 2 hours. Most patients need additional intravenous saline, at a rate of 1 liter every 3 to 6 hours for the next 24 hours. If an excessive amount of sodium chloride solution is infused, pulmonary or cerebral edema may occur.

If the blood pressure does not respond to the intravenous hydrocortisone and saline, it may be necessary to use a pressor amine, such as phenylephrine (Neo-Synephrine) or dopamine (Intropin) intravenously.

Treatment of Hyperkalemia

The hyperkalemia responds to the intravenous glucocorticoids and saline solution. If the serum potassium concentration is higher than 6.5 mEq/L and if cardiac arrhythmias are present, 1 or 2 ampuls of 44.5 mEq sodium bicarbonate (Chapter 38) can be given intravenously every 1 to 2 hours, until the serum potassium concentration falls and the arrhythmias disappear.

One should remember that high-dose glucocorticoid therapy may produce severe *hypo*kalemia by the second to the fourth day of therapy, which may require treatment with potassium chloride.

Treatment of Hypoglycemia

This usually responds to the intravenous infusion of dextrose in saline. If the patient has diabetes and is taking insulin, the blood sugar level should be checked repeatedly to prevent severe hypoglycemia.

Treatment of Hyperpyrexia

Fever usually disappears with the intravenous therapy described above. An alcohol sponge bath can be used if necessary. The fever may also be a sign of a bacterial or viral infection, which may require treatment. When adrenal crisis develops without an apparent cause, one should suspect that an infection has precipitated the crisis.

CLINICAL APPROACH TO A HYPONATREMIC PATIENT

This and the preceding two chapters have described in detail the multiple causes of hyponatremia. Because of the complexity and clinical importance of this subject, this final section is devoted to a review of the bedside and laboratory approaches to a hyponatremic patient.

First, it is important to remember that not all low serum sodium values indicate true hyponatremia. Laboratory error must always be ruled out. A useful way of checking the consistency of a laboratory report is to calculate the anion gap (Chapter 1). An anion gap of less than 9 mEq/L is unlikely and suggests that the "hyponatremia" is due to a laboratory error.

Next, hyperlipidemia or hyperproteinemia must also be excluded as a cause of pseudohyponatremia (Chapter 11).

A concomitant measurement of serum glucose concentration must always be obtained, because hyerglycemia will produce a misleading hyponatremia due to osmotic fluid shifts. Every elevation of the serum glucose concentration of 100 mg/dL will decrease the serum sodium concentration approximately 1.6 mEq/L (Appendix IV).

When true hyponatremia has been ascertained, the most important step is a clinical assessment of the patient's extracellular fluid volume. Hyponatremic patients can be divided as follows:

1. Patients with decreased extracellular fluid volume, due to sodium loss (indicated by decreased skin turgor, hypotension, shock, and so on; see above).
2. Patients with increased extracellular fluid volume due to water excess. These patients can be further subdivided into those with and those without edema.

In medical patients, the most important causes of hyponatremia with decreased extracellular fluid volume are adrenocortical insufficiency, gastrointestinal sodium loss syndromes (due to vomiting, diarrhea, and so on), excessive sweating, or excessive diuresis, with replacement of the losses with water rather than a sodium-containing solution. Salt-losing nephritis is rare (see above). Adrenocortical insufficiency is listed first because it is important to rule out an incipient Addisonian crisis in every patient with hyponatremia and a decreased extracellular fluid volume. The combination of a low serum sodium concentration and a high serum potassium concentration, a history of recent corticosteroid use, and the physical stigmata of Addison's disease (increased pigmentation, and so on) should be carefully sought.

The treatment of a hyponatremic patient with a decreased extracellular fluid volume requires the replacement of sodium ions and fluid, as has been discussed above.

Patients who show hyponatremia and *edema* indicate an excessive total body sodium content, in spite of the low serum sodium concentration. This problem is commonly encountered in patients with congestive heart failure, cirrhosis, or the nephrotic syndrome. The low serum sodium concentration can result from numerous factors, including excessive diuretic therapy, excessive water intake, and the inability of the kidneys to excrete water normally. The primary therapy in these patients is water restriction, in contrast to the sodium and volume replacement needed in patients with hyponatremia and a decreased extracellular fluid volume.

Patients with hyponatremia, no edema, and no signs of decreased extracellular fluid volume usually have evidence of water excess produced iatrogenically, inappropriate secretion of ADH syndromes (SIADH), or compulsive water drinking. The diagnosis of SIADH is made by finding a low serum sodium concentration and a low serum osmolality, usually a high urine sodium concentration and a high urine osmolality, and normal adrenal and renal functions. A workup for a suspected SIADH patient should include chest x-ray examination and sputum culture (to detect tuberculosis or pulmonary fungal infection, or pulmonary carcinoma), careful neurological assessment, thyroid studies (to rule out myxedema), and a careful listing of all medications the patient has been taking (see Chapter 7).

In the general assessment of the hyponatremic patient, urinary sodium determinations are valuable. (This can be done on a "spot" sample of urine and does not require 24-hour collection.) As mentioned above, SIADH is typically associated with an inappropriately high urine sodium concentration (usually more than 20 mEq/L), despite the hyponatremia. A high urine sodium concentration with hyponatremia can also be seen in adrenocortical insufficiency, salt-losing nephritis, and with excessive diuretic therapy.

Conversely, patients with hyponatremia and extracellular fluid loss due to gastrointestinal losses will have a low urine sodium concentration. Patients with hyponatremia and edema due to congestive heart failure, cirrhosis, and the nephrotic syndrome also typically retain sodium ions and show a low urine sodium concentration.

Finally, it is important to emphasize that hyponatremia may be due to more than one cause, or to a combination of sodium loss and water excess. For example, a patient with congestive heart failure may develop hyponatremia because of a low sodium intake, excessive water intake, excessive diuresis, vomiting, removal of a large pleural effusion, and so on. Treatment of hyponatremia associated with congestive heart failure includes an angiotensin converting enzyme inhibitor, such as captopril or enalapril, and furosemide.

Bibliography

Almufti, H, and Asrief, A: Captopril-induced hyponatremia with irreversible neurologic damage. Am J Med 79:769, 1985.

Ashraf, N, et al: Thiazide-induced hyponatremia associated with death or neurologic damage in outpatients. Am J Med 70:63, 1981.

Avery, MD, and Snyder, JD: Oral therapy for acute diarrhea. N Engl J Med 323:893, 1990.

Avus, JC, et al: Treatment of symptomatic hyponatremia and its relation to brain damage. N Engl J Med 317:1190, 1987.

Berry, REL: The "third kidney" phenomenon of the gastrointestinal tract. Arch Surg 81:193, 1960.

Cash, RA, Nalin, DR, Forrest, JN, and Abrutyn, E: Rapid correction of acidosis and dehydration of cholera with oral electrolyte and glucose solution. Lancet 2:549, 1970.

Carey, RJ, and Burbank, CB: Mucus-secreting villous adenoma of the colon presenting as circulatory collapse. N Engl J Med 267:609, 1962.

Carpenter, CCJ: Clinical studies in Asiatic cholera. Bull Johns Hopkins Hosp 118:165, 174, 197, 216, 243, 1966.

Carpenter, CCJ: Oral rehydration. Is it as good as parenteral therapy? Editorial. N Engl J Med 306:1103, 1982.

Cooke, RE, and Crowley, LG: Replacement of gastric and intestinal fluid losses in surgery. N Engl J Med 246:637, 1952.

Durr, JA, et al: Diabetes insipidus in pregnancy associated with abnormally high circulating vasopressinase activity. N Engl J Med 316:1070, 1987.

Dwek, JH, et al: Salt wasting bronchorrhea and its mechanisms. Arch Intern Med 137:791, 1977.

Griffen, KA, and Bidani, AK: How to manage disorders of sodium and water balance. J Crit Ill 5:1054, 1990.

Harrington, JT, and Cohen, JJ: Measurement of urinary electrolytes. Indications and limitations. N Engl J Med 293:1241, 1975.

Himathongkam, T, et al: Medical emergency management. Acute adrenal insufficiency. JAMA 230:1317, 1974. Also, Emergency Med, April 1976, page 71.

Hughes, JM: Salt-losing nephritis. Arch Intern Med 114:190, 1964.

Ishikawa, SE, et al: Hyponatremia responsive to fludrocortisone acetate in elderly patients. Ann Intern Med 106:187, 1987.

Kassirer, JP, and Gennari, FJ: Salt wasting. Consequence or functional adaptation? N Engl J Med 296:42, 1977.

Kerpel-Fronius, E: Uber die Beziehungen zwischen Salz- und Wasseraushalt bei experimentellen Wasserverlusten. Z Kinderheilk, 57:489, 1935.

Krumlovsku, FA: Hyponatremia. Rational Drug Ther 9:5, May 1975.

Leshin, M: Acute adrenal insufficiency. Recognition, management, and prevention. Urologic Clin N Am 9:229, 1982.

Lilly, LS: The clinical significance of hyponatremia in congestive heart failure. Practical Cardiol 12:53, 1986.

McCance, RA: III. Experimental salt deficiency. Lancet 1:823, 1936.

Medical Letter: Treatment of heat injury, 32: July 13, 1990.

Medical Letter on Drugs and Therapeutics: Gatorade and other oral electrolyte solutions, 2:71, 1969.

Nadal, JW, Pedersen, S, and Maddock, WG: Comparison between dehydration from salt loss and from water deprivation. J Clin Invest 20:691, 1941.

Nalin, DR, et al: Oral maintenance therapy for cholera in adults. Lancet 2:370, 1968.

Narins, RG: Therapy of hyponatremia. Does haste make waste? Editorial. N Engl J Med 314:1573, 1986.

Pierce, NF, and Hirschhorn, N: Oral fluid. A simple weapon against dehydration in diarrhoea. How it works and how to use it. WHO Chron 31:87, 1977.

Pierce, NF, et al: Replacement of water and electrolyte losses in cholera by an oral glucose-electrolyte solution. Ann Intern Med 70:1173, 1969.

Questions and Answers: Fluid and electrolyte replacement in sweating athletes. JAMA, 212:1713, 1970.

Sagnella, GA, Markandu, ND, Buckley, MG, et al: Hormonal responses to gradual changes in dietary sodium intake in humans. Am J Physiol 256:R1171, 1989.

Santosham, M, et al: Oral rehydration therapy of infantile diarrhea. N Engl J Med 306:1070, 1982.

Schrier, RW: Treatment of hyponatremia. Editorial. N Engl J Med 312:1123, 1985.

Schrier, RW, and Briner, VN: The differential diagnosis of hyponatremia. Hosp Practice Sept. 30, 1990, 29.

Schwachman, H, and Gahm, N: A simple test for the detection of excessive chloride on the skin. N Engl J Med 255:999, 1956.

Sherman, RA, and Eisenger, RP: The use (and misuse) of urinary sodium and chloride measurements. JAMA 247:3121, 1982.

Snyder, N, et al: Hypernatremia in elderly patients. Arch Int Med 107:309, 1987.

Stanbury, SW, and Mahler, RF: Salt-wasting renal disease. Quart J Med 28:425, 1959.

Taclob, LT, and Needle, MA: Hyponatremic syndromes. Med Clin N Am, 57:1425, 1973.

Westerman, RL: Oral electrolyte solutions for fluid and electrolyte replacement. Questions and Answers. JAMA 248:370, 1982.

9

SODIUM LOSS SYNDROMES (Continued)

BURNS

Burns can be classified as follows:

1. *Partial thickness.* The injury involves both the epidermis and the dermis, but does not destroy the dermis. Vesicles, bullae, and blebs occur with oozing. The skin is pink and reddened, and is painful. Second-degree burns usually result from contact with hot liquids or exposure to flashes of short duration.
2. *Full thickness.* The epidermis and the dermis are destroyed. The skin is pearly-white or charred, dry and anesthetic, because the nerve endings have been destroyed. Full thickness burns usually result from contact with a flash or flame of longer duration.

In this chapter, we will be concerned with the physiological disturbances caused by partial and full thickness burns.

PATHOPHYSIOLOGY

Burns can cause the following physiological disturbances:

1. Even partial thickness burns result in massive exudation of water, plasma, electrolytes, and plasma proteins into the burned and injured areas.

   The most rapid exudation of fluid occurs in the first 6 to 8 hours after the burn. However, the exudation may continue for a total of 48 to 96 hours. This causes a severe sodium loss syndrome (Chapter 8) and may require treatment with large amounts of water, electrolytes, and colloid solutions. Adults with a burn of 20% or more will almost always develop the sodium loss syndrome.

2. Extensive burns, especially third-degree burns, cause destruction of red blood cells. The anemia that results may be severe.
3. Hyperkalemia may occur due to the release of intracellular potassium ions from the burned cells. Similarly, a metabolic acidosis may result from the accumulation of organic acids from the burned cells. A moderate azotemia (BUN concentration 30 to 60 mg/dL) may also develop. Hypocalcemia, even with tetany, can develop 12 to 24 hours after a large deep burn, probably due to saponification of burned subcutaneous tissue.
4. The urine may contain hemoglobin from destruction of red blood cells.

From a physiological point of view, burns can be classified in the following stages:

1. *Stage of sodium loss and shock.* This occurs in the first 48 to 72 hours. Adequate therapy with water and electrolytes, with or without colloid solutions, usually causes the patient to gain from 8 to 10% weight during this period of time, after a severe burn.
2. *Stage of sodium and water reabsorption and diuresis.* This occurs from the third or fifth to the twelfth or fourteenth day because the edema fluid in the tissues surrounding the burn begins to be reabsorbed and excreted by the kidneys.
3. *Stage of anemia and malnutrition.* This occurs from the fifth day onward. In this stage, it is important to maintain the patient's blood count and to feed him or her adequately, in order to stop the negative nitrogen balance due to the destruction of tissue.

COURSE AND PROGNOSIS

Shock, oliguria, and fever are unfavorable signs. The prognosis of a person with a burn of less than 20% is uniformly good. However, at least one out of two patients will die when 50% or more of the body surface is burned. The cause of death is usually overwhelming infection that does not respond to antibiotic therapy.

TREATMENT
Stage of Sodium Loss and Shock

All investigators agree that burn patients at this stage require electrolytes with or without colloid solutions. However, there is no agreement about the types or volumes of the electrolyte or colloid solutions that should be used. It is interesting to note that very different treatments appear to be almost equally effective.

At the 1978 Consensus Development Conference on Supportive Therapy in Burn Care, the participants agreed on the following general principles of fluid treatment for severe burns (Schwartz):

1. In the initial 24-hour postburn period, an isotonic balanced (lactated Ringer's) salt solution is as adequate as colloid-containing solutions, and no other solution (neither colloid nor 5% dextrose in water) needs to be given at this time. The calculated dose of lactated Ringer's solution should range between 2 and 4 mL/kg/% body surface burned.
2. At approximately 24 hours post burn, colloid-containing solutions can be given to expand the plasma volume.
3. The total time required for resuscitation can be shortened by the rapid reconstitution of plasma volume as soon as leaky capillaries are sealed, i.e., between 24 and 32 hours post-burn.

The Parkland Hospital (Baxter) formula corresponds to these recommendations.

A burned patient can be treated like other patients with sodium loss syndrome, with merely oral or parenteral saline or similar sodium-containing solutions. The fluid and electrolyte requirements of a burned patient depend partly on the extent of the burn. This can be determined in a simple way by the following *rule of nines:*

Anterior head—4 1/2% of the body surface
Posterior head—4 1/2% of the body surface
Each upper extremity—9% of the body surface
Each lower extremity—18% of the body surface
Anterior thorax and abdomen—18% of the body surface
Posterior thorax and back—18% of the body surface

The Treatment of Limited Burns (10% to 15% of the body surface)

A patient with a burn of only 10% to 15% of the body surface can usually be treated by means of a sodium-containing electrolyte solution, given orally. The solution should be iced. The container can be placed in a pan of ice at the patient's bedside, so that the solution remains chilled. (However, if repeated vomiting or diarrhea occurs, oral therapy should be stopped.)

Many oral electrolyte solutions have been described, for example,

Moyer's solution, consisting of 1 level teaspoonful (approximately 3 g) sodium chloride, and 1 level teaspoonful (approximately 1.5 g) sodium bicarbonate (baking soda), to 1 liter of iced drinking water. (It is hypotonic and provides 69 mEq sodium ions, 52 mEq chloride ions, and 17 mEq bicarbonate ions per liter.)
Markley's solution, consisting of 5.5 g sodium chloride and 4.0 g sodium bicarbonate in 1 liter iced drinking water. (It is isotonic and provides

140 mEq sodium ions, 94 mEq chloride ions, and 47 bicarbonate ions per liter.)

The oral solution can be imbibed at a rate of 50 to 100 mL/hr, as tolerated: 1 to 2.5 liters can be imbibed in 24 hours. (The volume taken in the first 24 hours should not exceed 5% of the body weight.) The patient is also allowed soft food, occasionally broth or fruit juice, but *no* tap water.

The Treatment of Extensive Burns (20% or more of the skin surface)

A patient with an extensive burn can also be treated with a sodium-containing electrolyte solution, just as a less seriously burned patient, and just as other patients with sodium loss syndrome. However, the solution is usually given intravenously because of the large volume needed. Part (or even all) of the solution can be given orally, using one of the oral formulas described above, if the patient tolerates it.

The following discussions present widely used methods of giving fluids intravenously.

The Parkland Hospital or Baxter Formula (Table 9–1). In the first 24 hours, lactated Ringer's solution, 4 mL per kg body weight per % of total body surface burned, is given.

Example: Patient, 70 kg weight, with a 50% second-degree burn.

The total volume of lactated Ringer's solution needed during the first 24 hours is:

$$4 \times 70 \times 0.5 = 14 \text{ liters}.$$

One half of the calculated volume is given rapidly during the first 8 hours; one quarter is given in the next 8 hours; the final one quarter is given in the final 8 hours.

The goal of the intravenous fluid is to establish a urine flow of 50 to 70 mL/hr, a pulse rate less than 120 per minute, a normal pH and serum bicarbonate concentration, and a lucid patient with stable vital signs. (It may be difficult or impossible to measure blood pressure if the upper extremities are burned.) When a urine flow greater than 50 mL/hr has been established and the patient's clinical condition improves, the rate of flow of the infusion can be adjusted.

When most or all of the lactated Ringer's solution has been infused, 18 to 24 hours after the burn, a small amount of plasma or serum albumin (see Table 9–1) can be given intravenously if the patient does not show optimum vital signs.

After the first 24 hours, lactated Ringer's solution is not used. Instead, dextrose in water should be administered in an amount necessary to maintain a normal serum sodium concentration. Two (or more) liters of dextrose in water may be needed in this second 24-hour period.

TABLE 9–1
FORMULAS FOR ESTIMATING ADULT BURN PATIENT RESUSCITATION NEEDS*

Formula	Electrolyte Solution	Colloid Solution†	5% Dextrose in Water
FIRST 24 HOURS			
Parkland Hospital (Baxter)	Lactated Ringer's 4 mL/kg/% burn		
Brooke Army Med. Center	Lactated Ringer's 1.5 mL/kg/% burn	0.5 mL/kg/% burn	2000 mL
Hypertonic sodium chloride (250 mEq Na/L)	Volume to maintain urine output at 30 mL/hr		
SECOND 24 HOURS			
Parkland Hospital (Baxter)		20–60% of calcu- lated plasma volume‡	To maintain ade- quate urinary output
Brooke Army Med. Center	1/2 to 1/4 of first 24-hr needs	1/2 to 1/4 of first 24 hr needs	2000 mL
Hypertonic sodium chloride (250 mEq Na/L)	1/3 isotonic saline orally up to 3500-mL limit		

*Adapted from Pruitt.
†The usual colloid solutions are blood plasma or human serum albumin.
‡Calculated plasma volume is 39 mL/kg for men; 40 mL/kg for women.

The Brooke Army Medical Center Formula (Table 9–1). (This is a modification of the Evans formula.)

First 24 hours:

Colloid (plasma or human serum albumin): 0.5 mg per kg body weight per % of total body surface burned.

Lactated Ringer's solution: 1.5 mL per kg body weight per % of total body surface burned.

Dextrose in water solution: 2000 mL.

Second 24 hours:

Approximately one half the volumes of the lactated Ringer's solution and of the colloid solution.

Dextrose in water solution: 2000 mL.

One half of this amount is given in the first 8 hours after the burn. One quarter is given in the next 8-hour period; the final one quarter is given in the next 8-hour period.

Whole blood should not be used at first because of the presence of hemoconcentration. However, it can be given when the hematocrit falls below normal (usually on the second to seventh day after the burn). (If the patient shows an anemia but the central venous pressure is elevated, a packed red blood cell transfusion should be given instead.)

Dextran can be used as a plasma substitute, but not more than 1 liter a day should be given (Chapter 38).

(In the original Evans formula, isotonic saline solution was used instead of lactated Ringer's solution. However, a large amount of sodium chloride intravenously may cause a metabolic acidosis [Chapter 17], or it may aggravate the metabolic acidosis that is usually present in a severely burned patient.)

When the extent of the burn is more than 50% of the body surface, colloid and lactated Ringer's solutions should be given in an amount calculated for only a 50% burn. In this way, the patient will not receive an excessive amount of fluid (which can cause pulmonary edema when the burn edema fluid begins to be reabsorbed into the circulation on the third day or later).

In addition, not more than 10,000 mL of total fluids should be given in 1 day, regardless of the extent of the burn and the weight of the patient, except under unusual circumstances.

If the patient is able to tolerate oral fluids, plain water or sweetened tea can be considered as part of the daily water intake.

The urinary output should be maintained between 30 and 50 mL/hr, and vital signs should be stable. (It may be difficult or impossible to take blood pressure readings if the upper extremities are burned.)

If the urinary output falls below 30 mL/hr, it is a sign that more electrolyte and colloid solutions should be given. If the urinary output exceeds 50 mL/hr, this may be a sign of excessive fluid administration.

The hematocrit should be determined every 3 to 4 hours for the first 2 or 3 days. It should be maintained at approximately 45%.

When either the Parkland or the Brooke formula, or any other formula, is used, one must remember that a formula is only a guide to the treatment of the patient, and that changes in the clinical condition of the patient or in laboratory test reports may require extensive changes in the intravenous or oral therapy.

Patients with burns caused by high-voltage electricity require larger amounts of fluid during early resuscitative therapy.

Stage of Sodium and Water Reabsorption and Diuresis

Fluid intake should be decreased when the edema fluid begins to be reabsorbed and diuresis occurs. Too much fluid given at this time may cause pulmonary edema. However, the diuresis may be so great that a water loss syndrome with desiccation may occur. This situation is similar to the water loss syndrome that occurs with an excessive solute intake (Chapter 4). In addition, the patient may be losing a large amount of water from the burned skin, from fever, and from seepage into dressings.

The physician must observe the patient closely for clinical signs of water loss, such as thirst and dryness of the mucous membranes (Chapter 3). If these signs are present, water must be given freely. As much as 4 to 6 liters a day may be needed.

The best method of determining water needs in this stage in the serum sodium concentration. It should be maintained at about 136 mEq/L, or the hematocrit should be maintained at about 45%.

In addition, the patient may lose a large amount of potassium in this stage. To avoid this, potassium chloride can be added to the infusions in a daily dose of approximately 80 mEq/L (6 g KCl).

After the third to the fifth day, a vigorous attempt should be made to give the patient adequate nourishment. Nasogastric tube feedings of a high-protein solution are valuable (also see Chapter 4). In addition, repeated transfusions may be necessary.

Diet Requirements After Severe Burns

Curreri et al. have developed a simple formula for caloric food intake to minimize weight loss during the acute burn period, namely, daily calories needed are equal to the sum of the patient's weight in kg multiplied by 25, plus the % of the total body surface burn multiplied by 40.

Other treatment is outside the scope of this book.

Bibliography

Asch, MJ, White MG, and Pruitt, BA: Acid base changes associated with topical Sulfamylon therapy. Ann Surg 172:946, 1970.

Baxter, CR: Crystalloid resuscitation of burn shock. In Polk, HC, Jr, and Stone, HN, (eds.). Contemporary Burn Management. Boston, Little, Brown, 1971.

Baxter, CR: Guidelines for fluid resuscitation. J Trauma 21:687, 1981.

Boswick, JAJ (ed): The Art and Science of Burn Care. Aspen, Rockville, MD, 1987.

Burke, JF, et al: 1981—approach to burn therapy. Surg Annual 13:1, 1981.

Caldwell, FT, Jr, and Bowser, BH: Critical evaluation of hypertonic and hypotonic solutions to resuscitate severely burned children. A prospective study. Ann Surg 189:546, 1979.

Curreri, PW, et al: Dietary requirements of patients with major burns. J Am Diet Assoc 65:415, 1974.

Demling, RH: Fluid resuscitation after major burns. JAMA 250:1438, 1983.

Evans, EI, et al: Fluid and electrolyte requirements in severe burns. Ann Surg 135:804, 1952.

Guntheer, R, et al: Effects of hypertonic saline on post burn edema. Bull Clin Res Burns 10:51, 1984.

Hinton, P, et al: Electrolyte changes after burn injury and effect of treatment. Lancet 2:218, 1973.

Hutcher, N, and Haynes, BW: The Evans formula revisited. J Trauma 12:453, 1972.

Markley, K: Comparison of sodium salts and plasma therapy in burned patients in Peru. Ann New York Acad Sci 150:845, 1968.

Monafo, WW, et al: Hyertonic sodium solutions in the treatment of burn shock. Am J Surg 126:778, 1973.

Monafo, WW: The Treatment of Burns. St. Louis, Warren H. Green, 1971.

Moyer, CA, Margraf, HW, and Monafo, WW: Burn shock and extravascular sodium deficiency. Treatment with Ringer's solution with lactate. Arch Surg 90:799, 1965.

Peaston, MJT: Metabolic acidosis in burns. Br Med J 1:809, 1968.

Pruitt, BA, Jr: Fluid resuscitation for extensively burned patients. J Trauma 21:690, 1981.

Scheulen, H, and Munster, AM: The Parkland formula in patients with burns and inhalation injury. J Trauma 22:869, 1982.

Schwartz, SI: Consensus summary on fluid resuscitation. J Trauma 19:(Suppl II)876, 1979.

Shires, GT, and Black, EA, (eds): Consensus development conference supportive therapy in burn care. J Trauma 19:Suppl. II, Nov. 1979.

Warden, GD, et al: Hypernatremic state in hypermetabolic burn patients. Arch Surg 106:420, 1973.

10

SODIUM EXCESS SYNDROMES (EDEMA)

PATHOPHYSIOLOGY

In Chapter 8, it was pointed out that the serum sodium concentration and the total exchangeable body sodium do not vary proportionately. Therefore, a low serum sodium concentration may be associated with a low, normal, or high total exchangeable body sodium. Similarly, a high serum sodium concentration may be associated with a low, normal, or high total exchangeable body sodium.

An excessive total exchangeable body sodium is almost always associated with an excess of water, except possibly in certain patients with hypernatremia due to cerebral lesions. In other words, *an excess of total exchangeable body sodium is not manifested by hypernatremia, but by edema.*

Edema occurs in several ways:

Cardiac Edema

Cardiac edema occurs when the heart fails as a pump and the renal blood flow decreases as a result of this. This is followed by a retention of sodium ions and water.

The decreased renal blood flow stimulates the production of renin, which increases angiotensin II levels. This in turn stimulates the secretion of aldosterone. As a result, the distal renal tubules reabsorb an excessive amount of sodium ions (and water); therefore, the plasma volume increases, the venous pressure rises, and edema occurs.

It has been known for many years that dogs respond to a saline infusion with a prompt increase both in glomerular filtration rate and the excretion of sodium ions. This increase is caused by a decreased tubular reabsorption of sodium ions from the proximal renal tubules. A similar loss or "escape" of sodium ions from the kidneys occurs when a salt-retaining hormone such as aldosterone or 11-desoxycorticosterone is administered over a prolonged period of time to normal subjects. This escape appears to be mediated by the release of atrial natriuretic factor. This explains why patients with primary aldosteronism do not develop severe edema.

The decreased effective arterial blood volume may also stimulate the secretion of ADH (vasopressin), the antidiuretic hormone of the posterior pituitary. The ADH level in the blood may also become abnormally high when chronic passive congestion of the liver is present (caused by right-sided congestive heart failure) because the liver may not be able to degrade and inactivate the circulating ADH normally. If excessive ADH secretion occurs, water rather than sodium ions is retained and the serum sodium concentration will fall.

The relation of hormonal imbalances to the formation of edema is actually very complicated; for example, aldosterone secretion may be high only when edema formation starts. Congestive heart failure is also not usually associated with excessive ADH secretion. And, if it occurs, water rather than sodium ions is retained and the serum sodium concentration falls. In congestive heart failure there is also increased adrenocortical activity. As a result, the sodium content of sweat, saliva, and urine decreases.

Circulatory Edema

In this group of patients, the heart does not fail as a pump. However, other factors cause the continued secretion of aldosterone. This type of edema occurs, for example, in cirrhotic and nephrotic patients. The primary disturbance is a decreased circulating blood volume.

In *cirrhosis of the liver,* edema is associated with ascites, which is due essentially to obstruction of the lymphatic flow from the liver. This, in turn, is affected by any factor that interferes with the return of blood through the hepatic and portal veins. The ascites can occur as a result of the following factors:

1. Obstruction of the portal vein itself rarely causes ascites. However, obstruction of the hepatic vein is almost always associated with ascites. Conversely, if the inferior vena cava is ligated below the insertion of the hepatic veins, ascites will not develop.

    In cirrhosis, the inflammatory process in the liver obstructs both venous return through the hepatic veins and the portal venous return. Marked congestion of the lymphatics of the liver occurs. The transudation of fluid from the lymphatics on the surface of the liver is the direct cause of the ascites.

Ascites is associated with a marked increased secretion of aldosterone, which can occur in several ways. It has been shown that if the
hepatic veins of a dog are ligated, a marked increased aldosterone secretion occurs almost immediately, *before* ascites develops (Orloff and
associates). The mechanism by which this occurs is not known. Later,
when ascites has developed, the entrance of fluid into the abdominal
cavity may decrease the circulating blood volume and cause a secondary aldosteronism in this way.

2. When liver injury is present for a long time, the liver loses its capacity
to form serum albumin. When hypoalbuminemia develops, the osmotic pressure of the blood decreases. This enhances the effect of the
hydrostatic pressure of the blood and increases the ascites and the
edema.

3. In addition, cirrhotic patients may show an increased amount of ADH
in the blood, which causes water retention and also aggravates the ascites. The cause of the ADH secretion is not known.

4. Cardiac factors may also be present to cause the ascites and the edema,
because patients with chronic cirrhosis may show microscopic signs of
myocardial degeneration. (This may be due partly to malnutrition, and
partly to chronic potassium loss.) Another cardiac factor that may contribute to the development of the ascites and edema is the development
of abnormal vascular anastomoses in the liver and lungs, which may
cause an increased venous return and high-output type of heart failure.

(Ascites can of course occur not only in cirrhosis of the liver and in
severe right-sided congestive heart failure, but also in constrictive pericarditis, the nephrotic syndrome, pancreatitis, malignant disease of
the abdomen, intraabdominal infections, myxedema, and so on.)

The development of edema in the *nephrotic syndrome* is apparently related primarily to the increased glomerular permeability to albumin. Long-
continued loss of serum albumin decreases the oncotic pressure of the
blood and causes an increased flow of water from the blood to the tissue
spaces. As a result, the circulating blood volume decreases. This stimulates
aldosterone secretion, which in turn causes the retention of sodium and water that leads to edema, just as in a cardiac patient. In addition, some investigators believe that albuminuria directly disturbs tubular function so
that sodium is excessively reabsorbed.

Acute Glomerulonephritis

In acute glomerulonephritis (particularly poststreptococcal glomerulonephritis in children), sodium retention may be an early sign that appears
as hypertension and edema. In children the edema frequently is facially
predominant.

Hormonal Edema

In Cushing's syndrome and during ACTH or corticosteroid therapy with hydrocortisone or its derivatives, the edema that occurs may be due to increased aldosterone secretion as a result of either the disease process or the drugs.

Edema Associated With Excessive ADH Secretion

Cardiac edema is not ordinarily associated with an excessive secretion of ADH. However, under special circumstances, an excessive ADH secretion may develop, for example, postoperatively, during acute infections, and in other ways (see Chapter 7). If this occurs, a patient with congestive heart failure whose diet has been too low in sodium, or who has lost an excessive amount of sodium ions by vomiting, paracentesis, as a result of excessive administration of diuretics, or in any other way, and who has been drinking water freely, or has been given an excessive amount of water parenterally, may develop edema related to the abnormal retention of water. Such a patient will show an abnormally low serum sodium concentration (see Chapter 6).

Idiopathic Cyclic Edema

This consists of periodic nonpitting edema of the face, hands, and feet, and occurs in women who still have their menses. However, it is not related to premenstrual tension. Patients also complain of abdominal distention and a sense of fullness in the bladder. The edema is minimal when the patient awakens and becomes more marked during the day. This is due to fluid retention in the upright position. However, the way in which an upright position produces the fluid retention is not known. Some patients may gain as much as 12 pounds a day. The usual weight gain is 2 to 4 pounds. Many patients are emotionally disturbed. The syndrome may last for years. Diuretic dependency and abuse frequently compound the state.

Laboratory tests may show hypoalbuminemia, hyponatremia, hypokalemia, or hypomagnesemia. The loss of serum albumin may be due to abnormal transudation from the blood into the extracellular spaces as a result of abnormal capillary permeability. Hyponatremia, hypokalemia, and hypomagnesemia are usually the effects of the diuretics the patient has been given.

TREATMENT

The treatment of edema depends on the physiological mechanisms that have produced it. In cardiac patients, an attempt should be made to strengthen the force and efficiency of cardiac contractions. Digitalis is the drug of choice. In addition, a low-sodium diet tends to prevent the retention of sodium ions associated with cardiac edema.

A patient placed on a sodium-restricted diet must avoid not only salt but also processed and packaged foods, such as canned foods, delicatessen products, and most cheeses. (Further details of low-sodium diets are beyond the scope of this book.)

Diet lists describing the sodium content of foods may also be misleading. For example, the sodium content of foods can be expressed either as grams of sodium *ions,* or as grams of sodium chloride (salt). For example, 1 g of sodium ions is equivalent to 43 mEq sodium ions. However, 1 g of sodium chloride is equivalent to 17 mEq sodium ions. Therefore, a 2-g sodium (ion) diet and a 5-g sodium chloride diet contain approximately similar amounts of sodium ions.

Medications may be an inadvertent source of sodium intake. For example, each gram of carbenicillin disodium (Geopen-Roerig) contains approximately 5.9 mEq (136 mg) sodium ions. If a patient is given a daily dose of 24 g of carbenicillin, this will contain 142 mEq (6.2 g) of sodium ions. Each 2.5 g of sulfadiazine (Parke Davis) for parenteral use contains 9.3 mEq (215 mg) of sodium ions.

Widely used proprietary drugs that have a relatively high sodium content include Alka-Seltzer. Bisodol powder, Bromo-Seltzer, Metamucil instant mix, Sal Hepatica, and sodium bicarbonate. Fleet enema also has a high sodium content, although it is not totally absorbed from the rectum.

Another possible source of sodium is drinking water, because the water content may be more than 8.7 mEq (200 mg) sodium per liter in some cities. In addition, home water-softening units replace the magnesium and calcium salts that may be present in the water with sodium chloride. In Chicago, the water is moderately hard, and about 5.2 mEq (120 mg) sodium per liter is added when the water is processed.

Diuretics are also effective in treating cardiac edema. The commonly used diuretics are of two major types: (1) the *thiazides,* such as chlorothiazide (Diuril), hydrochlorothiazide (HydroDIURIL, Esidrix), trichlormethiazide (Metahydrin, Naqua), and similar nonthiazide diuretics such as the sulfonamyls (Hygroton), and the quinazolines (Hydromox and Zaroxolyn), and (2) the *loop* diuretics such as furosemide (frusemide, Lasix), ethacrynic acid (Edecrin), and bumetanide (Bumex).

The various diuretics can cause a urinary excretion of sodium, potassium, bicarbonate, and phosphate ions, and a urinary excretion of free water, depending on the site or sites of their action in the kidneys. Figure 10–1 is a schematic diagram of a nephron, showing the major sites of actions of the commonly used diuretics. The various diuretics act in the following ways:

Carbonic Anhydrase Inhibitors (Diamox)

Carbonic anhydrase inhibitors work in the following way. In the kidneys, all the bicarbonate ions that pass the glomeruli and enter the proximal tubules (glomerular filtrate) are reabsorbed. This occurs because hydrogen and bicarbonate ions are produced by the tubule cells by means of the enzyme carbonic anhydrase. The hydrogen ions pass into the tubular urine and react with sodium bicarbonate to form carbonic acid, which is excreted. The sodium ions pass back into the tubule cells, react with bicarbonate ions, and then pass back into the plasma as sodium bicarbonate. As a result, sodium ions are conserved by the kidneys.

When a carbonic anhydrase inhibitor is given, the formation of carbonic acid in the proximal tubule cells (Fig. 10–1 [1]) is inhibited, and a large amount of sodium bicarbonate and water is excreted in the urine. This causes a diuresis and also a rise in the hydrogen and chloride concentration in the blood and a tendency to a metabolic acidosis. The serum potassium concentration may fall because a large amount of potassium ions is also excreted in the urine. (There is an exchange mechanism for potassium and hydrogen ions in the kidney tubule cells. This causes hydrogen and potassium ions to be excreted in inverse proportional concentrations in the urine.)

A carbonic anhydrase inhibitor loses its effectiveness after 2 to 3 days. Therefore, it should be used only intermittently, for example, for 2 or 3

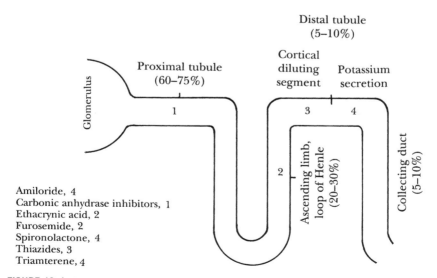

FIGURE 10–1. Sites of action of diuretics in the nephron. See text.

days, then a rest period of at least 2 days before it is started again. In the intervals when it is not given, the patient can receive a thiazide diuretic, or furosemide or ethacrynic acid. A carbonic anhydrase inhibitor can be given simultaneously with a thiazide diuretic or with ethacrynic acid. There is some evidence that it can interfere with the effectiveness of chlorthalidone (Hygroton).

Ethacrynic Acid (Edecrin)

Ethacrynic acid inhibits the reabsorption of sodium ions in the ascending limb of the loop of Henle (Fig. 10–1 [2]) and decreases distal tubular reabsorption of sodium and chloride ions. As a result, an increased amount of sodium and chloride ions and slightly less potassium and bicarbonate ions are excreted in the urine. Ethacrynic acid is effective when either a metabolic alkalosis or acidosis is present. However, it may aggravate either of these conditions.

Furosemide (Lasix)

The actions of furosemide are similar to those of ethacrynic acid (see Ethacrynic Acid above). It is particularly effective when renal insufficiency is present.

Spironolactone (Aldactone)

Spironolactone inhibits the physiological effects of the adrenocortical hormone aldosterone, on the distal renal tubules (Fig. 10–1 [4]), and in this way produces an increased excretion of sodium and chloride ions. It also increases the urinary excretion of free water. It characteristically decreases the urinary excretion of potassium ions and can cause hyperkalemia. It also increases the urinary excretion of ammonium and phosphate ions.

Because most of the sodium ions are reabsorbed in the proximal renal tubules, spironolactone is relatively ineffective when given alone, and a diuretic, such as a thiazide, ethacrynic acid, or furosemide, which blocks reabsorption of sodium ions in a region of the nephron proximal to the site of action of spironolactone, should be given concomitantly.

Thiazides and Related Diuretics

The thiazides and related sulfonamide diuretics, such as chlorthalidone (Hygroton), and quinethazone (Hydromox) inhibit the reabsorption of sodium ions in the distal renal tubules (Fig. 10–1 [3]) and in this way increase the urinary excretion of sodium ions. Hyponatremia can therefore develop. There is also an increased urinary excretion of chloride ions so that hypochloremia can also develop.

Hyponatremia and a sodium loss syndrome may develop with any of the above diuretics, particularly if the diuretic is given to a patient who is on a low-sodium diet. Hyperglycemia and/or hyperuricemia may also develop when a thiazide diuretic, ethacrynic acid, or furosemide is used.

When the diuretics (with the exception of spironolactone or triamterene) are given regularly for a long time, supplementary potassium chloride is needed to prevent both hypokalemia and hypochloremia and a metabolic alkalosis. Both spironolactone and triamterene cause a retention of potassium ions so that hyperkalemia may occur as a toxic effect. Therefore, when either of these is prescribed, the patient must not take supplemental potassium chloride. Otherwise, a severe and even fatal hyperkalemia can develop. In addition, congestive heart failure patients who are being treated with angiotensin converting enzyme inhibitors are particularly vulnerable to hyperkalemia.

The urinary excretion of potassium ions is also increased, so that hypokalemia often occurs. Plasma renin activity is also greatly increased by the thiazides, probably as a result of the decreased plasma volume produced by them. This causes an increased secretion of aldosterone, which may contribute to the hypokalemia.

The urinary excretion of magnesium ions also is increased. When given for a long time, the thiazides decrease the excretion of calcium ions and can raise the serum calcium level. The thiazides also have a slight carbonic anhydrase inhibitor activity (see Carbonic Anhydrase Inhibitors, above). The diuretic effect of the thiazides is not affected by the acid base balance of the patient.

Trimaterene (Dyrenium)

Triamterene has a weak action similar to spironolactone and depresses reabsorption of sodium ions in the distal renal tubules (Fig. 10–1 [4]) (also see Spironolactone, above). It also increases the urinary excretion of chloride ions, but slightly less than the urinary excretion of sodium ions. The urinary excretion of potassium ions is characteristically decreased, so that hyperkalemia may develop. The serum sodium level is lowered.

Amiloride (Mydamor)

Amiloride is an extremely potent blocker of distal tubular potassium excretion (Fig. 10–1 [4]), and is occasionally useful in refractory hypokalemia (e.g., Barrter's syndrome).

All the diuretics have side effects, some of which can be serious. Therefore, it is important to be familiar with the indications, contraindications, side effects and toxicity, reactions with other drugs, and dosages of each of these diuretics. (This statement also applies to the use of all drugs.) For example, if a patient who is on long-term lithium therapy receives a thiazide diuretic, or any diuretic that promotes the urinary excretion of both potassium and sodium ions, the serum lithium level may rise greatly and produce lithium toxicity. Therefore, the lithium dosage must be reduced and serum lithium levels must be checked constantly. (A potassium-sparing diuretic, such as spironolactone or triamterene, is safer for such patients.)

When diuretics are given to a patient on a low-sodium diet, a severe sodium loss syndrome (Chapter 8) may develop. Hyperglycemia and/or hyperuricemia may also develop when the thiazides, ethacrynic acid, or furosemide are used.

Spironolactone and triamterene are weak diuretics, as was mentioned above, and are rarely prescribed by themselves. Spironolactone is particularly effective as a diuretic when right-sided congestive heart failure (with congestion of the liver) is present.

When congestive heart failure and edema are severe, digitalis, the thiazides, ethacrynic acid or furosemide, and spironolactone or triamterene can be used concomitantly. Angiotensin converting enzyme inhibitors and certain calcium channel blockers may also be useful, by virtue of their hemodynamic and mildly natriuretic (salt-losing) effects.

Peritoneal dialysis, using a 4.25% dextrose solution, can also be used when edema and severe congestive heart failure do not respond to medical therapy.

The treatment of congestive heart failure associated with a retention of water, rather than a retention of sodium ions, is described on page 60. These patients often show a metabolic alkalosis, with low serum sodium, chloride, and potassium concentrations, associated with the excessive use of thiazide diuretics or with furosemide or ethacrynic acid. The treatment is described in Chapters 29 and 30.

Patients with *cirrhosis of the liver* and ascites can be treated with a low-sodium diet and with an aldosterone-antagonist such as spironolactone (Aldactone). Small doses of furosemide (Lasix), with or without supplemental potassium chloride, if indicated, can be used. (Excessive doses can precipitate hepatic coma or the hepatorenal syndrome.) If severe hypoproteinemia is present, infusions of salt-poor albumin may temporarily increase the colloid osmotic pressure and produce a diuresis.

Ammonium chloride or a carbonic anhydrase inhibitor (such as Diamox) should *not* be used, because it may precipitate hepatic coma.

Even when maximal diuresis is obtained, it is not possible to decrease the volume of ascitic fluid by more than 1000 mL a day. Therefore, a weight loss of 1 to 2 pounds a day is satisfactory. If excessive diuresis is produced, a low-sodium syndrome, hepatic coma, or progressive renal insufficiency (hepatorenal syndrome) may develop.

Discussion of use of the peritoneovenous shunt in the treatment of refractory ascites is outside the scope of this book.

Paracentesis should be performed cautiously, because it results in a loss of serum proteins, it decreases the effective blood volume, and increases the secretion of aldosterone and ADH. In addition, repeated paracentesis may produce a sodium loss syndrome with shock or renal failure. (Excessive diuretic therapy can also cause a similar syndrome.)

Patients with a *nephrotic syndrome* may or may not respond to corticosteroids. Approximately three fourths of children will respond; approximately three fourths of adults will not.

Rigid salt restriction and diuretics may be dangerous because they may cause a decrease in the circulating blood volume and a decrease in glomerular filtration rate. As a result, hypotension, shock, or hyperkalemia may result. If a diuretic is needed, a loop diuretic such as furosemide or a thiazide diuretic can be used. Spironolactone or triamterene should not be used because either one raises the serum potassium concentration.

Treatment of *idiopathic cyclic edema* is difficult. Spironolactone may be effective, although the increased aldosterone secretion that may be present is probably secondary to the decreased circulatory blood volume that results from the transudation of fluid out of the capillary walls, and from the decreased circulating blood volume that may result from excessive diuretic use. Small doses of a thiazide can also be used with or without spironolactone.

Supportive stockings or panty hose may be helpful in preventing some of the postural changes. Angiotensin converting enzyme inhibitors have been helpful in some patients. Counseling, combined with efforts to reduce self-administration of diuretics, is the favored approach.

Bibliography

Annotation: Drug therapy. Dietary sodium. Drug Therapy, August 1977, page 121.

Ascione, FJ: Lithium with diuretics. Drug Therapy, Sept 1977, page 125.

Baggenstoss, AH, and Wollaeger, EE: Portal hypertension due to chronic occlusion of the extrahepatic portion of the portal vein: Its relation to ascites. Am J Med 21:16, 1956.

Beyer, KH, Jr: The pharmacological basis for modern diuretic therapy. Rational Drug Ther 12:2, February 1978.

Coleman, M, Horwith, M, and Brown, JL: Idiopathic edema. Studies demonstrating protein-leaking angiopathy. Am J Med 49:106, 1970.

Davis, JO: Mechanisms of salt and water retention in congestive heart failure. The importance of aldosterone. Am J Med 29:486, 1960.

Edwards, OM, and Bayliss, RIS: Idiopathic edema of women. Q J Med 45:125, 1976.

Erstad, BL, Gales, BJ, and Rappaport, WD: The use of albumin in clinical practice. Arch Intern Med 151:901, 1991.

Espiner, EA, Jagger, PI, et al.: Effect of acute diuresis on aldosterone secretion in edematous patients. N Engl J Med 280:1141, 1969.

Feldman, HA, Jayakumar, S, and Puschett, JB: Idiopathic edema. A review of etiologic concepts and management. Cardiovasc Med 3:475, 1978.

Firth, BG: Southwestern Internal Medicine Conference: The multifaceted role of angiotensin converting enzyme inhibitors in congestive heart failure. Am J Med Sci 296(4):275–288, 1988.

Gill, JR, Jr, et al.: Idiopathic edema resulting from occult cardiomyopathy. Am J Med 134:253, 1965.

Gill, JR, Jr., Waldman, TA, and Bartter, FC: Idiopathic edema. I. The occurrence of hypoalbuminemia and abnormal metabolism in women with unexplained edema. Am J Med 52:444 and 452, 1972.

Ginsberg, AL: Cirrhotic diuresis. Questions and Answers. JAMA 247:2152, 1982.

Gonzales-Campoy, JM, Romero, JC, and Knox, FG: Escape from sodium-retaining effects of mineralocorticoids: Role of ANF and intrarenal hormone systems. Kidney Int 35:767, 1989.

Gregory, PB: The treatment of ascites. Rational Drug Ther, 12:no. 7, July 1978.

Liebowitz, HR: Pathogenesis of ascites in cirrhosis of liver. New York State J Med 69:1895, 1969.

Lipman, AG: Sodium content of commonly used parenteral antibiotics. Modern Med, May 30, 1977, page 83.

Lipman, AG: Sodium content of frequently used analgesics and gastrointestinal drugs. Modern Medicine, June 15, 1977, page 59.

Loon, NR, Wilcox, CS, and Unwin, RJ: Mechanism of impaired natriuretic response to furosemide during prolonged therapy. Kidney Int 36:682, 1989.

Maffly, RH: How to avoid complications of potent diuretics. JAMA 235:2526, 1976.

Mailloux, LV, et al: Peritoneal dialysis for refractory congestive heart failure. JAMA 199:123, 1967.

Martinez-Maldonado, M, and Garcia, A: A practical approach to the nephrotic syndrome. Drug Therapy, March 1981, p 79.

Mees, EJD, Geers, AB, and Koomans, HA: Blood volume and sodium retention in the nephrotic syndrome: a controversial pathophysiological concept. Nephron 36:201–211, 1984.

Porter, GA: The role of diuretics in the treatment of heart failure. JAMA 244:1614, 1980.

Reineck, HJ, and Stein, JH: Mechanisms of action and clinical use of diuretic drugs. In Brenner, BM, and Rector, FC, Jr (eds): The Kidney, vol 1, 2nd ed., Philadelphia, W.B. Saunders, 1981.

Riemer, AD: Application of the newer corticosteroids to augment diuresis in congestive heart failure. Am J Cardiol 1:488, 1958.

Rose, BD: Diuretics. Kidney Int 39:336, 1991.

Rubin, AL, et al: The use of 1-lysine monohydrochloride in combination with mercurial diuretics in the treatment of refractory fluid retention. Circulation 21:332, 1960.

Shashall, PD: Gross oedema in the nephrotic syndrome treated with furosemide in high dosage. BMJ 1:319, 1971.

Shear, L, Ching, S, and Gabuzda, GJ: Compartmentalization of ascites and edema in patients with hepatic cirrhosis. N Engl J Med 282:1391, 1970.

Sherlock, S, et al.: The complications of diuretic therapy in patients with cirrhosis. Ann New York Acad Sci 139:497, 1966.

Smith, FG, et al.: The nephrotic syndrome. Current concepts. Ann Intern Med 76:463, 1972.

Streeten, DHP: The role of posture in idiopathic edema. S Afr Med J 49:462, 1975.

11

SYNDROMES ASSOCIATED WITH DISTURBED OSMOLALITY

OSMOMETRY

Osmotic pressure was described in a general way in Chapter 2. In this chapter, the clinical uses of osmometry will be described. Measurement of the osmolality of the plasma (or serum) and the extracellular water is important because osmolality is related to the concentration of free particles, molecules, or ions in a solution. For example, when sodium or chloride ions, which are the chief ions in the extracellular water, are lost, the osmolality of the plasma and the extracellular water will decrease greatly. Similarly, when the concentration of glucose or blood urea nitrogen rises, this will tend to be associated with an increased osmolality of the extracellular water.

The terms "osmolarity" and "osmolality" are almost but not quite synonymous. For example, a *molar* solution contains a gram molecular weight of a substance dissolved in a solvent to make 1 liter. A *molal* solution, however, contains a gram molecular weight of a substance dissolved in 1000 g of a solvent. *Osmolality* is therefore more exact. It is determined by measuring the depression of the freezing point of a solution, compared to water, using an osmometer, and expressing the value in degrees Celsius below 0°. The value can also be expressed in milliosmoles, using the factor 1000 mOsm = 186°C or 1°C = 538 mOsm. Osmolality may be quickly and easily determined on serum or plasma, urine, saliva, cerebrospinal fluid, sweat, or gastric or other juices.

The normal range of serum osmolality, as measured, is 275 to 290 mOsm/kg of water. Females show values 5 to 10 mOsm/kg less than males.

THE FREEZING POINT OSMOMETER

When a substance is dissolved in a solution, it can change many of the physical characteristics of the solution; for example, the specific gravity, refractive index, conductivity, viscosity, turbidity, and freezing point, depending on the number of particles in solution; the size of the particles; their electrical charge; the number, size, and shape of undissolved particles; and the opacity of the solution.

Variations in the freezing point of the solution are dependent only on the number of the dissolved particles (that is, their osmotic concentration or osmolality) and not on their size or shape. This is why measurement of the depression of the freezing point is used to determine the osmolality of a solution.

An osmometer consists essentially of (1) a refrigerated bath to hold, cool, stir, and freeze body or other fluids; (2) an electric thermistor or probe to measure temperature; and (3) a Wheatstone bridge and galvanometer to convert variations in temperature into calibrated units of osmolality.

The sample is supercooled to several degrees below its freezing point and then is vibrated intensely for a moment. This causes many ice crystals to form, which releases their heat of fusion. The heat cannot be transferred to the surrounding ethylene glycol bath all at once and the trapped heat melts some of the new ice. The sample stays at equilibrium temperature for a few minutes while the ice is freezing and thawing. During this time the temperature measurement is made.

The electrical resistance of the thermistor probe varies directly with the temperature of the sample. This resistance is balanced with a Wheatstone bridge. The electrical resistance of the thermistor is also directly proportional to the osmolality of the sample. Therefore, the variable resistance dial of the Wheatstone bridge can be calibrated directly into mOsm/kg of the sample. The greater the concentration of solute in the solution, the lower the temperature, the greater the electrical resistance, and the higher the osmolality reading.

THE RELATIONS BETWEEN SERUM OSMOLALITY AND SERUM SODIUM CONCENTRATION

Two formulas have been used to interpret serum osmolality values:

1. *Calculated serum osmolality.* Serum osmolality can be calculated from the serum concentrations of sodium, BUN (blood urea nitrogen), and glucose, viz:

$$\text{Calculated mOsm/kg} = 1.86\ \text{Na} + \frac{\text{Glucose}}{18} + \frac{\text{BUN}}{2.8}$$

The constant 1.86 is obtained by assuming that both sodium and chloride ions have an osmotic coefficient of 0.93. The term *osmotic coefficient* describes the percent deviation from an ideal behavior of a substance. For example, ideal behavior would include complete dissociation in the solution, no water binding, and so forth. If sodium chloride completely dissociated in plasma, each molecule of the salt would yield two ions. However, if the osmotic coefficient of sodium chloride is 0.93, the effective osmolality of a solution of sodium chloride is $2 \times 0.93 = 1.86$.

Glucose is the plasma glucose concentration in milligrams per deciliter. The constant 18 is derived from the molecular weight of glucose, which is 180. (Therefore, each 180 mg% glucose in the blood will raise the serum osmolality by 10 mOsm/L.)

BUN is the plasma concentration of blood urea nitrogen in milligrams per deciliter. The constant 1/2.8 is derived from the mean nitrogen content of BUN, or urea. Urea contains two nitrogen molecules and thus has a molecular weight of $14 \times 2 = 28$. (Therefore, each 28 mg% BUN concentration in the blood will raise the serum osmolality by 10 mOsm/kg.)

Normally, the *calculated* serum osmolality is 5 to 8 mOsm/kg less than the osmolality measured by the freezing point depression method.

The above formula for the *calculated* serum osmolality can be simplified by multiplying the serum sodium concentration by 2, rather than by 1.86. The formula therefore becomes:

$$\text{Calculated serum osmolality, mOsm/kg} = 2\,\text{Na} + \frac{\text{Glucose}}{18} + \frac{\text{BUN}}{2.8}$$

Relations Between Measured and Calculated Osmolality

Normally, as was pointed out above, the *calculated* serum osmolality is less than 5 to 8 mOsm/kg of the *measured* osmolality. However, wide differences of more than 10 mOsm/kg can occur in two situations:

a. When the water content of the serum is decreased, due either to marked hyperlipidemia, or marked hyperproteinemia (paraproteinemia). (When such marked hyperlipidemia is present, the serum will be lipemic on observation. When such marked hyperproteinemia is present, the serum protein level will be 10 g/L or higher.)

The *measured* serum osmolality will be normal, but the *calculated* serum osmolality will be about 10 to 15 mOsm/kg lower, due to the fact that the increased lipids or proteins are associated with a spurious lowering of the serum sodium concentration.

The reason for this is that the serum sodium concentration is measured in terms of mEq/L of serum volume. However, osmolality is measured in terms of the concentration of a substance per kilogram of serum or plasma water. In hyperlipemic or hyperproteinemic serum, the lipid or the protein occupies volume but displaces serum water, so that the serum concentration of sodium (and all the other electrolytes) in terms of mEq/L (total volume) is spuriously low. However, if the lipid is removed by ultracentrifugation, or if the excess protein is removed, the concentration of sodium and other electrolytes in the subnatant fluid will be normal. Albrink describes a 16-year-old boy with mild diabetes and xanthoma diabeticorum. His serum sodium concentration was 102.5 mEq/L, and his serum chloride concentration was 74.5 mEq/L. The serum was markedly lactescent. When the insoluble lipids were removed by ultracentrifugation, the electrolyte concentrations of the clear subnatant fluid were essentially normal: sodium 135 mEq/L, and chloride 102.5 mEq/L. (This is one of the reasons that serum sodium concentrations in mEq/L of serum *water* correlate better, with serum osmolality than serum sodium concentration as usually measured per liter of serum volume.)

b. When nonmeasured low-molecular-weight substances (molecular weight less than 150), such as ethanol, methanol, ethylene glycol, paraldehyde, acetone, trichlorethylene, and so on, are present in the plasma. In such cases, the *measured* serum osmolality is almost always more than 300 mOsm/kg. When such low-molecular-weight substances accumulate, they greatly increase the osmolality of the plasma because osmolality depends on the number of particles in solution, rather than on their size.

2. *Effective serum osmolality.* Evaluation of the serum osmolality can also be done by calculating the *effective* osmolality (Gennari), using the following formula:

$$2Na + \frac{Glucose}{18}. \text{ Normally the value is 185 mOsm/kg.}$$

This is based on the fact that the sodium ions and glucose are the major solutes in the blood and extracellular water that do not permeate cells freely.

When the *effective* osmolality is increased, this generally indicates a relative water loss.

When the *effective* osmolality is decreased, this generally indicates a relative water excess.

Example: Patient with renal insufficiency.
Na 125 mEq/L
Glucose 90 mg/dL
BUN 90 mg/dL
Measured serum osmolality 290 mOsm/kg water
Effective serum osmolality 255 mOsm/kg water

In this case, the *measured* serum osmolality is essentially normal, 290 mOsm/kg water (due to the high BUN of 90 mg/dL) but the *effective* serum osmolality is low, 255 mOsm/kg water. The cause of the low effective serum osmolality was the renal insufficiency. As a result, the patient was imbibing more water than he could excrete through his kidneys. This produced a water excess.

Example: Patient with diabetic acidosis.
Na 134 mEq/L
Glucose 700 mg/dL
Measured serum osmolality 312 mOsm/kg water
Effective serum osmolality 306.9 mOsm/kg water

The *measured* serum osmolality is high, 312 mOsm/kg water. However, the *effective* serum osmolality is also high, 306.9 mOsm/kg water. This is related to the water loss due to the osmotic diuresis caused by the glucose filtering through the kidneys, lack of adequate water intake, loss of fluids by vomiting, and so on. As a result, a water loss developed.

THE CLINICAL SIGNIFICANCE OF SERUM OSMOLALITY VALUES

A high *measured* serum osmolality indicates a high osmolality of the extracellular water. Values as high as 400 mOsm/kg have been reported in adults, with higher values in children. Values above 350 mOsm/kg indicate a grave prognosis. A high serum osmolality can occur in water loss, rarely with sodium excess; or with hypernatremia produced by drugs or diseases in diabetes; azotemia; lactic acidosis; liver failure; sepsis; after intoxication with salicylates, barbiturates, alcohol, and, other substances; with high-protein nasogastric feedings or total parenteral nutrition; or a combination of the above conditions. Treatment should be directed to lower the high serum osmolality by the removal of the abnormal substances, if possible, and by increasing the oral or parenteral water intake.

A high *measured* serum osmolality can be associated with a normal, low, or high serum sodium concentration. These uncorrected serum sodium concentrations do not indicate whether sodium loss or sodium excess is present and these uncorrected values cannot be used as a basis for treatment. It is therefore necessary to calculate the *effective* serum osmolality (see above).

A low *measured* serum osmolality indicates a low osmolality of the extracellular water. Values as low as 230 mOsm/kg have been reported. In these patients, the serum sodium concentration is also low. A low *measured* serum osmolality can occur in water excess or sodium loss, or a combination of both conditions. Treatment consists of water restriction, increased salt in the diet, or the intravenous use of hypertonic sodium chloride solution when indications are present.

OTHER CAUSES OF A HIGH SERUM OSMOLALITY

When the pylorus does not function normally to restrain the rapid passage of partially digested food into the duodenum and jejunum, concentrated food substances may enter the circulation from the duodenum or jejunum, and may cause a sudden rise in plasma osmolality. This is associated with symptoms of sweating, flushing, warmth, tachycardia, and increased pulse pressure associated with peripheral vasodilation (the *dumping syndrome*).

A marked rise in serum osmolality occurs with intoxication due to ethanol, methanol, trichlorethylene, ethylene glycol, and other low-molecular-weight substances.

Methanol and ethylene glycol cause a metabolic acidosis with an elevated anion gap. Therefore, if there is a wide gap between the calculated and measured osmolalities, and if the anion gap is elevated and if alcoholic acidosis or diabetic coma are excluded, this indicates methanol or ethylene glycol poisoning.

URINE OSMOLALITY

The osmolality of the urine is a more accurate measurement of kidney function than specific gravity of the urine, because the kidneys respond to changes in the osmolality of the body fluids and not to changes in specific gravity. In addition, the specific gravity of urine depends on the weight of the substances dissolved in it, not on the concentration of these substances. Therefore, heavy molecules such as glucose or albumin will cause a rise in specific gravity out of proportion to their concentration in the urine. This can cause marked differences between urine specific gravity and urine osmolality. For example, at a specific gravity of 1.023, the urine osmolality can vary from 722 to 1166 mOsm/kg urine.

If an adult is on a medium-protein diet with an average salt intake, about 1200 mOsm of solute are excreted a day. Urea comprises about 500 mOsm of this. The remainder is due mostly to sodium, potassium, and ammonium salts. If a patient receives only glucose, the urinary osmolality may fall to 200 mOsm a day. If he or she is on a high-protein diet with water restriction, the daily urine osmolality may even reach 1700 mOsm.

Normally, after a 14-hour fast, a person will show a concentrated urine with an osmolality of 850 mOsm/kg urine, or higher.

When moderate renal insufficiency is present, the urine osmolality may vary from 400 to 600 mOsm a day. When severe renal insufficiency is present, the daily urinary osmolality may be less than 400 mOsm.

THE URINE-SERUM OSMOLALITY RATIO

Normally, this ratio is greater than 1 and is usually 3 or higher. In chronic renal disease it falls to 1. In diabetes insipidus it is less than 1 because of the excretion of a large volume of water. In compulsive water drinking, the urine-serum ratio is also less than 1. However, when a patient with diabetes insipidus is deprived of water, the urine-serum ratio will continue to remain below 1 although the urine osmolality rises slightly. In compulsive water drinking, the urine-serum ratio will rise to 1 or higher after water deprivation.

In inappropriate ADH secretion syndromes, the urine osmolality is characteristically higher than the serum osmolality in spite of the presence of hyponatremia.

Bibliography

Abele, JE: The physical background of freezing point osmometry and its medical-biological applications. Am J Med Electronics 2:32, 1963.

Albrink, MJ, Hald, PM, Man, EB, and Peters, JP: The displacement of serum water by the lipids of hyperlipemic serum. A new method for the rapid determination of serum water. J Clin Invest 34:1483, 1955.

Boyd, DR, et al.: Utilization of osmometry in critically ill surgical patients. Arch Surg 102:363, 1971.

Champion, HR, et al.: Alcohol intoxication and serum osmolality. Lancet 1:1402, 1975.

Dashe, AM, et al: A water deprivation test for the differential diagnosis of polyuria. JAMA 185:699, 1963.

Galambos, JT, Herndon, EG, and Reynolds, GH: Specific gravity determination. Fact or fancy? N Engl J Med 270:506, 1964.

Gennari, FJ: Serum osmolality. Uses and limitations. N Engl J Med 310:102, 1984.

Glasser, L, et al.: Serum osmolality and its applicability to drug overdose. Am J Clin Path 60:695, 1973.

Holmes, JH: Measurement of osmolality in serum, urine and other biologic fluids by the freezing point determination. Pre-workshop manual of the workshop on urinalysis and renal function studies. Am Soc Clin Path 1962.

Jacobsen, D, et al.: Anion and osmolal gaps in the diagnosis of methanol and ethylene glycol poisoning. Acta Med Scandinav 212:17, 1982.

Jacobson, MH, et al.: Urine osmolality. A definitive test of renal function. Arch Intern Med 110:121, 1962.

Jamison, RL: The renal concentrating mechanism. Kidney Int 32(suppl 21):S-43, 1987.

Ladenson, JH, Apple, FS, and Koch, DD: Misleading hyponatremia due to hyperlipemia. A method-dependent error. Ann Intern Med 95:707, 1981.

Olmstead, EG, and Roth, DA: The relationship of serum sodium to total serum osmolarity. A method of distinguishing hyponatremic states. Am J Med Sci 233:392, 1957. Also Surg Gynecol Obstet 106:41, 1958.

Robinson, AG, and Loeb, JL: Ethanol ingestion—commonest cause of elevated plasma osmolality. N Engl J Med 284:1253, 1971.

Rodrigo, F, et al.: Osmolality changes during hemodialysis. Ann Intern Med 86:554, 1977.

Sklar, AH, and Linas, SL: The osmolal gap in renal failure. Ann Intern Med 98:481, 1983.

Warhol, RM, Eichenholz, A, and Mulhausen, RO: Osmolality. Arch Intern Med 116:743, 1965.

Weinberg, LS: Pseudohyponatremia: A reappraisal. Am J Med 86:315, 1989.

SYNDROMES DUE TO DISTURBANCES IN ACID-BASE BALANCE

12

THE PRINCIPLES OF ACID-BASE CHEMISTRY AND PHYSIOLOGY

The subject of acid-base balance is confusing because of its terminology. For example, a cation such as sodium and an anion such as bicarbonate have been called "bases" but the chloride anion has been called an "acid" by some investigators. Others have loosely called cations bases and anions acids. Much of the confusion can be eliminated if we accept the following chemical definitions of an acid and of a base:

An acid is a hydrogen ion (proton) donor.

A base is a hydrogen ion (proton) acceptor (Brønsted). For example,

Acid	H⁺	+	Base
(Hydrogen ion donor)	(Hydrogen ion)		(Hydrogen ion acceptor)
H_2CO_3	H^+	+	HCO_3^-
H_3PO_4	H^+	+	$H_2PO_4^-$

An alkali can produce hydroxyl (OH) ions (base) in aqueous solution, for example, $NaOH$, NH_4OH.

THE MEANING OF pH

Any acid, such as HCl, in a water solution dissociates wholly or partly into its component ions: $HCl \rightleftharpoons H^+ + Cl^-$. The strength of the acid depends on the degree to which it becomes dissociated in the solution and on the concentration of the hydrogen ions that it contains.

In 1909, S.P.L. Sorensen, a Danish biochemist, noted that enzyme activity was related to minute changes in the hydrogen ion concentration of a solution, for example, 0.01 to 0.0000001 mole per liter. Mathematically, these numbers can be rewritten as 10^{-2} to 10^{-7}. He called the -2 and the

-7 the hydrogen ion exponent or power, or *puissance hydrogen* (the paper was written in French), then eliminated the negative signs and further shortened in the term to pH.

pH therefore represents the negative logarithm of the hydrogen ion concentration in moles (gram molecules) per liter of solution.

For example, in a 0.01 molar solution of HCl (which is almost completely dissociated), the hydrogen ion concentration is approximately 0.01 molar, or $[H^+] = 0.01 = 1 \times 10^{-2}$. The logarithm of the hydrogen ion concentration is therefore -2; and the negative logarithm, or pH, is 2.

(A molar solution contains 1 gram-molecular weight of the solute in a liter of solution. A 0.01 molar solution of HCl therefore contains 0.01 of 36.5 g [the molecular weight of HCl] in a liter of water.)

Water dissociates into H and OH ions, as follows: $H_2O \rightleftharpoons H^+ + OH$. The equilibrium of this reaction at room temperature has been found to be $[H^+] \times [OH^-] = 10^{-14}$. Since pure water yields equivalent amounts of H and OH ions, it follows that the hydrogen ion concentration of pure water is 10^{-7}, and the pH of water is 7.

Since acids have a greater hydrogen ion concentration than water, the pH of an acid will be lower than 7. Since bases have a lower concentration of hydrogen ions than water, the pH of a base will be greater than 7. Since the normal pH of the blood is 7.4, this means that the blood normally has a faintly basic or alkaline reaction.

Hydrogen ion concentration can also be described in terms of its actual concentration rather than in terms of pH. Since the hydrogen ion concentration in plasma or other body fluids is very low, measurements are made in terms of *nanoequivalents* (or nanomoles) per liter. One nanoequivalent equals 10^{-9} equivalent per liter. The relationship between nanoequivalents per liter (nEq/L) (or nanomoles per liter, nM/L) and pH is shown in Figure 12–1.

Kassirer and Bleich have described the following simple rule to correlate pH and H^+ (hydrogen ion) concentrations: A pH of 7.40 is equivalent to a H^+ concentration of 40 nEq/L. Each increase (or decrease) in pH of 0.01 unit from 7.40 corresponds to a decrease (or increase) of 1 nEq/L of H^+ concentration of 1 nEq/L.

For example, a pH of 7.37 is 0.03 unit more acid than 7.40. Therefore, the equivalent H^+ concentration is 43 nEq/L (3 more than 40). A pH of 7.44 is 0.04 more alkaline than 7.40. Therefore, the equivalent H^+ concentration is 36 nEq/L (4 less than 40).

This rule is approximately accurate between pH values of 7.28 and 7.45. However, when the pH falls below 7.28 or rises above 7.45, the estimated H^+ concentration is always lower than its actual value (see Fig. 12–1).

Theoretically, it is preferable to use an nEq/L rather than pH to describe changes in acidity or alkalinity. One reason is that a decrease of 1 unit pH below 7.4 indicates a much larger change in hydrogen ion concentra-

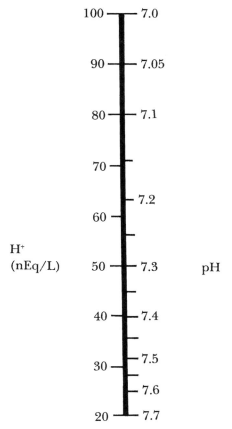

FIGURE 12–1. Relationship between hydrogen ion activity (nEq/L) and pH.

tion (expressed in nEq/L) than an equal rise of pH above 7.4. For example, a decrease of pH from 7.2 to 7.1 represents a large increase in hydrogen ion concentration of 17 nEq/L, but a rise in pH from 7.5 to 7.6 represents only a small decrease in hydrogen ion concentration of 7 nEq/L (Fig. 12–1). However, the term pH is so well known that we shall continue to use it.

THE CHEMICAL AND PHYSIOLOGICAL REGULATION OF THE pH OF THE BODY

In the past century, physiologists have learned that the reaction of the extracellular water must be maintained slightly to the base side of the neutral point in order for an organism to live. In other words, the pH of the extracellular water must be slightly above 7.

Three factors help maintain this pH:

1. Chemical buffers of the body fluids and cells can neutralize strong acids and bases that are produced within the body, or which enter the body. Extracellular chemical buffering occurs instantaneously. Cellular buffering (which consists of the diffusion of hydrogen ions into the cells and their neutralization) occurs in a period of several hours.
2. Respiratory regulatory mechanisms help eliminate and regulate the concentration of carbonic acid, which is the major acid end product of metabolism. Respiratory buffering occurs in a period of minutes.
3. The kidneys also help eliminate excess acids and bases. The kidneys are the most important of these three mechanisms, because they compensate for any defects in the action of the buffer salts, or of respiratory action. The sulfuric and phosphoric acids produced by the catabolism of proteins and phospholipids, as well as any acid that cannot be metabolized to carbonic acid, can be eliminated from the body only by the kidneys. Renal buffering occurs in a period of hours to days.

The Chemical Buffers of the Body

The term *buffer* describes a chemical substance that, by its presence in a solution, decreases the pH change caused by the addition of an acid or a base. A buffer is a mixture either of a weak acid and its alkali salt or of a weak base and its acid salt. In the body, the buffers of physiological importance are mixtures of weak acids and their alkali salts—carbonic acid and sodium (or potassium) bicarbonate; monohydrogen and dihydrogen phosphate salts and the proteins with their alkali salts, H protein and B protein. The B represents a cation such as sodium or potassium.

The importance of buffers can be appreciated when one realizes that all of the base that is available for the immediate neutralization of acid of the body is in the form of buffer salts. Salts of strong acids, such as sodium chloride, have no neutralizing power, and a strong alkali, such as sodium hydroxide, cannot exist in the living body.

There are four main buffer systems in the body that help maintain the constancy of the pH:

1. The bicarbonate-carbonic acid buffer system. This is quantitatively the largest in the body. It operates in the extracellular water.
2. The phosphate buffer system. This is important in the red blood cells and in other cells, especially in the cells of the kidney tubules, where it enables the kidneys to excrete hydrogen ions.
3. The protein buffer system. This is predominant in the tissue cells. It also operates in the plasma.
4. The hemoglobin buffer system of the red blood cells.

The Bicarbonate-Carbonic Acid Buffer System

During the course of the normal metabolic activities of the body, most of the organic and inorganic acids that are formed are stronger than carbonic acid. This causes the following type of reaction:

$$HCl + NaHCO_3 \rightarrow H_2CO_3 + NaCl \cdot H_2CO_3 \rightarrow H_2O + CO_2 \uparrow$$

The bicarbonate ion is not the only one that is able to neutralize acids, as we have already pointed out. However, bicarbonate is unique because its acid is volatile. Therefore, when the bicarbonate salt reacts with an acid, the carbon dioxide set free from the reaction can be removed from the body at once by the lungs. A foreign acid can therefore be completely neutralized by bicarbonate. The foreign acid is converted into a neutral salt and carbon dixoide, which is expelled in the expired air.

On the other hand, when a base such as sodium hydroxide enters the body, or is formed in the body, it combines with carbon dioxide to form bicarbonate in the following way:

$$NaOH + H_2CO_3 \rightarrow NaHCO_3 + H_2O$$

Carbon dioxide is continually produced in the body by the processes of metabolism and is always available. Therefore, any base that enters the body can be immediately and automatically converted into bicarbonate.

Because of the importance of bicarbonate ions and carbon dioxide in the regulation of acid or base excesses or deficits, the pH of the blood is dependent on the bicarbonate–carbonic acid ratio in the plasma and extracellular water. Under normal conditions, the bicarbonate–carbonic acid ratio is 20/1 and the pH is 7.4. This value is derived as follows.

Henderson, Hasselbalch, and others have shown that the pH of the body fluids can be expressed by the following equation:

$$pH = 6.1 + \log \frac{HCO_3^-}{H_2CO_3 + CO_2}$$

where HCO_3^- represents bicarbonate. The CO_2 and H_2CO_3 represent the concentrations of dissolved carbon dixoide plus carbonic acid. For example, at a pH of 6.1, the concentrations of bicarbonate and carbonic acid in the body are equal (and the logarithm of $1/1 = 0$).

Normally, the concentration of bicarbonate in the plasma and extracellular water is 27 mEq/L, and the concentration of carbonic acid is 1.35 mEq/L.

The pH can now be calculated as follows:

$$pH = 6.1 + \log \frac{27}{1.35}$$

Since $27/1.35 = 20$, the equation becomes pH $= 6.1 + \log 20$.

Using a calculator, one finds that the logarithm of 20 is 1.3. Therefore, the pH is $6.1 + 1.3 = 7.4$.

When the bicarbonate concentration of the blood rises, or the carbonic acid concentration falls, the bicarbonate–carbonic acid ratio increases, and the pH becomes greater than the normal value of 7.35 to 7.45. This is described as alkalosis.

When the bicarbonate concentration of the blood falls, or the carbonic acid concentration rises, the bicarbonate–carbonic acid ratio decreases, and the pH becomes less than the normal value of 7.35 to 7.45. This is described as acidosis, even though the pH is still slightly on the alkaline side of neutrality.

The Phosphate Buffer System

This is important in red blood cells and in other cells, especially in the cells of the kidney tubules, where it enables the kidneys to excrete hydrogen ions.

Phosphate ions exist in the body in two forms, monohydrogen phosphate ions, HPO_4^-, and dihydrogen phosphate ions, $H_2PO_4^-$. At the normal pH of 7.4, there is about five times as much monohydrogen phosphate as dihydrogen phosphate in the body. Therefore, if a strong acid such as hydrochloric acid is introduced into the body, the following reaction would occur: $HCl + Na_2HPO_4 \rightarrow NaCl + NaH_2PO_4$. In other words, a strong acid is converted to a neutral salt, sodium chloride, by a phosphate buffer salt, which undergoes a change from a mildly basic form to a mildly acid form.

Similarly, if a strong base such as sodium hydroxide is introduced into the body, the following reaction would occur: $NaOH + NaH_2PO_4 \rightarrow Na_2HPO_4 + H_2O$. In other words, a strong base is converted into water by a phosphate buffer salt, which undergoes a change from a mildly acid form to a mildly basic form.

The Protein Buffer System

This is predominant in the tissue cells. It also operates in the plasma. The proteins of the body act as anions in the alkaline pH of the body. They may exist in the form of acids (H protein), or as alkaline salts (B protein). In this way they are able to bind or release excess hydrogen ions as needed.

The Hemoglobin Buffer System

Only about 5% of the carbon dioxide is carried in the plasma in simple solution. Another 20% is transported in the red blood cells as a carbamino compound with hemoglobin. The remaining 75% of the carbon dioxide is carried by the blood as bicarbonate. The process by which this occurs can be briefly described as follows.

Carbon dioxide is formed during the processes of cellular metabolism. It then diffuses into the tissue spaces and into the plasma. As its concentration in the plasma increases, it diffuses into the red blood cells. Here the enzyme carbonic anhydrase (ca) converts the carbon dioxide to carbonic acid: $CO_2 + H_2O \rightarrow H_2CO_3$. This immediately dissociates into H^+ and HCO_3^- ions. The H^+ ion reacts with reduced hemoglobin, namely, $H^+ + Hb^- \rightarrow HHb$.

The bicarbonate ion accumulates within the red blood cells. When its concentration increases above that in the plasma, it diffuses into the plasma and is replaced by a chloride ion, to form potassium chloride to maintain electroneutrality.

$$\text{Red blood cell: } KHCO_3 \rightarrow K^+ + (HCO_3^-) \text{ to plasma}$$
$$\text{Plasma: } Cl \rightarrow \text{ to red blood cell} \rightarrow KCl$$

In the alveolar capillaries of the lungs, the reduced hemoglobin, HHb, is oxygenated and becomes $HHbO_2$. It reacts with bicarbonate salts to form carbonic acid ($HHbO_2 + KHCO_3 \rightarrow H_2CO_3 + KHbO_2$). As the carbonic acid is formed, the chloride that had previously entered the cells passes back into the plasma again, and the potassium ion reacts with bicarbonate to form potassium bicarbonate again. The carbonic acid that has been formed is converted into carbon dioxide and water by means of carbonic anhydrase. The carbon dioxide then passes from the red blood cells to the plasma and into the alveolar capillaries where it is eliminated.

Respiratory Regulation of pH

The chemical and physiological actions of a gas depend on the pressure it exerts. This pressure is called the *partial pressure* of the gas. It is usually represented by the symbol P. Thus, P_{CO_2} represents the partial pressure of carbon dioxide. The partial pressure of a gas depends only on the number of moles of the gas in a given volume and on the temperature. It is completely independent of the presence or absence of other gases in the same volume.

The partial pressure of a gas may be determined by chemical or physical means. When physical means are used, the result is given as millimeters of mercury (mm Hg) pressure. When chemical means are used, the result is given as volumes % (vol %). At normal (760 mm Hg) barometric pressure, the following formula can be used to convert vol. % CO_2 to mm Hg CO_2:

$$1 \text{ vol \% } CO_2 = 7 \text{ (approx.) mm Hg pressure}$$

The term *torr* is a unit of pressure, named in honor of Torricelli, the inventor of the barometer. It can be used to describe P_{CO_2}, P_{O_2}, blood pressure, or other pressure measurements. A torr is the unit of pressure equal to 1/760 of normal atmospheric pressure or the pressure necessary to support a column of mercury 1 mm high at 0°C and standard gravity. Therefore, pressure values can be described as either mm Hg or torr.

Respiration is regulated by sensors located in the central nervous system (CNS) and in the systemic circulatory system. The CNS receptors located in the medulla, which are in contact with the CSF (cerebrospinal fluid), are sensitive to small changes in pH and PCO_2. Small increments in PCO_2 or decrements in pH result in dramatic increases in ventilation triggered by these CNS receptors. Since the CSF is far more permeable to CO_2 than to HCO_3, acute changes in PCO_2 are sensed within minutes, whereas changes in HCO_3 concentration may not be sensed for hours.

The peripheral chemoreceptors located in the aortic arch and carotid sinus are also stimulated by an increase in PCO_2 or decrease in pH. In addition, hypoxemia stimulates the carotid sinus. Stimulation of these chemoreceptors results in increased ventilation, so that an acid load, a rise in PCO_2, or hypoxemia will be counteracted by a rapid ventilatory response.

Conversely, an alkaline load or a decline in PCO_2 will result in reduced ventilation mediated by the central and peripheral chemoreceptors.

It should be stressed that these respiratory compensations are capable of returning the pH of the blood toward normal, but do not result in complete restoration of normal pH.

Carbon dioxide excess or lack is the most important stimulant of the respiratory center. However, if the PCO_2 of the alveolar air rises above 9 vol % (approximately 65 mm Hg), this acts as a CNS depressant and can result in *carbon dioxide narcosis*. This occurs in patients with severe respiratory acidosis.

Oxygen does not normally act as a stimulus for the respiratory center as long as normal oxygenation occurs in the alveoli. However, if anoxemia is present and the amount of available oxygen is reduced, the decreased oxygen concentration of the blood acts as a respiratory stimulant, and hyperventilation results. If a patient with cor pulmonale, who may show such a condition, is given excessive concentrations of oxygen to inhale (more than 50%), the inhaled oxygen can cause the respiratory center to stop functioning. As a result, excessive carbon dioxide accumulates in the body and the patient may become comatose and die (see carbon dioxide narcosis, Chapter 16).

Changes in pH also affect respiration. For example, marked hyperventilation occurs when the pH falls to 7.2. This becomes maximal when a pH of about 7 is reached. However, when the pH falls below 7, the hyperventilation disappears. This is one reason that so-called *air hunger* (the Kussmaul type of hyperventilation with exaggerated respiratory action, particularly an exaggerated depth of respiration) is not always present in patients with acidosis.

The partial pressure carbon dioxide in the alveolar air is in equilibrium with the partial pressure of the carbon dioxide of the arterial blood, and this is in equilibrium with the carbonic acid content of the blood. Therefore, a change in the P_{CO_2} of the alveolar air will cause a corresponding change in the P_{CO_2} and in the H_2CO_3 content of the blood.

Normally, the P_{CO_2} of the alveolar air is about 40 mm Hg (5.5 vol %). If the concentration of carbonic acid in the blood increases, this will cause an increase in the P_{CO_2} of the alveolar air, and will stimulate the respiratory center. Hyperventilation will occur and will lower the P_{CO_2} of the alveolar air by causing carbon dioxide to be exhaled faster than it is produced. The most extreme voluntary hyperventilation can lower the P_{CO_2} to about 15 mm Hg.

Hyperventilation can also affect the P_{CO_2} of the alveolar air in the following way. The partial pressure of a gas is proportional to the volume in which it is enclosed. Minute ventilation can increase by means of deep respiration. As a result, the P_{CO_2} of the alveolar air and the CO_2 content of the arterial blood will decrease, even though the rate of respiration remains unchanged. Conversely, a decreased depth of respiration causes a decreased lung volume, an increased P_{CO_2} of alveolar air, and an increased CO_2 content of arterial blood.

Primary changes in the bicarbonate concentration of the blood can also be regulated by the respiratory mechanisms. For example, a patient is given a massive dose of sodium bicarbonate, and the bicarbonate concentration rises substantially. The respiratory center responds by decreasing the respiratory rate and depth. In this way, the lung volume is decreased and the P_{CO_2} of the alveolar air increases from the normal value of 40 mm Hg. The carbonic acid content of the blood, which is normally 1.35 mEq/L, will also rise substantially. In this way the bicarbonate–carbonic acid ratio and the pH are less severely changed by the change in P_{CO_2}.

Conversely, if the bicarbonate concentration of the blood decreases, the respiratory rate and depth will increase. This causes the lung volume to increase and the P_{CO_2} of the alveolar air and the carbonic acid content of the blood to decrease. As a result, the pH change is minimized.

Since the partial pressure of carbon dioxide in the plasma (P_{CO_2}) is proportional to the concentration of carbonic acid and dissolved carbon dioxide in the plasma, the Henderson-Hasselbalch equation (page 123) can be rewritten

$$pH = 6.1 + \log \frac{HCO_3^-}{P_{CO_2} \times 0.03}$$

where 0.03 represents a constant. (This is the basis for the Astrup method of describing acid-base disturbances—see Chapter 15.)

At this point it should be stressed again that both the buffer and respiratory compensations are essentially temporary mechanisms. They are often not completely successful in restoring or maintaining the pH of the blood and extracellular water. The kidneys, however, are able to make permanent adjustments.

Regulation of pH by the Kidneys

During the course of normal metabolism, the kidneys contribute to acid-base homeostasis in two ways. The bicarbonate ions that are filtered by the glomeruli must be reabsorbed by mechanisms described below. Over 24 hours, in a person with a normal GFR (glomerular filtration rate) of 120 mL/min, and a normal serum HCO_3 concentration of 24 mEq/L, over 4000 mEq of HCO_3 must be reabsorbed. Secondly, during normal metabolism, the body produces approximately 1 mEq/kg body weight per day of nonvolatile acids (such as phosphoric and sulfuric). This excess acid is excreted by the kidneys by acidification of buffer salts and by the excretion of NH_4^+. These two processes, which are also described below, account for the acid pH of the urine. The capacity of these processes can be dramatically increased during abnormal states of excess metabolic acid production (e.g., diabetic ketoacidosis or lactic acidosis).

The Reabsorption of Bicarbonate Ions

Normally, all the bicarbonate ions that pass the glomeruli and enter the tubular urine (glomerular filtrate) are reabsorbed. This occurs by means of an exchange of hydrogen ions (which the renal tubular cells secrete) for sodium ions in the tubular urine.

Hydrogen ions are available in the tubular cells because the enzyme carbonic anhydrase (ca) is able to convert carbon dioxide (which is present in all cells) and water into carbonic acid. This ionizes into H^+ and HCO_3^+ ions, namely,

$$CO_2 + H_2O \xrightarrow{\text{ca}} H_2CO_3 \rightarrow H^+ + HCO_3^-.$$

In the tubular urine, the hydrogen ions combine with the bicarbonate ions of the tubular urine to form carbonic acid. This then forms water and carbon dioxide. The water is excreted and the carbon dioxide is reabsorbed by the tubular cells. At the same time, sodium ions pass from the tubular urine into the tubular cells, where they unite with the bicarbonate ions there to form sodium bicarbonate. The bicarbonate then passes into the plasma and extracellular water where its concentration is maintained (Fig. 12–2).

Acidification of Buffer Salts

A similar exchange mechanism occurs between hydrogen ions of the renal tubular cells and the (sodium) salts of various buffer anions, which appear in the urine. Quantitatively, monohydrogen phosphate, Na_2HPO_4 is overwhelmingly the major buffer. This salt dissociates into Na and $NaHPO_4$ ions. As a sodium ion is reabsorbed, a hydrogen ion moves into the tubular urine to unite with the $NaHPO_4$ ion to form a dihydrogen phos-

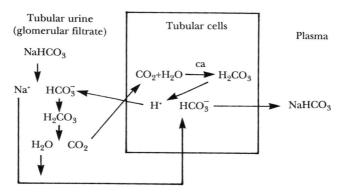

FIGURE 12–2. The mechanism by which bicarbonate ions are conserved by the kidneys. See text.

phate salt, NaH_2PO_4, which is excreted. In this way, a hydrogen ion is removed from the body.

(The term *titratable acid* is used to describe the amount of hydrogen ions in the urine that are bound to phosphate and organic buffers. Its value is measured by determining the milliequivalents of sodium hydroxide that have to be added to urine to raise the pH to 7.4, which is the pH of the plasma from which the glomerular filtrate originated.)

The Secretion of Ammonia

Ammonia, NH_3, is formed in the renal tubular cells from the oxidation of the amino acid glutamine by the enzyme glutaminase and by oxidation of other amino acids. The free ammonia is converted into an ammonium ion, NH_4^+, by uniting with a hydrogen ion and is excreted as ammonium chloride, NH_4Cl. In this way, another hydrogen ion is removed from the body. (The ammonia can also be converted to urea by the liver and then excreted by the kidneys.)

In acidosis, all these renal regulatory mechanisms are exaggerated. For example, the urine shows a pH that may be as low as 4.5. Bicarbonate excretion may diminish or disappear. Titratable acid and ammonium excretion increase dramatically.

On the other hand, in alkalosis, these regulatory mechanisms either decrease or stop. The urine shows a pH that may rise as high as 7.8. (In alkalosis due to potassium deficiency, the urinary pH may remain low [see Chapter 30].) Bicarbonate ion secretion increases. Ammonium salt excretion decreases, and the excretion of cations such as sodium and potassium increases. Titratable acid and chloride ion excretion also decrease and chloride ions may disappear from the urine.

Bibliography

Baker, ES, and Elkinton, JR: Hydrogen ions and buffer base. Am J Med 25:1, 1958.

Bates, RG: *Determination of pH. Theory and Practice.* New York, John Wiley & Sons, 1964.

Bear, RA, and Gribik, M: Assessing acid-base imbalances through laboratory parameters. Hosp Pract 9:157, 1974.

Brønsted, JN: Acid and base catalysis. Chem Rev 5:231, 1928.

Brown, EB, Jr: Blood and tissue buffers. Arch Intern Med 116:665, 1965.

Campbell, EJM: R I pH, Lancet 1:681, 1962.

Christensen, HN: Anions versus cations? Am J Med 23:163, 1957.

Christensen, HN: *Body Fluids and the Acid-Base Balance.* Philadelphia: WB Saunders, 1964.

Cohen, JJ, and Kassirer, JP: Acid-base metabolism. In Maxwell, MH, and Kleeman, CR (eds): *Clinical Disorders of Fluid and Electrolyte Metabolism,* 3rd ed. New York, McGraw-Hill, 1980.

Creese, R, Neil, MW, Ledingham, JM, and Vere, DW: The terminology of acid-base regulation. Lancet 1:419, 1962.

Davenport, HW: *The ABC of Acid-Base Chemistry,* 6th ed. Chicago: The University of Chicago Press, 1974.

Finston, HL, and Rychtman, AC: *A New View of Current Acid-Base Theories.* New York: Wiley-Interscience, 1982.

Gamble, JL, Jr: *Acid-Base Physiology: A Direct Approach.* Baltimore: Johns Hopkins University, 1982.

Gamble, JL, Jr: Sodium and chloride and acid-base physiology. Bull Hopkins Hosp 105:247, 1960.

Garfinkel, HB, and Gelfman, NA: Bicarbonate, not CO_2. Editorial. Arch Intern Med 143:2063, 1983.

Hood, I, and Campbell, EJM: Is pK OK? Editorial. N Engl J Med 306:864, 1982.

Kassirer, JP, and Bleich, HL: Rapid estimation of plasma carbon dioxide tension from pH and total carbon dioxide content. N Engl J Med 272:1067, 1965.

Kaufman, HE, and Rosen, SW: Clinical acid base regulation—the Brønsted schema. Surg Gynecol Obstet 103:101, 1956.

Peters, JP, and Van Slyke, DD: *Quantitative Clinical Chemistry,* vol I: Interpretations. Baltimore: Williams & Wilkins, 1932.

Pitts, RF: Mechanisms for stabilizing the alkaline reserves of the body. Harvey Lect 48:72, 1952–1953.

Seal, US: The chemistry of buffers. Arch Intern Med 116:658, 1965.

13

ACIDOSIS AND ALKALOSIS

The terms *acidosis* and *alkalosis* are used to describe changes in acid-base balance of the body fluids. The normal range of the plasma (or serum) pH is 7.36 to 7.44. The extreme range of pH compatible with life is 6.7 to 7.9.

ACIDOSIS

Acidosis is a term used to describe patients with an increased hydrogen ion concentration in the blood—in other words, with a pH below 7.36.

The increased hydrogen ion concentration may occur as a result of a primary respiratory disturbance (*primary respiratory acidosis, carbonic acid excess*), or as a result of primary metabolic disturbance (*primary metabolic acidosis, primary nonrespiratory acidosis*). Here it may be due to an excess of inorganic or organic acids, or to a decreased amount of base in the body.

ALKALOSIS

Alkalosis is a term used to describe patients with a hydrogen ion concentration in the blood below normal—in other words, with a pH above 7.44.

The decreased hydrogen ion concentration may occur as a result of a primary respiratory disturbance (*primary respiratory alkalosis, carbonic acid loss*), or as a result of a primary metabolic disturbance (*primary metabolic alkalosis, primary nonrespiratory alkalosis*). Here it may be due to an increased amount of base, or a loss of acid from the body.

UNCOMPENSATED AND COMPENSATED ACIDOSIS AND ALKALOSIS

In the previous chapter, the chemical and physiological mechanisms by which the pH of the body is maintained at a more or less constant level

131

were described. When an acidosis or an alkalosis develops, these compensatory mechanisms help restore the pH toward its previous normal level. However, in the process, marked changes in the concentrations of carbonic acid, partial pressure of carbon dioxide (PCO_2) and bicarbonate may occur, even though the pH is restored to normal.

These changes can be demonstrated in four main types of acid-base disturbances.

Respiratory Acidosis

In a patient with respiratory acidosis, an accumulation of carbonic acid occurs due to hypoventilation. This causes the PCO_2 of the plasma to rise, and the bicarbonate–carbonic acid ratio and the pH to fall. This can be called an *uncompensated* respiratory acidosis (Table 13–1).

However, as a result of the compensatory mechanisms described in Chapter 12, bicarbonate is retained in the body, and the bicarbonate–carbonic acid ratio and the pH rise and may return to normal, even though the concentration of both carbonic acid and bicarbonate are now greater than normal. The PCO_2 remains high and unchanged. This can be called a *compensated* respiratory acidosis (Table 13–1).

Respiratory Alkalosis

In a patient with respiratory alkalosis, there is a loss of carbonic acid due to hyperventilation. As a result, the PCO_2 falls, and the bicarbonate–carbonic acid ratio and the pH rise. This can be called an *uncompensated* respiratory alkalosis (Table 13–2).

However, as a result of compensatory mechanisms described in Chapter 12, bicarbonate is excreted by the kidneys, and the bicarbonate–car-

TABLE 13–1
UNCOMPENSATED AND COMPENSATED RESPIRATORY ACIDOSIS

	Normal	Uncompensated Respiratory Acidosis	Compensated Respiratory Acidosis
Bicarbonate	24 mEq/L	24 mEq/L*	38 mEq/L
Carbonic acid	1.2 mEq/L	2.7 mEq/L	2.7 mEq/L
Bicarbonate–carbonic acid ratio	20:1	8.8:1	14:1
PCO_2	40 mm Hg	90 mm Hg	90 mm Hg
pH	7.4	7.04	7.32

*The bicarbonate is presented here as unchanged for didactic simplification. In fact, even in uncompensated respiratory acidosis, a modest increase in bicarbonate level occurs as a result of cellular buffering.

TABLE 13–2
UNCOMPENSATED AND COMPENSATED RESPIRATORY ALKALOSIS

	Normal	Uncompensated Respiratory Alkalosis	Compensated Respiratory Alkalosis
Bicarbonate	24 mEq/L	24 mEq/L*	20 mEq/L
Carbonic acid	1.2 mEq/L	0.6 mEq/L	0.6 mEq/L
Bicarbonate–carbonic acid ratio	20:1	40:1	33.3:1
P_{CO_2}	40 mm Hg	20 mm Hg	20 mm Hg
pH	7.4	7.55	7.50

*The bicarbonate is presented here as unchanged for didactic simplification. In fact, a modest decrease in bicarbonate level occurs as a result of cellular buffering.

bonic acid ratio and the pH fall toward normal, even though the concentrations of bicarbonate and carbonic acid are now less than normal. The P_{CO_2} remains low and unchanged. This can be called a *compensated* respiratory alkalosis (Table 13–2).

Metabolic Acidosis

In a patient with metabolic acidosis, an excess of acid or a loss of base is present. This causes the bicarbonate–carbonic acid ratio and the pH to fall. No change occurs in the P_{CO_2} (*uncompensated* metabolic acidosis, Table 13–3).

However, compensatory mechanisms described in Chapter 12 may occur. As a result, carbonic acid is excreted by the lungs in the form of carbon dioxide, and bicarbonate is retained by the kidneys. Therefore, the P_{CO_2} falls, and the bicarbonate–carbonic acid ratio and the pH rise toward normal, even though the concentrations of bicarbonate and carbonic acid are now less than normal (*compensated* metabolic acidosis, Table 13–3).

TABLE 13–3
UNCOMPENSATED AND COMPENSATED METABOLIC ACIDOSIS

	Normal	Uncompensated Metabolic Acidosis	Compensated Metabolic Acidosis
Bicarbonate	24 mEq/L	15 mEq/L	15 mEq/L
Carbonic acid	1.2 mEq/L	1.2 mEq/L	0.75 mEq/L
Bicarbonate–carbonic acid ratio	20:1	12.5:1	20:1
P_{CO_2}	40 mm Hg	40 mm Hg	25 mm Hg
pH	7.4	7.2	7.3

Metabolic Alkalosis

In a patient with metabolic alkalosis, there is an excess of base or a loss of acid. This causes the bicarbonate–carbonic acid ratio and the pH to rise. No change occurs in the P_{CO_2} (*uncompensated* metabolic alkalosis, Table 13–4).

However, compensatory mechanisms described in Chapter 12 may develop. The compensatory respiratory acidosis may be so marked that the P_{CO_2} may rise higher than 55 mm Hg (see Chapter 29). In addition, bicarbonate ions are excreted by the kidneys. This is associated with a decrease in the bicarbonate–carbonic acid ratio and the pH, even though the serum concentrations of bicarbonate and carbonic acid are still greater than normal (*compensated* metabolic alkalosis, Table 13–4).

IMPORTANCE OF COMPENSATION

These observations are important for several reasons. Notice that in a severe respiratory acidosis, a normal bicarbonate concentration may be present. In addition, the bicarbonate rises to an abnormal value when compensation occurs and the pH returns toward normal (Table 13–1). Conversely, in a severe metabolic acidosis, the bicarbonate concentration is low and it remains very low even when compensation occurs and the pH rises toward normal (Table 13–3). Similar observations can be made for respiratory and metabolic alkalosis.

Overcompensation may also develop. For example, the respiratory compensation that occurs in a diabetic acidosis may continue after the metabolic acidosis has been corrected, so that a respiratory alkalosis, with a high pH and a low P_{CO_2}, may develop. Similarly, the metabolic compensation that occurs in a chronic respiratory acidosis may be so marked that a metabolic alkalosis with a high pH occurs.

In other words, an acid-base disturbance must be described in terms of both the primary or compensatory *respiratory* changes and the primary or compensatory *metabolic* changes that may occur, in addition to changes in pH. Clinically, the *respiratory* changes are indicated by the P_{CO_2} and other

TABLE 13–4
UNCOMPENSATED AND COMPENSATED METABOLIC ACIDOSIS

	Normal	Uncompensated Metabolic Acidosis	Compensated Metabolic Acidosis
Bicarbonate	24 mEq/L	28 mEq/L	34.5 mEq/L
Carbonic acid	1.2 mEq/L	1.2 mEq/L	1.35 mEq/L
Bicarbonate–carbonic acid ratio	20:1	31.6:1	25.6:1
P_{CO_2}	40 mm Hg	40 mm Hg	45 mm Hg
pH	7.4	7.6	7.55

measurements. The *metabolic* changes are indicated by the serum bicarbonate concentration and other measurements (see Chapters 14 and 15).

Some physicians have used the terms *acidemia* or *alkalemia* to describe an abnormally low or high pH, *hypocapnia* or *hypercapnia* to describe an abnormally low or high PCO_2, and *hypobasemia* or *hyperbasemia* to describe an abnormally low or high serum bicarbonate concentration.

Ordinarily, a hospital laboratory technician will determine the serum bicarbonate concentration indirectly by means of the CO_2 content test. However, this test merely indicates the metabolic component of an acid-base disturbance (see Chapter 14).

Simple methods of obtaining the PCO_2, serum bicarbonate concentration, and pH are described in Chapters 14 and 15.

THE USE OF 95% CONFIDENCE BANDS

Investigators have found that when they have studied large groups of patients with acidosis and alkalosis, the pH-PCO_2 changes of 95% of these patients are located within certain limits (95% confidence bands) (Fig. 13–1). These confidence bands have been used as guides, particularly in the

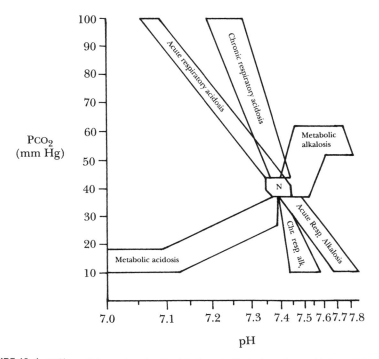

FIGURE 13–1. 95% confidence bands of acidosis and alkalosis patients. (Adapted from Goldberg et al.)

computer diagnosis of acid-base disturbances. They are generally helpful, but the fact that the pH-Pco_2 values of a patient are located within a confidence band does not necessarily indicate that the patient has only a simple, uncomplicated acid-base disturbance. One must consider pH-Pco_2 values in terms of a patient's history, clinical course, medication, or other therapy that has been used, and other previous and present laboratory data.

Bibliography

Camien, MN, Simmons, DH, and Gonick, HC: A critical reappraisal of "acid-base" balance. J Clin Nutr 22:786, 1969.

Campbell, EJM: R I pH. Lancet 1:681, 1962.

Creese, R, Neil, MW, Ledingham, JM, and Vere, DW: The terminology of acid-base regulation. Lancet 1:419, 1962.

Davenport, HW: *The ABC of Acid-Base Chemistry,* 6th ed. Chicago: The University of Chicago Press, 1974.

Goldberg, M, et al: Computer-based instruction and diagnosis of acid-base disorders. A systemic approach. JAMA 223:269, 1973.

Huckabee, WE: Henderson vs. Hasselbalch. Clin Res 9:117, 1961.

MacConnachie, HF: An old-fashioned approach to acid-base balance. Am J Med 49:504, 1970.

Masoro, EJ, and Siegel, PD: *Acid-Base Regulation.* Philadelphia: WB Saunders, 1971.

Nahas, GG, et al: Current concepts of acid-base measurement. Ann New York Acad Sci 133:1, 1966.

Weisberg, HF: Water and electrolyte balance. Bull Mt Sinai Hosp 2:65, 85, 112, 154, 1950.

14

CLINICAL MEASUREMENT OF ACID-BASE BALANCE

In Chapter 12, it was pointed out that

$$pH = 6.1 + \log \frac{bicarbonate}{carbonic + carbon \atop acid \quad dioxide}$$

This can be rewritten by stating that the pH is proportionate to the bicarbonate–carbonic acid ratio. To express this schematically,

$$pH \; ; \; \frac{bicarbonate}{carbonic \; acid}$$

Similarly,

$$pH \; ; \; \frac{bicarbonate}{P_{CO_2}}$$

Therefore, in order to describe an acid-base disturbance accurately and completely, it is necessary to know the pH, the serum bicarbonate concentration, and the serum carbonic acid concentration, or P_{CO_2}. When any two of these values are known, the third can be determined from an appropriate nomogram. When the physician measures only one value, such as the serum bicarbonate concentration (which is indicated indirectly in the CO_2 content), he or she may make serious errors in diagnosis. For example, Tables 13–2 and 13–3 show that a low bicarbonate concentration may occur in a patient with respiratory alkalosis with a high pH, or in a patient with metabolic acidosis with a low pH.

MEASUREMENT OF THE pH

The pH can be measured directly, using a pH meter equipped with a glass electrode. Theoretically, the pH should be determined on heparinized arterial blood, or arterialized blood, such as from a warmed ear lobe or fingertip. Venous blood, drawn without stasis, can also be used. The determination should be done as quickly as possible to prevent changes in pH due to loss of carbon dioxide and to the formation of lactic acid from the breakdown of glucose. The latter can be prevented by adding sodium fluoride to the blood.

Normally, the pH varies from 7.36 to 7.44. The ideal pH is 7.40. pH determinations should also be done at body temperature, 37 or 38°C, to obtain accurate results because the pH becomes more basic when blood is drawn at one temperature and the pH is measured at a lower temperature, such as room temperature and vice versa. Rosenthal has described the following formula to indicate this difference: pH (38°) = pH_t − 0.0147 (38° − t), or pH (37°) = pH_t − 0.0147 (37° − t), where t is the temperature at which the pH is measured. However, other investigators have noted variations from this formula.

The reverse situation occurs in patients who are undergoing surgical operations under hypothermia. Here, the true pH of the patient's blood will be different from the measured pH. The relations between the true and measured pHs are: True pH = pH (37°) + (37° − t) × 0.0147, where t is the patient's temperature.

Edmark has pointed out that when cardiac and other surgical procedures are done under hypothermia, a pH of 7.4 is not optimal. He has therefore suggested that the patient's pH should be reduced 0.0147 of a pH unit for each degree Celsius below 37°. Carson has varied the percentage of carbon dioxide in the pump–oxygenator gas mixture to obtain and maintain a desired pH. Frequent pH measurement should be done during the operation, and the necessary correction factors used, because, as was pointed out above, the measured pH is not identical with the true pH of the patient. The following illustrates this.

Example

Patient's body temperature 25°C. Measured pH (at 37°C) 7.0. The true pH of the patient is therefore:

$$\text{True pH} = \text{pH} (37°) + (37 − t) \times 0.0147$$
$$= 7.00 + (37 − 25) \times 0.0147$$
$$= 7.176$$

Since the patient's temperature has been lowered 12° (37° − 25°), the pH should be decreased to 7.40 − 12 (0.0147) = 7.22. However, the patient's true pH is now 7.176. Therefore, it should be raised slightly.

MEASUREMENT OF THE PLASMA CARBONIC ACID CONCENTRATION AND THE P_{CO_2}

The carbonic acid concentrations cannot be measured directly in a hospital laboratory. However, the concentration of carbonic acid in the blood is proportional to the partial pressure of the carbon dioxide (PCO_2) in the blood and in alveolar air. This can be measured with suitable PCO_2 meters.

In addition, when the pH and plasma bicarbonate (or the total carbon dioxide content) are known, the PCO_2 can be determined from an appropriate nomogram (Fig. 14–1).

MEASUREMENT OF THE PLASMA BICARBONATE ION CONCENTRATION

The plasma bicarbonate ion concentration is not measured directly. However, it can be calculated from the nomogram in Figure 14–1. The approximate bicarbonate ion concentration can also be determined by subtracting 1 mEq/L from the CO_2 content value (see below). The bicarbonate ion concentration can also be obtained from the following formula: Bicarbonate = CO_2 content − $(0.03 \times PCO_2)$. Similarly, the CO_2 content = bicarbonate + $(0.03 \times PCO_2)$.

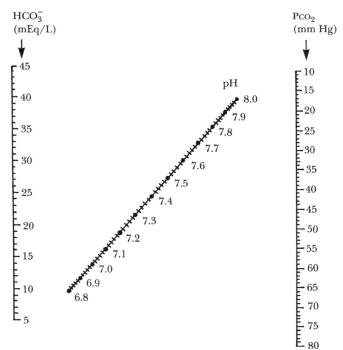

FIGURE 14–1. Nomogram by which the PCO_2 can be determined from the pH and the serum bicarbonate concentration. (After McLean.)

MEASUREMENT OF THE CO$_2$ CONTENT

The CO$_2$ content is the total carbon dioxide that is liberated by acidification of the plasma or serum. It therefore represents the sum of all forms of carbon dioxide in the blood, namely, the carbon dioxide dissolved in the plasma, the carbon dioxide derived from bicarbonate, and the carbon dioxide derived from plasma carbonic acid. It is measured on true plasma, that is, plasma obtained from blood that is collected anaerobically. Venous blood should be collected without stasis, allowed to clot, and centrifuged without exposure to air.

If the CO$_2$ content is measured on whole blood, higher values will be obtained because the whole blood has a greater buffering capacity than either plasma or serum.

Measurement of the CO$_2$ content is valuable, for example, when one is trying to determine wither a diuretic is producing a metabolic alkalosis as a side effect. This will be noted by a rise in CO$_2$ content (and a fall in serum potassium and chloride concentrations). However, one must be constantly aware that the CO$_2$ content merely measures the sum of the bicarbonate (HCO$_3^-$) ions and the carbonic acid (H$_2$CO$_3$) concentration in the blood and extracellular water, and that a value for the CO$_2$ content may indicate a high bicarbonate ion concentration with a low or normal carbonic acid concentration, a normal bicarbonate ion and normal carbonic acid concentration, or a low bicarbonate ion concentration with a normal or high carbonic acid concentration. Therefore, determining the value of the CO$_2$ content without measuring the value of the pH is like trying to interpret the meaning of a white blood cell count without determining the differential cell count (Gambino).

THE CO$_2$ CAPACITY AND THE CO$_2$ COMBINING POWER

Each of these tests measures the carbon dioxide concentration of plasma or serum that has been equilibrated with 5.5% carbon dioxide, which has a partial pressure of 40 mm Hg. However, there are important differences between these two tests.

The CO$_2$ Capacity Test

In this test, whole blood is equilibrated at 38°C (body temperature) with a 5.5% carbon dioxide gas mixture. (This has a partial pressure [P$_{CO_2}$] of 40 mm Hg, which is identical with the P$_{CO_2}$ of alveolar air.) Then the plasma (true plasma) is separated from the red blood cells anaerobically so that no carbon dioxide is lost in the process. The carbon dioxide concentration is then determined. This method is not used now. The CO$_2$ content test is used instead.

The CO_2 Combining Power Test

In this test, plasma or serum is separated from the red blood cells (separated plasma), and then is equilibrated at room temperature with the technician's alveolar air, which presumably has a P_{CO_2} of 40 mm Hg. The carbon dioxide concentration is then determined. This is the method that had been used in hospital laboratories, and what is meant when the term "carbon dioxide combining power," or "alkali reserve" is mentioned in the literature.

The CO_2 combining power is less accurate than the CO_2 capacity because the test is done on separated plasma rather than on the true plasma, at room temperature rather than at body temperature, and with the technician's air, which may not represent true alveolar air, rather than with a 5.5% carbon dioxide gas mixture.

For these reasons, the carbon dioxide combining power test is not used and the CO_2 content test is used instead.

In most patients, the history and clinical course are usually sufficient to determine whether the respiratory or metabolic disturbance is primary. However, if a complex problem is present, the pH must be measured.

MEASUREMENT OF P_{CO_2}

The P_{CO_2} of arterial or arterialized blood (or alveolar air) can now be easily and quickly determined with special P_{CO_2} meters. In addition, the P_{CO_2} can be determined from the pH and CO_2 content (or the bicarbonate concentration) using the nomogram in Figure 14–1.

The normal P_{CO_2} varies from 35 to 48 mm Hg. The ideal P_{CO_2} is 40 mm Hg.

DESCRIPTION OF AN ACID-BASE DISTURBANCE IN TERMS OF THE RELATIONS AMONG P_{CO_2}, pH, AND CO_2 CONTENT

A high P_{CO_2} indicates underventilation and a respiratory acidosis. A low P_{CO_2} indicates overventilation and a respiratory alkalosis. A normal P_{CO_2} represents *respiratory balance*. It may be present normally, or with a metabolic acidosis or alkalosis, or may occur as the result of respiratory acidosis which has been superimposed on a respiratory alkalosis, or *vice versa*.

An uncompensated respiratory acidosis is characterized by a low pH, a high CO_2 content, and a high P_{CO_2}.

An uncompensated respiratory alkalosis is characterized by a high pH, a low CO_2 content, and a low P_{CO_2}.

An uncompensated metabolic acidosis is characterized by a low pH, a low CO_2 content, and a normal P_{CO_2}.

An uncompensated metabolic alkalosis is characterized by a high pH, a high CO_2 content, and a normal Pco_2.

When a respiratory acidosis is compensated by a metabolic alkalosis, the pH tends to return to normal, but the CO_2 content becomes higher. The Pco_2 remains unchanged.

When a respiratory alkalosis is compensated by a metabolic acidosis, the pH tends to become normal, but the CO_2 content becomes lower. The Pco_2 remains unchanged.

When a metabolic acidosis is compensated by a respiratory alkalosis, the pH tends to return to normal, but the CO_2 content becomes lower, and the Pco_2 becomes low.

When a metabolic alkalosis is compensated by a respiratory acidosis, the pH tends to return to normal, but the CO_2 content becomes higher, and the Pco_2 becomes high. However, this does not ordinarily occur (Chapter 29).

Another method of describing the respiratory component of an acid-base disturbance in terms of Pco_2 and pH is described in Chapter 15.

THE USE OF VENOUS BLOOD TO MEASURE pH, Pco$_2$, AND CO$_2$ CONTENT

Theoretically, arterial or capillary blood should be used. However, venous blood drawn without stasis can also be used. The difference between the pH of arterial and venous blood ranges from 0.01 to 0.03 unit.

A tourniquet should be placed lightly around the extremity to avoid compressing the artery. If the arm or hand is cold, warm towels will improve the reliability of the blood sample. The tourniquet should be kept in place while the blood is drawn, and the first tube of blood should be used for measuring the pH. If the tourniquet is removed, one should wait 2 minutes before drawing the blood. The blood is drawn preferably into heparinized vacuum tubes.

Capillary blood from a warmed surface can also be used. If an ear or finger is heated with 40° to 45°C water or a lamp for 3 to 5 minutes, the capillary blood will become arterialized. The skin can be punctured with a #11 blade. Drops of blood can then be collected into a large heparinized capillary blood collecting tube, or into a heparinized Astrup capillary tube.

If the blood is kept at a room temperature below 27°C, the pH will change less than 0.015 pH unit in one-half hour. However, if the blood has to stand more than one-half hour, it should be placed in ice water, where it can be kept as long as 4 hours. If blood is placed in ice water, it should not be centrifuged when it is ice cold, if the pH is to be measured, because a pH reading too alkaline will be obtained. The error may be greater than 0.1 pH unit.

Studies by Phillip and Peretz indicate that measurements from central venous blood give reliable values for metabolic disturbances, but are not as reliable in determining respiratory disturbances.

Bibliography

American Society of Clinical Pathologists: Workshop Manual on Blood pH, pCO_2 Oxygen Saturation and pO_2, 1963.

Bedford, RH, and Woolman, H: Questions and answers. Arterial puncture for blood gas studies. Sites, complications, personnel. JAMA 228:763, 1974.

Campbell, EJM, and Howell, JBL: The determination of mixed venous and arterial CO_2 tension by rebreathing techniques. In Woolmer, RF (ed): A Symposium on pH and Blood Gas Measurement: Methods and Interpretation. Boston: Little, Brown, 1959.

Chung, TO: Central venous versus arterial blood gas values. Ann Intern Med 71:870, 1969.

Davenport, HW: *The ABC of Acid-Base Chemistry*, 3rd ed. Chicago: University of Chicago Press, 1950.

Fagan, TJ: Estimation of hydrogen ion concentration. N Engl J Med 288:915, 1973.

Faulkner, WR: Evaluation of error in measurement of pH in blood at room temperature. Cleveland Clin Q 28:116, 1961.

Fuh, Y-J: Acid-base disorders. JAMA 223:330, 1973.

Gambino, SR: Workshop Manual on Blood pH, pCO_2, Oxygen Saturation and pO_2. Am Soc Clin Path, 1963.

Gambino, SR: Comparison of pH in human arterial, venous, and capillary blood. Am J Clin Path 32:298, 1959. Also Ann New York Acad Sci 133:235, 1966.

Gleason, DF: pH measurements. Arch Intern Med 116:649, 1965.

Hills, AG, and Reid, EL: More on pH. Ann Intern Med 66:238, 1967.

Hofford, JM, Dowling, AS, and Pell, S: More about arterialized capillary blood measurements. JAMA 224:1297, 1973.

Huckabee, WE: Henderson vs. Hasselbalch, Clin Res 9:116, 1961.

Henderson, LJ: *Blood.* New Haven: Yale University Press, 1929.

Kaufman, HE, and Rosen, SW: Clinical acid-base regulation—the Bronsted schema. Surg Gynecol Obstet 103:101, 1956.

Long, AP: Venous or arterial blood gas measurements. JAMA 217:1706, 1971.

McLean, FC: Application of law of chemical equilibrium (law of mass action) to biological problems. Physiol Rev 18:495, 1938.

Morganroth, ML: An analytic approach to diagnosing acid-base disorders. J Crit Illness 5:138, 1990.

Olivia, JV, et al: Earlobe capillary blood for estimating arterial oxygen tension. JAMA 223:1388, 1973.

Paine, EG, Boutwell, JH, and Stoloff, LA: The reliability of "arterialized" venous blood for measuring arterial pH and pCO_2. Am J Med Sci 242:431, 1961.

Paulsen, L: Comparison between total carbon dioxide content in plasma or serum from blood collected with or without paraffine oil. Scand J Clin Lab Invest 9:402, 1957.

Peters, JP, and Van Slyke, DD: *Quantitative Clinical Chemistry,* vol. 1 and 2. Baltimore: Williams & Wilkins, 1932.

Petty, TL, Cheng, TO, Sharp, JT, Peretz, DI, and Grossfeld, JI: Questions and Answers. Source of blood samples for blood gas studies in critically ill patients. JAMA 216:1042, 1971.

Phillips, B, and Peretz, DI: A comparison of central venous and arterial blood gas values in the critically ill. Ann Intern Med 70:745, 1969.

Rosenthal, TB: The effect of temperature on the pH of blood and plasma in vitro. J Biol Chem 173:25, 1948.

Severinghaus, JW: Recent developments in blood O_2 and CO_2 electrodes. In Woolmer, RF (see below).

Singer, RB, and Hastings, AB: Improved clinical method for estimation of disturbances of acid-base balance of human blood. Medicine 27:223, 1948.

Stadie, WC, and Van Slyke, DD: Studies on acidosis. XV. Content and capacity in arterial and venous blood plasma. J Biol Chem 41:191, 1920.

Ullian, RB, Kogos, IG, Golub, M, and Stein, M: Calculation of pH with the use of venous blood. N Engl J Med 265:235, 1961.

Van Slyke, DD, and Cullen, GE: Studies on acidosis. I. J Biol Chem 30:289, 1917.

Weisberg, HF: pH of venous blood. Queries and minor notes. JAMA 194:688, 1968.

Wilson, RF, and Walt, AJ: Differences in acid base levels and oxygen saturation between central venous and arterial blood. Lancet 2:748, 1967.

Woolmer, RF, Editor: *A Symposium on pH and Blood Gas Measurement: Methods and Interpretation.* Boston: Little, Brown, 1959.

15

CLINICAL MEASUREMENT OF ACID-BASE BALANCE
(Continued)

THE ASTRUP METHOD OF DETERMINING ACID-BASE DISTURBANCES

Astrup and his colleagues invented an apparatus (manufactured by the Radiometer Co., Copenhagen), with which one can determine the pH and PCO_2 of blood quickly and simply. They also developed several ways of describing acid-base disturbances and introduced the terms *standard bicarbonate concentration* and *base excess concentration*. Although some experts have objected to the use of base excess values, the Astrup method is still used in some facilities. Accordingly, we show below how these objections can be overcome in interpreting base excess data.

PRINCIPLES OF THE ASTRUP METHOD

In Chapter 12 it was pointed out that

$$pH = 6.10 + \log \frac{HCO_3}{H_2CO_3 + CO_2}$$

However, when a gas such as carbon dioxide dissolves in a liquid, the concentration of the gas in the liquid is directly proportional to the partial pressure of the gas PCO_2. In addition, the concentration of carbonic acid (H_2CO_3) is proportional to the concentration of the dissolved carbon dioxide. Therefore, the term PCO_2 can be substituted for the denominator of the above equation, which becomes

$$pH = 6.10 + \log\frac{HCO_3^-}{PCO_2 \times 0.03}$$

where 0.03 represents a proportionality constant between dissolved CO_2 and PCO_2. The pH, therefore, varies with the PCO_2.

If pH values are plotted against PCO_2 values on fully oxygenated blood with a normal hemoglobin concentration, their relations will be denoted by a curved line. However, when pH values are plotted against the logarithms of PCO_2 values, a straight (diagonal) line results. (The actual slope of this line will vary with the hemoglobin concentration of the blood sample.)

Therefore, if a sample of blood is equilibrated with two known CO_2 tensions, the pH for each of these tensions is measured, and these values are plotted on a graph, as in Figure 15–1. The line joining these two pH values describes the relations between all pH and PCO_2 values of this particular blood sample. This can be called the pH–log PCO_2 line.

If the actual pH of the blood sample is then determined, the PCO_2 of this sample can be read directly from the graph (Fig. 15–1). In addition, the

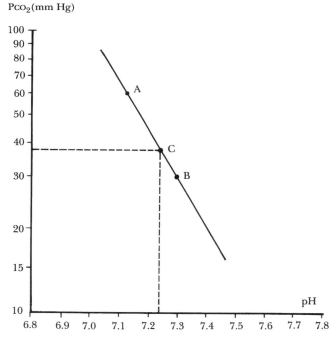

FIGURE 15–1. The pH–log PCO_2 line for a blood sample. (After Astrup.) Point A indicates the measured pH value of 7.12 after equilibration of the blood at a PCO_2 tension of 60 mm Hg. Similarly, point B indicates a pH of 7.30 at a PCO_2 tension of 30 mm Hg. The line between points A and B is the pH–log PCO_2 line. Because the actual pH of the anaerobically drawn blood is 7.24 (point C), the actual PCO_2 of this blood sample is 38 mm Hg (see text for details).

pH–log P_{CO_2} line itself intersects several scales that give values for buffer base concentration, actual bicarbonate concentration, standard bicarbonate concentration, and base excess concentration. The total CO_2 concentration can also be obtained by adding actual bicarbonate concentration to ($P_{CO_2} \times 0.03$).

INTERPRETATION OF THE DATA OBTAINED WITH THE ASTRUP METHOD AND THE SIGGAARD-ANDERSEN NOMOGRAM

The values of P_{CO_2}, buffer base concentration, actual bicarbonate concentration, and total CO_2 concentration can be interpreted in the usual way, regardless of whether these values are obtained directly or indirectly, with any macro or micro methods. However, Astrup has described two new measurements that are obtained from the Siggaard-Andersen nomogram, namely, standard bicarbonate concentration and base excess. These are related to the buffer base in the following way.

The term *whole blood buffer base* was first used in 1948 by Singer and Hastings. They defined it as the sum of the concentrations of the buffer anions (in mEq/L) that were contained in whole blood. These buffer anions include the bicarbonate in plasma and in red blood cells, hemoglobin, plasma proteins, and the phosphates in plasma and red blood cells. Nearly all of this buffering action is due to the hemoglobin and the bicarbonate. The total quantity of these buffer anions in normal blood (determined by the titration of whole blood with strong acid) is about 45 to 50 mEq/L.

If respiration is impaired and CO_2 accumulates, it dissolves in the blood and forms carbonic acid (H_2CO_3). However, this excess acid can be buffered by hemoglobin, for example, to form acid hemoglobin and bicarbonate:

$$H_2CO_3 + Hb \rightarrow HHb + HCO_3^-$$

The decreased amount of hemoglobin buffer that results from this reaction is equal to the increased amount of bicarbonate ions that are released by the reaction. Therefore, the total buffer anion content of the whole blood will not be altered by changes in CO_2 content or P_{CO_2}. *Buffer base changes, therefore, represent the effect of metabolic (nonrespiratory) disturbances in the body.* Buffer base can be determined using Singer and Hasting's original nomogram, or the Siggaard-Andersen nomogram.

Astrup's terms *standard bicarbonate* and *base excess* represent these metabolic changes in a slightly different way. Standard bicarbonate represents the bicarbonate concentration in the plasma of blood which has been equilibrated at a P_{CO_2} of 40 mm Hg, and with oxygen, in order to fully saturate the hemoglobin. Since most of the buffering of blood is carried out by the hemoglobin, unsaturated blood will show a deficient buffering activity. The normal value of standard bicarbonate is 24 (22 to 26) mEq/L. Base excess describes the presence in the blood of an excess of base (or deficit of fixed acid), or a deficit of base (or an excess of fixed acid). (Fixed acid does not include carbonic acid.) It is defined as zero for blood with a pH of 7.4 at a P_{CO_2} of 40 mm Hg. *Positive* values indicate an excess of base (or deficit of fixed acid). *Negative* values indicate a deficit of base (or an excess of fixed acid).

Base excess represents the amount of strong base or acid per liter of blood that has been added as a result of metabolic disturbances (which may be primary or compensatory). Its value is determined from the Siggaard-Andersen nomogram. It is derived by multiplying the deviation in standard bicarbonate from normal by an empirical factor of 1.2. This factor represents the greater buffer action of red blood cells, compared to plasma. The exact correction actually depends on the hemoglobin concentration of the blood sample, but relatively large changes in hemoglobin cause small changes in this value. The normal value of base excess is 0 (+ 2.5 to − 2.5) mEq/L.

There are two advantages of using standard bicarbonate and base excess rather than buffer base values: these values can be rapidly and accurately determined with the Astrup method, and they are not influenced by the oxygen saturation of the original blood sample, unlike buffer base.

Astrup has suggested that the values of base excess can be used not only for diagnosis but also for the treatment of metabolic acidosis or alkalosis patients using the following formula:

mEq base required to correct a metabolic acidosis = body weight (kg) × 0.3 × − base excess, where 0.3 represents a factor which Astrup and his associates determined experimentally.

Similarly: mEq acid required to correct a metabolic alkalosis = body weight (kg) × 0.3 × − base excess.

Clinically, this formula has been found useful in treating metabolic acidosis or alkalosis. However, these values can be misleading when used to treat respiratory acidosis or respiratory alkalosis.

We have already pointed out (Chapter 13) that a patient with uncompensated respiratory acidosis or respiratory alkalosis may show a normal actual bicarbonate concentration. Similarly, such a patient will show a normal standard bicarbonate concentration and a normal base excess value. In addition, a patient who shows a primary *respiratory* acidosis complicated by a primary (independent) *metabolic* acidosis, or a patient with primary *respiratory* alkalosis who develops a primary (independent) *metabolic* alkalosis, may also show normal actual bicarbonate, standard bicarbonate, and base excess concentrations (Table 15–1), despite the serious acidosis or alkalosis which is present. In such patients, the normal base excess concentration cannot be used as a guide to treatment. This difficulty of understanding the significance of base excess values can be resolved if one remembers the following.

TABLE 15–1
COMPLICATED ACID-BASE CHANGES WHICH MAY THEORETICALLY OCCUR

	pH	Pco_2	Actual Bicarbonate	Standard Bicarbonate	Base Excess
1	7.18	80	29	24	0
2	7.58	20	18	24	0

1. Chronic primary respiratory acidosis (emphysema) with a complicating primary (independent) (diabetic) metabolic acidosis.
2. Primary respiratory alkalosis induced by a mechanical respirator, with a complicating primary (independent) metabolic alkalosis, induced by severe vomiting.

In Chapter 12, it was pointed out that a disturbance in pH can be associated with compensatory changes that occur in three different regulatory systems, namely, buffer compensation, respiratory compensation, and renal compensation. As a result of the interaction of these three systems, a pH abnormality seldom indicates a simple disturbance, but, instead, represents the interaction of primary or compensatory metabolic disturbances, associated with primary or compensatory respiratory disturbances.

Similarly, a Pco_2 value that is obtained represents a *balance* between respiratory acidosis and alkalosis processes that may be present simultaneously in a patient. For example, a patient with respiratory acidosis will usually develop a compensatory metabolic alkalosis. However, if for any reason a metabolic acidosis develops independently, there will be a tendency for a compensatory respiratory alkalosis to develop. Also, a patient with chronic respiratory acidosis may be placed in a respirator. A "normal" Pco_2 in such a patient, therefore, merely indicates that *respiratory balance* is present and does not necessarily indicate that no respiratory disturbance is present.

Similarly, the standard bicarbonate and base excess values represent a *balance* between metabolic acidosis and metabolic alkalosis processes that may be present simultaneously in a patient. For example, a patient with metabolic acidosis will usually develop a compensatory respiratory alkalosis. However, if for any reason a respiratory acidosis develops independently, there will be a tendency for a compensatory metabolic alkalosis to develop. "Normal" standard bicarbonate and base excess values in such a patient, therefore, merely indicate that *metabolic balance* is present, and do not necessarily indicate that no metabolic disturbance is present (see Table 15–1).

The importance of this is that a physician must always use the base excess value in association with a description of the *patient*, the Pco_2 and pH, to obtain a full description of the total acid-base balance (in the extracellular water).

DESCRIPTION OF AN ACID-BASE DISTURBANCE IN TERMS OF THE RELATIONS BETWEEN THE ACTUAL BICARBONATE AND THE STANDARD BICARBONATE CONCENTRATIONS

In previous editions of the book, we described how the relationships between the values of the CO_2 content and the CO_2 capacity could be used to describe various acid-base disturbances. Since the CO_2 capacity is infrequently calculated now, we have deleted discussion of the CO_2 capacity from this edition. However, similar information can be obtained by using the values of the standard bicarbonate and actual bicarbonate, popularized by Astrup, because the CO_2 capacity is similar to that of the standard bicarbonate, and the CO_2 content is similar to that of the actual bicarbonate.

Under ideal conditions, the standard bicarbonate and the actual bicarbonate concentrations should show equal values. The reason for this is that normally the pCO_2 of the blood is 40 mm Hg, and the standard bicarbonate value represents the bicarbonate value when the blood plasma has been equilibrated at a pCO_2 of 40 mm Hg.

If a respiratory acidosis is present, the actual bicarbonate concentration will be higher than the standard bicarbonate value for the following reason: standard bicarbonate concentration is determined from a pCO_2 of 40 mm Hg. When a respiratory acidosis is present, the pCO_2 is higher than 40 mm Hg. Therefore, when the blood is equilibrated with a gas mixture of 40 mm Hg, some of the carbon dioxide will leave the blood as equilibration occurs. As a result, the actual bicarbonate value will be higher than the standard bicarbonate value.

If a respiratory alkalosis is present, the actual bicarbonate value will be lower than the standard bicarbonate value for the following reason: standard bicarbonate concentration is determined from a pCO_2 of 40 mm Hg. When a respiratory alkalosis is present, the pCO_2 is lower than 40 mm Hg. Therefore, when the blood is equilibrated with a gas mixture of 40 mm Hg, the blood will absorb some of the carbon dioxide as equilibration occurs. As a result, the actual bicarbonate value will be lower than the standard bicarbonate value.

When these relationships are used, one should remember that normally the standard and actual bicarbonate values may vary as much as ± 2 mEq/L.

1. The standard bicarbonate indicates a metabolic acidosis or alkalosis.
   a. When the standard bicarbonate is low, this is a sign of a metabolic acidosis.
   b. When the standard bicarbonate is high, this is a sign of a metabolic alkalosis.
2. The difference between the actual bicarbonate and the standard bicarbonate concentrations indicates a respiratory acidosis or alkalosis.
   a. When the actual bicarbonate is higher than the standard bicarbonate, this is a sign of a respiratory acidosis.

b. When the actual bicarbonate is lower than the standard bicarbonate, this is a sign of respiratory alkalosis.

3. When the actual bicarbonate and standard bicarbonate are equal, this indicates respiratory balance.

    a. When the actual bicarbonate and standard bicarbonate are low and equal, this indicates an uncompensated metabolic acidosis.

    b. When they are high and equal, this indicates an uncompensated metabolic alkalosis.

4. When the standard bicarbonate is high or low, the actual bicarbonate must also be high or low. However, a low, normal, or high actual bicarbonate may occur with a normal standard bicarbonate concentration.

Bibliography

Astrup P: Acid-base disorders. Correspondence. N Engl J Med 268:817, 1963.

Astrup P: A new approach to acid-base metabolism. Clin Chem 7:1, 1961.

Astrup, P, Jørgensen, K, Siggaard-Andersen, O, and Engle, K: Acid-base metabolism. New approach. Lancet 1:1035, 1960.

Maas, AHJ, and van Heijst, ANP: A comparison of the pH of arterial blood with arterialized blood from the ear lobe with Astrup's microglass electrode. Clin Chim Acta 6:31, 34, 1961.

McDonald, JS, Laughlin, DE, and Bedell, GN: Direct approach to evaluation of patients with acid-base imbalance. JAMA 188:9, 1964.

Nahas, GG: Consulting Editor: Current concepts of acid-base measurement. Ann New York Acad Sci 133:1, 1966.

Relman, AR, and Schwartz, WB: Primum pH. N Engl J Med 272:541, 1965.

Schwartz, WB, and Relman, AS: A critique of the parameters used in the evaluation of acid-base disorders. N Engl J Med 272:541, 1963.

Siggaard-Andersen, O: A graphic representation of changes of the acid-base status. Scand J Clin Lab Invest 12:311, 1960.

Siggaard-Andersen, O: Sampling and storing of blood for determination of acid-base status. Scand J Clin Lab Invest 13:196, 1961.

Siggaard-Andersen, O: The pH-log pCO$_2$ blood acid-base nomogram revised. Scand J Clin Lab Invest 14:598, 1962.

Siggaard-Andersen, O: The Acid-Base Status of the Blood, 2nd ed. Baltimore: Williams & Wilkins, 1964.

Siggaard-Andersen, O, and Engle, K: A new acid-base nomogram. Scand J Clin Lab Invest 12:186, 1960.

Singer, RB, and Hastings, AB: Improved clinical method for estimation of disturbances of acid-base balance of human blood. Medicine 27:223, 1948.

16

PRIMARY RESPIRATORY ACIDOSIS

Primary respiratory acidosis is due to the accumulation of carbon dioxide and carbonic acid in the body. This can occur in one of two ways: (1) when the patient breathes air with a carbon dioxide content above normal, or (2) most commonly, when a pulmonary or neuromuscular lesion is present that interferes with respiration and with the elimination of carbon dioxide by the lungs.

Synonym: Carbonic acid excess, hypercapnia.

PATHOPHYSIOLOGY

The primary characteristic of respiratory acidosis is an increase (above 46 mm Hg) in the partial pressure of CO_2 in arterial blood. As a result of this, the normal bicarbonate–carbonic acid ratio of 27:1.35 (20:1) decreases, because the carbonic acid concentration may rise to 2.70 or higher. The pH of the blood may therefore fall to 7.0 or lower, as the P_{CO_2} rises (see Chapter 13).

When this happens, the following compensatory mechanisms develop:

1. The blood buffers react with the carbonic acid and form more basic salts (Chapter 12).
2. The following compensatory mechanisms develop in the kidneys (Chapter 12).
   a. An increased secretion and excretion of hydrogen ions occur.
   b. Ammonium formation is stimulated, and ammonium ions are excreted.
   c. Bicarbonate is retained, and chloride ions are excreted instead. This causes an increased serum bicarbonate concentration and a decreased serum chloride concentration. The increase in serum bi-

carbonate concentration is approximately the same as the decrease in serum chloride concentration. Therefore, respiratory acidosis does not affect the anion gap (see Chapter 1).

    d. There is also a slight decrease in sodium excretion because of the conservation and retention of bicarbonate.

    e. Monohydrogen phosphate is converted into dihydrogen phosphate and is excreted.

As a result of these compensatory changes, the bicarbonate concentration and the pH rise toward normal to produce a partially compensated respiratory acidosis (see Chapter 13). However, compensation is always incomplete with severe respiratory acidosis (when the PCO_2 is 80 mm Hg or higher).

Many patients may actually overcompensate so that the pH rises above normal. Such patients therefore show a respiratory acidosis (with a high PCO_2) and an overcompensatory metabolic alkalosis, associated with a decreased serum potassium concentration, and the other characteristics of a metabolic alkalosis, namely, high standard bicarbonate concentration, a positive base excess, and a pH above 7.46.

An overcompensatory metabolic alkalosis with an elevated pH can occur in patients with chronic respiratory acidosis in several ways:

1. It has already been pointed out that the respiratory acidosis causes a decreased serum chloride concentration because the kidneys excrete chloride ions at the same time as bicarbonate ions are retained. When the PCO_2 falls to normal, the lost chloride ions must be replaced before the serum bicarbonate concentration can also fall to normal. If this does not occur, a metabolic alkalosis will develop. This condition of posthypercapneic metabolic alkalosis is generally transient.

2. A metabolic alkalosis can also develop because of the loss of potassium ions after the PCO_2 has been lowered, especially in patients who have received corticosteroids or thiazide or other diuretics.

3. Normally the PCO_2 rises during sleep and falls when one wakens in the morning. When the PCO_2 falls, it decreases the renal tubular reabsorption of bicarbonate ions, which are excreted in the urine. However, this mechanism may be absent in patients with chronic respiratory acidosis.

ETIOLOGY

Acute respiratory acidosis can be caused by acute pulmonary lesions such as acute pulmonary edema; severe pulmonary infections; bronchial obstruction; foreign bodies; mechanical respirators; atelectasis; pneumothorax; hemothorax or open chest wounds; severe abdominal distension; positions on an operating room table that interfere with respiration; central nervous system lesions involving the respiratory center in the medulla; poliomyelitis; rarely, extreme loss of potassium or phosphorus ions that interferes with the function of the respiratory muscles; an overdosage of opiates, anesthetics, alcohol, sedatives that depress respiration; or hypothyroidism.

Acute respiratory acidosis can also result if air with a high carbon dioxide content is inhaled for any length of time. This can occur during surgical anesthesia.

Chronic respiratory acidosis can be caused by chronic pulmonary lesions, such as pulmonary fibrosis; emphysema; bronchiectasis; multiple pulmonary embolizations; bronchial asthma; kyphoscoliosis; and chronic cor pulmonale from any cause. Hypoventilation also occurs in some obese patients as part of the pickwickian syndrome, which is characterized by hypercapnia, cyanosis, somnolence, polycythemia, and cor pulmonale. Chronic respiratory acidosis can also occur in brain tumors and when the respiratory nerves are damaged, as in poliomyelitis.

SYMPTOMS AND SIGNS
Acute Respiratory Acidosis

There may not be any evident signs of an acute respiratory acidosis. For example, during an operation, a patient who has a normal color and apparently good oxygenation may develop acute respiratory acidosis if respiratory movements are not sufficient to cause the elimination of carbon dioxide from the lungs. The first sign of respiratory acidosis may therefore be the development of ventricular fibrillation. Ventricular fibrillation may also occur if an acute respiratory acidosis is suddenly corrected.

Carbon dioxide narcosis may occur as a sign of acute respiratory acidosis when a patient with chronic pulmonary disease is given an excessive amount of oxygen.

Carbon Dioxide Narcosis

This syndrome is due to the development of acute respiratory acidosis in a patient with chronic pulmonary disease. It is serious and may be fatal. It is produced in the following way.

The respiratory center is normally sensitive to changes in arterial carbon dioxide content. However, when the partial arterial carbon dioxide pressure (PCO_2) rises above approximately 65 mm Hg, the respiratory center becomes insensitive to carbon dioxide. As a result, hypoxia (anoxia) becomes the main stimulus to respiration, by way of aortic and carotid chemoreceptors, which respond to the lowered arterial *oxygen* saturation. When oxygen is given in a sufficient concentration to raise the arterial oxygen saturation (PaO_2), this stimulus is removed. Ventilation decreases, and the rate of carbon dioxide elimination is decreased. As a result, increased amounts of carbon dioxide are retained in the blood. This causes the carbon dioxide concentration and carbonic acid concentration of the blood to rise, and the pH to fall. Therefore, the respiratory acidosis deepens, and coma and death may occur. Inspired oxygen may also produce hypercapnia as a consequence of worsened pulmonary ventilation perfusion mismatching.

(The mechanism for carbon dioxide narcosis is probably more complex than this, because it has been shown that patients with emphysema with a normal PCO_2 may show a decreased respiratory response when they inhale carbon dioxide.)

The clinical signs of carbon dioxide narcosis are varied. Psychological disturbances are common. There is impairment of consciousness, ranging from drowsiness to deep coma. The patient may be irritable, depressed, euphoric, manic, show paranoid tendencies, or have hallucinations.

Common neurological findings include muscle twitching and tremors of the face or limbs. Flaccid or spastic paralysis of the extremities may occur, as may myoclonus or generalized convulsions. The deep tendon reflexes may be unequal, diminished, or absent. *Asterixis* (an abnormal involuntary jerking movement of the hands that occurs when the patient is asked to put the wrist in dorsiflexion and then extend and spread the fingers) is common. The electroencephalogram may show increased or decreased voltage with prominent theta waves or abnormal alpha waves.

The corneal reflexes may disappear during deep coma. The pupils may be small or dilated, unequal, or sluggish in reaction. Blurring of vision may occur in association with increased cerebrospinal pressure (pseudotumor cerebri).

Slight respiratory depression, or even apnea, may be present. Cardiovascular signs such as tachycardia and a warm flushed skin with excessive perspiration (due to acidosis) may be present. The blood pressure varies. It may be elevated, or hypotension or signs of shock may appear.

When carbon dioxide narcosis develops slowly, coma does not usually appear until the PCO_2 is 80 mm Hg or higher, and extreme levels of hypercapnia may be well tolerated as long as pH is well compensated. However, if it develops rapidly, coma may develop when the PCO_2 is only 60 mm Hg.

Chronic Respiratory Acidosis

A patient with chronic respiratory acidosis usually has severe chronic pulmonary disease, especially bronchiectasis, chronic bronchitis, or pulmonary fibrosis. He or she may show hyperpnea, a chronic productive cough, cyanosis, polycythemia, and a typical emphysematous barrel chest. However, the decreased oxygenation of the blood (low PaO_2) that is present, or even cyanosis that may be present, does not itself indicate that respiratory acidosis (high PCO_2) is also present in these patients.

General symptoms, such as weakness and a dull headache, may also be present. When the respiratory acidosis becomes acute, stupor or coma may develop (see Carbon Dioxide Narcosis, above).

The depression of the central nervous system that occurs in acidosis is due more to a decreased pH of the spinal fluid than to a decreased pH of the blood. Therefore, symptoms are more common and more profound in respiratory acidosis than in metabolic acidosis because respiratory acidosis is associated with a retention of carbon dioxide, which quickly and easily diffuses across the blood-brain barrier. (A metabolic acidosis is not primarily associated with a retention of carbon dioxide, but with the retention of hydrogen ions from metabolic disturbances. In these patients, the increased hydrogen ions do not easily move across the blood-brain barrier.)

Cardiac arrhythmias, such as shifting pacemaker, atrial tachycardia, or atrial or ventricular premature beats, may occur.

LABORATORY FINDINGS

These depend on whether the respiratory acidosis is acute or chronic.

Acute Respiratory Acidosis

The typical compensatory changes are not yet apparent. Therefore, the characteristic findings are:

pH. This falls to the lower level of normal. However, it may reach 7 or lower, in a few minutes.

PCO_2. This is above the upper level of normal (about 46 mm Hg) and may rise to 120 mm Hg or higher.

CO_2 content. This rises to the upper normal level of 28 mEq/L and may exceed this.

Standard bicarbonate and base excess. These remain normal.

Actual bicarbonate. This rises to the upper limit of normal (26 mEq/L) and may reach 29 mEq/L, but it does not exceed this. Notice that the actual bicarbonate value is higher than the standard bicarbonate value. This is a characteristic finding in respiratory acidosis. The normal base excess indicates that metabolic balance is present.

95% Confidence Bands

Figure 13–1, page 135, shows the pH and PCO_2 ranges in both acute and chronic respiratory acidosis. Notice that the high PCO_2 values of acute respiratory acidosis are associated with lower pH values than occur in chronic respiratory acidosis.

These confidence bands can be used for diagnosis. For example, if a patient with respiratory acidosis shows a pH of 7.2 and a PCO_2 of 70 mm Hg, and if these values are plotted on Figure 13–1, they meet within the confidence band of acute respiratory acidosis. This highly suggests that the patient has an acute respiratory acidosis.

Serum Electrolytes

The cation-anion balance is normal. The serum sodium concentration may rise slightly as a result of the respiratory acidosis. The serum potassium concentration generally remains normal. If the PCO_2 is lowered by treatment, the serum potassium concentration may fall below normal and signs of hypokalemia may develop.

Example: Acute respiratory acidosis in a patient during surgical anesthesia.
pH, 7.22
PCO_2, 80 mm Hg
CO_2 content, 33.9 mEq/L
Standard bicarbonate level, 26 mEq/L
Actual bicarbonate level, 31.5 mEq/L
Base excess, +2.5 mEq/L
Serum potassium concentration, 6 mEq/L

The pH is low, indicating an acidosis. The PCO_2 is high, indicating that a respiratory acidosis is present. Similarly, the actual bicarbonate level is higher than the standard bicarbonate level, because of the respiratory acidosis. The base excess is normal, indicating that metabolic balance is present.

Chronic Respiratory Acidosis

The changes in pH, PCO_2, and CO_2 content described for acute respiratory acidosis patients are present in chronic respiratory acidosis. However, the kidneys have been able to retain bicarbonate so that the CO_2 capacity and the pH rise. This is associated with a reciprocal fall in serum chloride concentration. The serum sodium concentration may be slightly elevated, and the serum potassium concentration is also elevated.

The 95% confidence band of chronic respiratory acidosis patients is discussed in Chapter 13.

Example: Patient with chronic respiratory acidosis.
pH, 7.4
PCO_2, 66 mm Hg
CO_2 content, 33.9 mEq/L
Standard bicarbonate level, 31 mEq/L
Actual bicarbonate level, 39.5 mEq/L
Base excess, +8 mEq/L

The pH is normal. This indicates that if any acid-base disturbance is present, it is compensated. The PCO_2 is high. This indicates a respiratory acidosis. Similarly, the actual bicarbonate level is higher than the standard bicarbonate level. The base excess is high. This indicates that a metabolic alkalosis is present.

However, these values do not indicate whether the respiratory acidosis or the metabolic alkalosis is primary. One indirect clue is the PCO_2 of 66 mm Hg because it is rare for the PCO_2 to rise higher than 55 or 60 mm Hg when a compensatory respiratory acidosis develops in a patient with a primary metabolic alkalosis (see Chapter 29). In most patients, a knowledge of the history and clinical course is necessary to determine whether the respiratory or the metabolic disturbance is primary (or whether two independent acid-base disturbances are present; see Chapter 32).

Cation-Anion Balance:
Na 140   K 4.5 HCO_3 39.5   Cl 89 mEq/L

$$\begin{aligned}
\text{Anion gap} &= (\text{Na} + \text{K}) - (HCO_3 + \text{Cl}) \\
&= (140 + 4.5) - (39.5 + 89) \\
&= 144.5 - 128.5 \\
&= 16 \text{ mEq/L (normal)}
\end{aligned}$$

DIAGNOSIS

Respiratory acidosis (PCO_2 above 50 mm Hg) is almost always associated with hypoxemia (PaO_2 below 60 mm Hg) unless a patient with normal ventilation has been inhaling carbon dioxide. However, hypoxemia can exist with or without respiratory acidosis, for example, hypoxemia *with* respiratory acidosis (*ventilatory failure*) occurs in patients with chronic obstructive pulmonary disease (COPD), neuromuscular diseases affecting the respiratory muscles, as a result of the depressant effect of drugs on breathing, and so on.

Hypoxemia *without* respiratory acidosis (*gas exchange failure*) occurs in patients with acute pulmonary edema, shock, massive pulmonary embolism, interstitial fibrosis and other causes of alveolar-capillary block, and so on. (Discussion of hypoxemia without respiratory acidosis is outside the scope of this book.)

Normally, the arterial oxygen content is more than 80 mm Hg (corresponding to a hemoglobin oxygen saturation of approximately 95%). Normal elderly persons have slightly lower values. Hypoxemia is minimal until the PaO_2 falls to approximately 55 mm Hg, but becomes serious when the PaO_2 falls below 45 mm Hg, and dangerous to life when it falls to approximately 30 mm Hg.

Acute respiratory acidosis should be suspected or anticipated when inadequate respiratory ventilation or signs of shock occur in any acutely ill or injured patient, or during an operation. The patient may show good color and is usually not cyanosed.

Characteristic laboratory findings of the respiratory acidosis are a low pH and a high PCO_2. However, metabolic compensation often occurs in a chronic respiratory acidosis. The pH may not only return to normal but may even become high due to the metabolic alkalosis that has developed. However, this does not occur in patients with severe respiratory acidosis who show a PCO_2 greater than 80 mm Hg (also see page 132).

COURSE AND PROGNOSIS

If pulmonary obstruction is suddenly released by tracheotomy, for example, in an acute respiratory acidosis, the patient may begin to hyperventilate and may eliminate a large amount of carbon dioxide. However, bicarbonate concentration may remain temporarily high. As a result, an acute respiratory alkalosis and tetany may develop. Death in acute respiratory acidosis is often due to ventricular fibrillation.

In patients with chronic respiratory acidosis, most of the pulmonary changes are chronic and irreversible. Therefore, the prognosis for such a patient is poor.

TREATMENT

Acute Respiratory Acidosis

If acute respiratory acidosis is suspected in a surgical patient, assisted respiration or intubation should be used. Moore has pointed out that there is no time to wait for chemical confirmation, because pH can be lowered to 7.2 within 8 minutes of rebreathing, or breathing a carbon dioxide–enriched mixture, even in a normal subject.

ACUTE RESPIRATORY ACIDOSIS COMPLICATING CHRONIC OBSTRUCTIVE PULMONARY DISEASE (COPD)

This can be treated in the following way:

1. Treat hypoxemia if necessary. If the PaO_2 is 50 mm Hg or higher, oxygen therapy is generally not needed (Keighley and Mithoefer). If the PaO_2 is less than 50 mm Hg, oxygen should be given with a Venturi type of mask rather than with nasal cannulas to ensure sustained adequate oxygenation. A flow rate of 28% (rarely 35%) is adequate. The PaO_2 should be raised only to 60 mm Hg, to prevent carbon dioxide narcosis.

   Oxygen can also be given at a concentration not exceeding 40%, using nasal catheters or cannulas, at a flow rate of 1 to 2 L/min or less. However, this requires a special flowmeter.

The PCO_2 should be checked periodically. If it rises when oxygen is given, this may be a sign of impending carbon dioxide narcosis. Stop the oxygen.

2. Eliminate thick secretions. An increased fluid intake (oral or parenteral) helps decrease the viscosity of bronchial secretions. In addition, the inspired air should be humidified to 100% saturation with water. A solution of acetylcysteine can also be given, either with a nebulizer or with intermittent positive pressure breathing apparatus, to help liquefy the thick mucus. (Acetylcysteine must be used cautiously in patients with bronchial asthma because it can induce bronchospasm.)

   If the patient's cough reflex is adequate, deep breathing exercises and postural drainage may also be helpful. If the cough reflex is ineffective, nasotracheal suctioning or bronchoscopy may be indicated.

3. Treat bronchospasm. Bronchodilators such as albuterol can be given by nebulizer. Aminophylline can be given intravenously. Oral bronchodilators such as theophylline or other xanthines or terbutaline, a beta-2 agonist; albuterol; isoetharine; metaproterenol; or isoproterenol are also of value. Corticosteroids can be used if life-threatening bronchospasm persists. Some patients may require long-term therapy with oral corticosteroids.

4. Treat respiratory infection, if present, with an appropriate antibiotic.

5. Maintain an adequate airway. Endotracheal intubation or tracheostomy may be needed if the PaO_2 does not rise with medical treatment. Mechanical ventilation should be used only if the patient is apneic or has not responded to treatment.

Chronic Respiratory Acidosis

The treatment of chronic respiratory acidosis depends on many factors—the degree of hypoxemia, presence of infection, bronchospasm, and so on.

Oxygen therapy is not needed in every patient with chronic respiratory acidosis. For example, a patient with COPD can continue to be ambulatory even when the PaO_2 is persistently 40 mm Hg and the PCO_2 50 mm Hg or higher. However, when oxygen is indicated, it should be used as described above.

General therapy is as follows. The patient must stop smoking. Antihistamines should be avoided because they cause thickening of the bronchial mucus. Sedatives should also be avoided because they may depress respiration. Bronchial or pulmonary infections should be treated promptly with appropriate antibiotics. Bronchospasm can be treated with theophylline or other preparations described above. Corticosteroids should be avoided unless other medication is not effective; then they should be given in minimally effective doses. When given on a long-term basis, the patient may also need isoniazid to prevent reactivation of a quiescent tuberculosis infection. Intermittent positive pressure breathing has been used in patients with COPD, but its value has been questioned. Cough and thick bronchial secretions can be treated by adequate hydration and by the use of water vapor inhalation, postural drainage, and physical therapy with chest percussion. Potassium iodide drops have also been used to loosen thick bronchial secretions.

One should remember that chronic respiratory acidosis itself does not require treatment. However, severe hypoxemia must always be treated.

Vigorous treatment of chronic respiratory acidosis patients with mechanical ventilation may be associated with the development of generalized convulsions and other signs of central nervous system excitation, and coma, along with the development of alkalosis. Because of this, the elevated PCO_2 should be decreased slowly.

A carbonic anhydrase inhibitor such as Diamox may be helpful, with small doses of digitalis if the patient has chronic cor pulmonale and congestive heart failure. A metabolic acidosis may develop from the use of the drug and this may stimulate ventilation.

If a metabolic alkalosis with a high pH is present in chronic respiratory acidosis, the patient should be given potassium chloride to correct the alkalosis in addition to the other treatment for the respiratory acidosis.

Bibliography

Aberman, A, and Fulop, M: The metabolic and respiratory acidosis of acute pulmonary edema. Ann Intern Med 76:173, 1972.
Beale, HD, Schiller, IW, Halperin, MH, Franklin, W, and Lowell, FC: Delirium and coma precipitated by oxygen in bronchial asthma complicated by respiratory acidosis. N Engl J Med 244:710, 1951.
Bedon, GA, Block, AJ, and Ball, WC, Jr: The "28%" Venturi mask in obstructive airway disease. Arch Intern Med 125:106, 1970.
Campbell, EJM: Respiratory failure. BMJ 1:1451, 1965.
Carter, NW, Seldin, DW, and Teng, HC: Tissue and renal response to chronic respiratory acidosis. J Clin Invest 38:949, 1959.
Comroe, JH, Jr, Bahnson, ER, and Coates, EO, Jr: Mental changes occurring in chronically ill anoxemia patients during oxygen therapy. JAMA 143:1044, 1950.
Editorial: Convulsions after therapy for alveolar hypoventilation JAMA 189:993, 1964.
Editorial: Carbon dioxide in body fluids. N Engl J Med 280:162, 1969.
Haynie, GD, et al: Recovery from chronic hypercapnia. The critical role of chloride in restoration of normal acid-base equilibrium. J Clin Invest 40:1047, 1961.
Hunter, CC: Errors in management of patients dying of chronic obstructive lung disease. JAMA 199:488, 1967.
Keighley, JVH, and Mithoefer, JC: The management of arterial hypoxia in chronic obstructive pulmonary disease. Chest 62:45S, 1972.
Kettel, LJ: Acute respiratory acidosis. Hospital Med 12:31, 1976.
Kettel, LJ, et al: Treatment of acute respiratory acidosis in chronic obstructive lung disease. JAMA 217:1503, 1971.
Levitin, H, Branscome, W, and Epstein, EH: The pathogenesis of hypochloremia in respiratory acidosis. J Clin Invest 37:166, 1958.

MacDonald, FM: Respiratory acidosis. Arch Intern Med 116:681, 1965.

Makoff, D: Compensatory patterns in acid-base disorders. Geriatrics 26:107, 1971.

McCurdy, DK: Mixed metabolic and respiratory acid-base disturbances. Diagnosis and treatment. Chest 62:35S, 1972.

Miller, A, Bader, R, and Bader, ME: The neurologic syndrome due to marked hypercapnia with papilledema. Am J Med 33:309, 1962.

O'Donohue, WJ, Jr, and Baker, JP: Controlled low-flow oxygen in the management of acute respiratory failure. Chest 63:818, 1973.

Pitt, B, et al: Respiratory failure with focal neurological signs. Arch Intern Med 115:714, 1965.

Rastegar, A, and Thier, SO: Physiological consequences and bodily adaptations to hyper- and hypocapnia. Chest 62:28S, 1972.

Vandenberg, R, et al: Oxygen therapy in acute respiratory failure. Med J Aust 2:874, 1970.

Weinberger, SE, Schwartzenstein, RM, and Weiss, JW: Hypercapnia. N Engl J Med 321:1223, 1989.

17

METABOLIC ACIDOSIS SYNDROMES

The term *metabolic acidosis* describes acidosis resulting from a relative excess of inorganic or organic acids that are not freely excreted by the kidneys or from a loss of base from the body.

Synonyms: Base deficit, bicarbonate deficit.

PATHOPHYSIOLOGY

We know that a metabolic acidosis develops because of an increased amount of acid or a decreased amount of base in the body. As a result of this, the normal bicarbonate–carbonic acid ratio of 27/1.35 (20/1) decreases, and the pH falls below 7.36 and may fall to 7.0 or lower.

The decreased pH stimulates the respiratory center, and increased depth and rate of respiration occur in an attempt to lower the carbonic acid concentration and restore the pH to its normal value. (Pulmonary compensation is usually not complete.) In addition, the renal compensatory mechanisms described in Chapter 16 for respiratory acidosis may develop with enhanced renal ammonium and titratable acid excretion and renal bicarbonate retention.

As a result of these compensatory changes (i.e., the pulmonary elimination of carbon dioxide and augmented renal acid excretion), the bicarbonate–carbonic acid ratio and the pH rise toward normal.

When renal insufficiency is the cause of the acidosis, the renal compensatory mechanisms will be inadequate. In addition, pulmonary compensation may be markedly inadequate if the patient has chronic pulmonary disease and a respiratory acidosis. Such a patient will not be able to hyperventilate sufficiently to remove the excess carbonic acid.

The compensatory hyperventilation that occurs as a result of the metabolic acidosis may persist even after the patient is no longer acidotic. The reason for this is not known. However, this observation is important because the patient who is recovering from metabolic acidosis can develop a serious respiratory alkalosis due to the hyperventilation that continues.

This can lead to great confusion, particularly if an alkaline salt such as sodium bicarbonate or sodium lactate has been given to correct the metabolic acidosis. The reason for this is as follows: The original metabolic acidosis causes a low actual bicarbonate and standard bicarbonate level. The sodium bicarbonate or lactate causes the pH and the bicarbonate values to rise. However, the compensatory respiratory alkalosis due to hyperventilation persists even when the metabolic acidosis is corrected. This causes the pH to rise and the actual bicarbonate level to fall. The standard bicarbonate also tends to remain low to compensate for the respiratory alkalosis that has developed. Therefore, if the patient's progress is being checked only by determination of the CO_2 content, it will be noted that, as the alkalinizing salt is given, the rise in CO_2 values will be deceptively low in relation to the rise in pH and will be deceptively high in relation to the rise in PCO_2.

The following example illustrates this. Block, Field, and Adair described a 14-year-old boy (case 4) who was admitted to the hospital with typical signs of diabetic acidosis and stupor. Immediate treatment consisted of small doses of insulin, subcutaneous saline, and orange juice by mouth. After 6 hours, his condition was only slightly improved. Therefore, he was given 4 g of sodium bicarbonate in a rectal enema of 6 ounces of 5% dextrose every 3 hours, a total of 32 g/day. This was continued for 3 days. The following are some of the electrolyte concentrations:

Date	CO_2 Content	PCO_2	pH
Jan. 29	4.37 mmEq/L	9.7 mm Hg	7.03
Jan. 31	16.0	21.4	7.46

Notice that the CO_2 content had risen more than three times, but that the PCO_2 had risen less than three times its previous value. The rise in the CO_2 content indicates that the patient's metabolic acidosis was being corrected. Theoretically, when this happened, the compensatory hyperventilation and the respiratory alkalosis should have stopped and the PCO_2 should have risen almost to normal. This did not occur. The hyperventilation and the respiratory alkalosis continued, even though the original stimulus, namely, the low pH of 7.03, was no longer present, and even though an alkalosis with a pH of 7.46 had developed.

ETIOLOGY

Patients with metabolic acidosis can be classified in several ways. For example, they can be divided into two groups: those with a normal anion gap $(Na + K) - (HCO_3 + Cl)$ of approximately 16 mEq/L or less (Chapter 1), and those with an abnormally large anion gap (22 mEq/L or more), due to the accumulation of abnormal acid anions.

The serum bicarbonate concentration is reduced in both groups of patients. However, when the anion gap is normal, the serum chloride concentration becomes reciprocally elevated to fill the gap produced by the decreased serum bicarbonate concentration (hyperchloremic metabolic acidosis). When the anion gap is increased, unmeasured anions fill this gap.

Metabolic Acidosis Associated with a Normal Anion Gap

These patients show an increased serum chloride concentration (*hyperchloremic metabolic acidosis*).

1. Administration of ammonium chloride or other chloride salts (see below).
2. Carbonic anhydrase inhibitor administration (see below).
3. Other drugs, such as sulfamylon, cholestyramine.
4. "Dilution" acidosis (see below).
5. Diarrheas or draining gastrointestinal (particularly pancreatic) fistulas (see below).
6. Proximal or distal renal tubular acidosis (Chapter 18).
7. Intravenous hyperalimentation.
8. Post-hypocapnia.

Metabolic Acidosis Associated with an Abnormal (Large) Anion Gap

These patients show a normal serum chloride concentration, but an accumulation of unmeasured acid anions.

1. Diabetic ketoacidosis (Chapter 24)
2. Azotemia (Chapters 20, 21, 22, 23)
3. Lactic acidosis (Chapter 19)
4. Salicylate (salicylic acid) intoxication (Chapter 25)
5. Alcoholic ketoacidosis (Chapter 27)
6. Starvation ketoacidosis (usually mild)
7. Intoxication due to the accumulation of other acids, such as methanol (methyl alcohol), formic acid, paraldehyde, various organic acids, boric acid, ethylene glycol, and oxalic acid.

Further, patients with metabolic acidosis can be described based on the presence of an acid excess or a base (bicarbonate ion) deficit.

Metabolic Acidosis Due to Acid Excess (Acid Gain Acidosis)

This occurs from an increase in the absolute amount of acids in the blood. Normally, the catabolism of proteins and nucleic acids produces amino acids, phosphoric, sulfuric and uric acids. Similarly, lactic, pyruvic, and succinic acids are produced in the course of carbohydrate catabolism, and ketone and fatty acids are produced from the hydrolysis and oxidation of fats. However, these acids may accumulate in the body in the following way:

1. Diabetic acidosis (Chapter 24).
2. Starvation. When there is a deficient intake of carbohydrate, an increased catabolism of body protein and fat occurs, causing an increase in ketone acids.
3. Lactic acidosis (Chapter 19).
4. Rare metabolic disorders (D-lactic acidosis associated with short bowel syndrome, inherited aminoacidemias).

Metabolic Acidosis Due to Dietary or Parenteral Intake of Excessive Acids

Chloride Acidosis

This condition is the result of the oral or parenteral administration of acids, such as hydrochloric acid, or salts containing chloride ions, such as calcium chloride, ammonium chloride, cation exchange resins, or arginine HCl.

Ammonium Chloride

Ammonium chloride acidosis occurs as the ammonium ion NH_4 reaches the liver and is converted to ammonia (NH_3), releasing a hydrogen ion and producing an acidosis. The ammonia is later converted to urea and excreted. Part of the chloride is also excreted by the kidneys with sodium and water. (In this way it acts as a diuretic.)

Sodium Chloride

Large doses of sodium chloride parenterally (especially in the form of hypertonic saline) can cause a metabolic acidosis in the following way: Normally, the extracellular water contains more sodium ions than chloride ions, Na, 142 mEq/L to Cl, 100 Eq/L. Isotonic saline solution contains approximately 150 mEq of sodium and chloride per liter. Therefore, when a large amount of sodium chloride is administered and kidney function is not normal, an excess of chloride ions is added to the body. The sodium ions are excreted as sodium bicarbonate and the chloride ions are retained with hydrogen ions. This can produce a mild metabolic acidosis.

An increased volume of extracellular water can itself produce a metabolic acidosis in the following way: If one adds some neutral fluid, such as isotonic saline solution, to a buffer solution that contains sodium bicarbonate and carbonic acid in a normal bicarbonate–carbonic acid ratio of 20:1 (see Chapter 12), the buffering capacity of the solution per unit volume will decrease, but the pH will not change because the bicarbonate–carbonic acid ratio does not change. However, if a large volume of isotonic saline solution is infused into a patient and the extracellular water volume is increased in this way, the pH will fall because carbon dioxide and carbonic acid are constantly being produced in the body and the bicarbonate–carbonic acid ratio becomes smaller. The metabolic acidosis produced in this way has been called a *dilution (or expansion) acidosis.*

Calcium Chloride

When calcium chloride is given orally, the calcium is not able to penetrate the intestinal mucosa. But the chloride ions are absorbed as hydrochloric acid; calcium is excreted in the stool with bicarbonate.

Boric Acid Poisoning

This condition may cause metabolic acidosis.

Salicylic Acid Poisoning (Chapter 25)

Methanol Poisoning

Acidosis occurs as a result of the formation of formic and other organic acids.

Ethylene Glycol Poisoning

Ethylene glycol is the active ingredient in permanent antifreeze solutions. If it is imbibed, a metabolic acidosis, acute renal failure, and death may develop. The metabolic acidosis is due to the breakdown of the ethylene glycol to oxalic acid, which crystallizes in the kidneys. In addition, other metabolic acids are formed.

Metabolic Acidosis Due to Retention of Acids Normally Produced

This occurs in renal disease where sulfuric and phosphoric acids particularly, as well as other metabolic acids, are retained in the body (see Chapter 20).

Metabolic Acidosis Due to Loss of Base (Bicarbonate Ions)

This can occur with loss of intestinal secretions due to severe diarrheas, small bowel fistulas, or severe biliary fistulas. (This type of acidosis can also occur in patients with renal tubular acidosis [Chapter 18].)

When diarrhea occurs, large amounts of bicarbonate are secreted into the gut and excreted. As a result, the bicarbonate concentration and the bicarbonate-carbonic acid ratio fall, causing a decreased pH and an acidosis. Sodium ions are also excreted into the gut along with bicarbonate as sodium bicarbonate. Therefore, the serum sodium concentration may be lowered.

Ureterosigmoidostomy patients also may develop hyperchloremic acidosis, as the colonic mucosa in contact with urine may reabsorb chloride ions and secrete bicarbonate ions, which are lost from the body. Ureterosigmoidostomy is very rarely performed, but patients with ileal conduits occasionally develop a similar acidosis, particularly if the conduit drains urine sluggishly into an external collecting appliance.

Carbonic Anhydrase Inhibitors

On page 128 it was pointed out that all the bicarbonate ions that pass the glomeruli and enter the tubular urine (glomerular filtrate) are reabsorbed. This occurs because the hydrogen and bicarbonate ions are produced in the tubule cells by means of carbonic anhydrase. The hydrogen ions pass into the urine and react with sodium bicarbonate to form carbonic acid, which is excreted. The sodium ions pass back into the tubular cells, react with the bicarbonate, and then pass back into the plasma as sodium bicarbonate.

When a carbonic anhydrase inhibitor such as Diamox is given, carbonic acid is not formed in the kidney tubule cells, and a large amount of sodium bicarbonate and water is excreted in the urine. This causes a diuresis and also an acidosis, due to the loss of bicarbonate. In addition, a large amount of potassium ions is also excreted in the urine.

SYMPTOMS AND SIGNS

A mild metabolic acidosis may be asymptomatic. Symptoms usually appear when the CO_2 content falls to 18.2 mEq/L or lower. The patient may complain of weakness or general malaise or dull headache. In addition, nausea, vomiting, and abdominal pain may be present. Characteristic *deep* respirations (Kussmaul breathing, air hunger) are often present. This is more common in acute metabolic acidosis than in chronic metabolic acidosis. The respiratory rate is also usually increased, but may be slow. The increased depth of respiration is more characteristic of acidosis than the increased respiratory rate. Occasionally, patients are aware of their increased ventilation and complain of shortness of breath.

These signs are usually present when the CO_2 content falls below 9.1 mEq/L and the pH is 7.2 or lower. When the pH falls to 7.0, respiratory depression may occur.

Peripheral vasodilatation may be present. This produces a warm and flushed skin, a wide pulse pressure with a bounding pulse, and active apical impulse.

Osteomalacia may develop as a complication of chronic metabolic acidosis, because calcium salts may be withdrawn from bone for use as buffers to neutralize the excessive hydrogen ions.

The clinical picture also depends on the cause of the acidosis. Diabetic acidosis patients may have a fruity, acetone odor to the breath, and may show signs of severe water loss, such as thirst and dry mucous membranes, or signs of severe sodium loss, such as loss of skin turgor and shock. In addition, hyperglycemia, ketonemia, ketonuria, and glycosuria are present.

Uremic patients also have a fruity odor to the breath and may show signs of water or sodium loss. Muscle twitching may occur because of a decreased concentration of ionized serum calcium. Convulsions may occur, usually due to hypertensive encephalopathy and not to uremia or acidosis.

When the pH falls below 7.0, the cardiac output decreases and bradycardia may develop; the circulatory system becomes unresponsive to catecholamines. This is particularly important when a patient develops metabolic acidosis associated with cardiogenic shock, or particularly cardiac arrest. In such a patient, it is imperative to raise the pH to 7.30 if possible, in association with other treatment.

When the pH in a diabetic acidosis patient decreases to 7.0 or less, the acidosis interferes with carbohydrate metabolism and with the effectiveness of insulin. The pH in such a patient should also be raised with intravenous sodium bicarbonate.

Electrocardiogram

Hyperkalemia is often associated with acidosis for reasons already discussed. However, the electrocardiogram may or may not show signs of hyperkalemia (Chapter 26). Patients with diabetic acidosis may show signs of hypokalemia (Chapter 30), and these signs may become more marked with treatment (if the serum potassium concentration becomes lowered). When azotemic acidosis is present, the electrocardiogram may show signs of hypocalcemia as well as hyperkalemia (prolongation of the QT interval and peaked T waves).

Severe acidosis can cause ST deviations of the type usually found in myocardial injury.

LABORATORY FINDINGS

The laboratory findings are somewhat different in uncompensated and compensated metabolic acidosis.

Uncompensated Metabolic Acidosis

In a patient with uncompensated metabolic acidosis, renal and pulmonary compensatory mechanisms have not developed. Therefore, the pH is low and the PCO_2 is normal. The standard bicarbonate is low and equal to the actual bicarbonate, and the base excess shows a negative value (Chapter 15).

Serum electrolytes may show a low bicarbonate and a reciprocal elevation of chloride. Serum sodium concentration may be normal, high, or low, depending on the cause of the acidosis.

A large abnormal anion gap may or may not be present, depending on the cause of the acidosis (see above).

Compensated Metabolic Acidosis

When compensation occurs, the pH rises slightly but remains lower than normal. The PCO_2 falls as a result of the hyperventilation. This produces a compensatory respiratory alkalosis. The bicarbonate concentration (the standard bicarbonate) may also rise toward normal if the kidneys are able to conserve bicarbonate ions. The actual bicarbonate also rises but also remains below normal.

Because of the respiratory alkalosis the actual bicarbonate is lower than the standard bicarbonate.

Serum electrolytes show a low bicarbonate and a normal, low, or high chloride concentration. Serum sodium may be normal or low. It will be low when sodium loss is associated with the development of the acidosis, as in diarrheas, diabetic acidosis, or renal disease. Serum potassium concentration is elevated because of the acidosis (Chapter 26). However, if a severe potassium depletion is present, the serum potassium concentration may be normal.

(A normal or low potassium concentration in the presence of acidosis is a sign of potassium depletion.)

A large abnormal anion gap may or may not be present, depending on the cause of the acidosis (see above).

White Blood Count

A leukocytosis may be present.

Urine

The urine has a high ammonia content and is acid (pH 4.6 to 6.2). However, in acidosis due to chronic kidney disease, the renal compensatory mechanisms for combatting acidosis are not effective. In such patients, the urinary pH may be normal in spite of the acidosis.

Example: Partially compensated metabolic acidosis in chronic nephritis.
pH 7.28

P_{CO_2} 26.4 mm Hg
CO_2 content 12.8 mEq/L
Standard bicarbonate 15 mEq/L
Actual bicarbonate 12 mEq/L
Base excess -13 mEq/L

The pH is low. This indicates an acidosis. The negative base excess and the low standard bicarbonate indicate that a metabolic acidosis is present. The low P_{CO_2} and the fact that the actual bicarbonate is lower than the standard bicarbonate indicate that a respiratory alkalosis is present. Therefore, a primary metabolic acidosis is present with a partially compensatory respiratory alkalosis (see Chapter 15).

Cation-Anion Balance:
Na 132   K 6   Cl 102 HCO_3 12 mEq/L
$$\begin{aligned}
\text{Anion gap} &= (Na + K) - (HCO_3 + Cl) \\
&= (132 + 6) - (12 + 102) \\
&= 138 - 114 \\
&= 24 \text{ mEq/L. This is abnormal and is due to the retention} \\
&\quad \text{of sulfuric, phosphoric, and other metabolic acids.}
\end{aligned}$$

Example: Partially compensated metabolic acidosis due to ammonium chloride poisoning.
pH 7.3
P_{CO_2} 30 mm Hg
CO_2 content 14.9 mEq/L
Standard bicarbonate 16.5 mEq/L
Actual bicarbonate 14 mEq/L
Base excess -10.5 mEq/L

The pH is low, indicating an acidosis. The negative base excess and the low standard bicarbonate indicate that a metabolic acidosis is present. The low P_{CO_2} and the fact that the actual bicarbonate is lower than the standard bicarbonate indicate that a respiratory alkalosis is present. Therefore, a primary metabolic acidosis is present with a partially compensatory alkalosis (Chapter 15).

Cation-Anion Balance:
Na 131   K 4.5 HCO_3 14   Cl 111 mEq/L
$$\begin{aligned}
\text{Anion gap} &= (Na + K) - (HCO_3 + Cl) \\
&= (131 + 4.5) - (14 + 111) \\
&= 135.5 - 125 \\
&= 10.5 \text{ mEq/L. This is normal.}
\end{aligned}$$

The serum sodium concentration is low, because sodium has been excreted as a result of the diuresis produced by diuretics and the ammonium chloride.

COURSE AND PROGNOSIS

This depends on the cause of the metabolic acidosis. If it occurs in a patient with chronic renal disease, it may continue for months or years. However, if it occurs in a diabetic patient, for example, or as a result of salicylic acid poisoning, it may cause death quickly unless the patient is energetically treated.

TREATMENT

The aims of treatment are to stop the metabolic disturbance that has produced the acidosis and to restore the electrolytes that have been lost. When this is done, the acid-base balance is automatically restored.

If the acidosis is due to chloride excess, the chloride salt should be stopped immediately. In most patients the kidneys will be able to excrete the excessive amount of chloride. In patients with diabetic acidosis, insulin, sodium chloride solutions, and often potassium chloride will be needed (see Chapter 24). In acute renal failure, water excess should be avoided, sodium balance should be maintained, and hyperkalemia should be treated (see Chapter 21). In metabolic acidosis due to severe losses of intestinal fluids, sodium, potassium, and other electrolytes and water must be replaced.

One should always remember that as the metabolic acidosis is treated, the serum potassium concentration will usually decrease, due to the movement of potassium ions out of the extracellular water and into the cells (Chapter 24). As a result, serious hypokalemia may develop in some patients, and it may be necessary to give potassium chloride, as has been mentioned above. However, this should be done only after the metabolic acidosis has started to improve, and in conjunction with serial observations of the serum potassium concentration (also see Chapter 24).

Detailed therapy of metabolic acidosis is described in the chapters that follow.

The Use of Alkalinizing Salts

The use of an alkalinizing salt, such as sodium bicarbonate or sodium lactate, is usually not necessary and may be dangerous because it may cause a complicating metabolic alkalosis, and it can aggravate the respiratory alkalosis that usually is present (see Chapter 24). Alkalinizing solutions should be reserved for seriously ill patients or when the etiological agent that has caused the acidosis cannot be directly treated.

Type of Solution Needed

Alkalinizing solutions, such as sodium bicarbonate or sodium racemic lactate, are used. The lactate is rapidly oxidized to carbonic acid (by the liver), allowing the sodium to react with the carbonic acid to form sodium bicarbonate. The lactate solution also provides a small amount of calories. It cannot be used if shock, severe congestive heart failure, or respiratory alkalosis is present, or in any patient with impaired liver function. In such cases, the blood lactate concentration is high, and the liver is not able to metabolize the lactate.

Either isotonic sodium bicarbonate or lactate is usually used. However, if the water intake must be kept low, hypertonic sodium bicarbonate or lactate can be used (Chapter 38).

Volume of Solution Needed

When sodium bicarbonate or lactate is given, part of the sodium will remain in the extracellular water space to correct the acidosis. An unpredictable part of the sodium will pass into the cells. For this reason, no completely satisfactory formula for determining the volume of needed sodium bicarbonate or lactate has yet been devised.

In order to prevent the development of a metabolic alkalosis from the bicarbonate or lactate, we suggest that the CO_2 content should be raised to only 18 mEq/L.

The following methods of calculating the necessary volume of sodium bicarbonate or lactate are satisfactory.

METHOD 1. Calculate the unit CO_2 content deficit, and multiply by the volume of extracellular water (which is 20% of the body weight). (Similar calculations can be made using the serum HCO_3^- concentration.)

Example: Patient weighing 70 kg; CO_2 content 10 mEq/L
It is desired to raise the CO_2 content to 18 mEq/L
  Extracellular water: $70 \times 0.2 = 14$ liters
  Unit CO_2 deficit: $18 - 10 = 8$ mEq/L
  Total CO_2 deficit: $8 \times 14 = 112$ milliequivalents

Therefore, treatment consists of giving 112 mEq bicarbonate ions, either as sodium bicarbonate or sodium lactate, intravenously. The following solutions can be used: (1) The volume of hypertonic (7.5%) sodium bicarbonate needed to supply 112 mEq CO_2 is $112 \times 50/45 = 124$ mL. (2) The volume of isotonic (1.5%) sodium bicarbonate needed to supply 112 mEq CO_2 is $112/178 \times 1000 = 630$ mL. (3) The volume of 1/6 molar sodium lactate needed to supply 112 mEq CO_2 is $112/167 \times 1000 = 670$ mL. (4) The volume of molar (11%) sodium lactate needed to supply 112 mEq CO_2 is 112 mL.

Experiments by Singer, Garella, and others have indicated that when sodium bicarbonate is administered, it is distributed intracellulary as well as extracellulary in a space equivalent to 50% or more of the body weight (particularly if the metabolic acidosis is severe and the serum HCO_3^- concentration is less than 5 mEq/L). If this is correct, one would have to multiply the body weight (in kg) by the constant 0.5, and then multiply this value by the unit HCO_3^- or CO_2 content deficit instead of using the constant 0.2.

It is preferable to multiply by the lower constant of 0.2 for the following reasons. When a metabolic acidosis is present, a compensatory respiratory alkalosis develops (due to hyperventilation). Both the metabolic acidosis and the respiratory alkalosis produce a low serum HCO_3^- concentration and low CO_2 content. Therefore, the measured HCO_3^- concentration or CO_2 content represents the combined effects of an acidosis (metabolic) and an alkalosis (respiratory). If enough sodium bicarbonate (or lactate) is given to control the metabolic acidosis and to raise the HCO_3^- or CO_2 content to normal, a severe alkalosis may develop because the compensatory respiratory alkalosis often persists for several hours or longer after the metabolic acidosis disappears. The respiratory alkalosis does not primarily affect the serum HCO_3^- concentration. However, if the HCO_3^- concentration is raised to normal, and the respiratory alkalosis persists, a severe alkalosis may develop.

Therefore, one should try to raise the serum HCO_3^- concentration or the CO_2 content to approximately 18 to 20 mEq/L, instead of to a normal value of 27 mEq/L, or the pH should be raised only to 7.30 with sodium bicarbonate or lactate.

METHOD 2. To raise the CO_2 content 1 mEq/L, give 1.2 mL of 1/6 molar sodium lactate per kg body weight.

Example: Patient weighing 70 kg; CO_2 content 10 mEq/L
It is desired to raise the CO_2 content 8 mEq/L to 18 mEq/L
Volume of 1/6 molar sodium lactate need is 70 × 8 (the CO_2 deficit) × 1.2 = 672 mL

This rule is derived as follows: The extracellular water content of an adult is 20% of the body weight. Therefore, there is 0.2 kg, or 0.2 liter, of extracellular water for every 1 kg body weight. If an ion such as lactate has a concentration in the extracellular water of 1 mEq/L, this represents 0.2 mEq/kg body weight.

If one uses a solution of 1/6 molar sodium lactate, which contains 167 mEq/L, 1 mL of the solution contains 0.167 mEq of the lactate ions. Therefore, 1.2 mL of the 1/6 molar solution contains 0.2 mEq.

If 1.2 mL of the 1/6 molar sodium lactate solution per kg body weight is given, this raises the lactate concentration 0.2 mEq/kg body weight, or 1 mEq/L of extracellular water. The bicarbonate concentration is raised similarly, because 1 mEq sodium lactate is converted into 1 mEq sodium bicarbonate.

METHOD USING NEGATIVE BASE EXCESS VALUES. Astrup's original formula is described on pages 151–152. However, if the extracellular water is considered to be 20% of the body weight, the formula can be modified as follows:

$$mEq\ base\ needed = body\ weight\ (kg) \times 0.2 \times -base\ excess\ (mEq/L)$$

Route of Administration of the Solution

A mild metabolic acidosis can be treated with oral sodium bicarbonate in a dose of 5 g a day (one level teaspoonful contains 1.5 to 2 g). However, in a patient seriously ill with metabolic acidosis, sodium bicarbonate or lactate should be given intravenously. If gastric lavage is done, 200 ml of a 5% sodium bicarbonate solution can be placed in the stomach.

Rate of Administration of the Solution

Isotonic sodium bicarbonate or lactate can be given at a rate that does not exceed 1 L/hr. Hypertonic sodium bicarbonate or lactate should be diluted with at least an equal volume of water or glucose in water and given at a rate that does not exceed 100 mL/hr.

When alkalinizing salts are given to an acidotic patient, calcium gluconate should be given in a dose of 1 to 3 g daily intravenously to prevent tetany.

Bibliography

Altschule, MD, and Sulzbach, WM: Tolerance of the human heart to acidosis: Reversible changes in RS-T segment during severe acidosis caused by administration of carbon dioxide. Am Heart J 33:453, 1947.

Battle, DD, et al: The use of the urinary anion gap in the diagnosis of hyperchloremic metabolic acidosis. N Engl J Med 318:594, 1988.

Block, AV, Field, H, Jr, and Adair, GS: The acid-base equilibrium in diabetic coma, being a study of five cases treated with insulin. J Metab Res 4:27, 1923.

Chazan, JA, Stenson, R, and Kurland, GS: The acidosis of cardiac arrest. N Engl J Med 278:360, 1968.

Fernandez, PC, Cohen, RM, and Feldman, GM: The concept of bicarbonate distribution space: The crucial role of body buffers. Kidney Int 36:747, 1989.

Fraley, DS, et al: Metabolic acidosis after hyperalimentation with casein hydrolysate. Occurrence in a starved patient. Ann Intern Med 88:352, 1978.

Garella, S, Dana, CL, and Chazan, JA: Severity of metabolic acidosis as a determinant of bicarbonate requirements. N Engl J Med 289:121, 1973.

Green, J, and Kleeman, CR: Role of bone in regulation of systemic acid-base balance. Kidney Int 39:9, 1991.

Halperin, ML, and Jungas, RL: The metabolic production and renal disposal of hydrogen ions: An examination of biochemical processes. Kidney Int 24:709, 1983.

Peters, JP, and Van Slyke, DD: *Quantitative Clinical Chemistry*, vol 1, Interpretations. Baltimore: Williams & Wilkins, 1931.

Russell, CD: Response to bicarbonate in severe acidosis. N Engl J Med 289:755, 1973.

Shires, GT, and Holman, J: Dilution acidosis. Ann Intern Med 28:557, 1948.

Shugoll, GI: Transient QRS changes simulating myocardial infarction associated with shock and severe metabolic stress. Am Heart J 74:402, 1967.

Singer, RB, and Hastings, AB: An improved clinical method for the estimation of disturbances of the acid-base balance of human blood. Medicine 27:223, 1948.

Wang, F, Butler, T, Rabbani, GH, and Jones, PK: The acidosis of cholera: Contributions of hyperproteinemia, lactic acidemia and hyperphosphatemia to an increased anion gap. N Engl J Med 315:1591, 1986.

Winter, SD, et al: The fall of the serum anion gap. Arch Intern Med 150:311, 1990.

18

METABOLIC ACIDOSIS SYNDROMES (Continued)

RENAL TUBULAR ACIDOSIS

Most patients with acidosis due to renal failure have either acute renal tubular failure or chronic renal disease. In these patients, glomerular function and tubular function are both decreased. Since glomerular function is decreased more than tubular function, the patient becomes not only acidotic but also azotemic. This common type of renal acidosis has been called *uremic* or *azotemic acidosis.* However, there is a less common type of renal acidosis known as *renal tubular acidosis* (RTA). Here the renal tubular function is decreased even though glomerular function is normal or only moderately reduced.

The renal tubules are capable of reabsorbing numerous ions and substances from the tubular urine (glomerular filtrate), including water, glucose, phosphate, bicarbonate, calcium, and amino acids such as cystine. Any one or several of these functions may become disturbed. For example, a genetic defect in tubular reabsorption of water causes the *renal diabetes insipidus syndrome.* A genetic deficiency of renal tubular reabsorption of glucose causes the *renal glycosuria syndrome,* which is asymptomatic except for the glycosuria. A genetic defect of tubular reabsorption of the amino acid cystine causes *cystinuria,* with recurrent renal calculi composed of cystine. A genetic defect in the tubular reabsorption of phosphate may cause vitamin D–resistant hypophosphatemic rickets. A genetic defect of tubular reabsorption of glucose, cystine, other amino acids, and phosphate produces the classic *Fanconi syndrome.* A deficient renal tubular reabsorption of bicarbonate ions and/or a deficiency in tubular ability to excrete hydrogen ions causes the syndrome of *renal tubular acidosis.*

ETIOLOGY

In adults, renal tubular acidosis may occur in many ways and may be associated with either functional or pathological changes in either the distal or proximal renal tubules.

Distal renal tubular acidosis (type I, classic) can occur in the following common conditions (adapted from Morris and Sebastian):

1. Metabolic syndromes: hyperthyroidism with nephrocalcinosis, primary hyperparathyroidism with nephrocalcinosis.
2. Drug-induced problems: amphotericin B, vitamin D–induced nephrocalcinosis.
3. Hypergammaglobulinemic syndromes: cryoglobulinemia, Sjögren's syndrome, lupoid hepatitis, lupus erythematosus, and so on.
4. Pyelonephritis (rare).
5. Rejection of renal transplant.

Proximal renal tubular acidosis (type II) can occur in the following conditions (adapted from Morris and Sebastian):

1. Syndromes associated with disturbances of protein metabolism: nephrotic syndrome, multiple myeloma, Sjögren's syndrome, amyloidosis, and so on.
2. Drug-induced problems: from deteriorated (outdated) tetracycline, from 6-mercaptopurine, sulfonamides, and so on.
3. Heavy metals: lead, cadmium.
4. Metabolic syndromes: vitamin D deficiency, secondary hyperparathyroidism.
5. Medullary cystic disease.
6. Rejection of renal transplant.
7. Genetically transmitted syndromes (adult Fanconi syndrome, hereditary or acquired, and other rare syndromes).

Type III shows signs of both distal and proximal renal tubular acidosis.

Hyperkalemic RTA—type IV (frequently with associated hyporeninemia and hypoaldosteronism) can occur in the following:

1. Chronic interstitial nephritis of any cause.
2. Obstructive uropathy.
3. Lead nephropathy.
4. Sickle hemoglobinopathies.
5. SLE (systemic lupus erythematosus).

PATHOPHYSIOLOGY

Renal tubular acidosis is characterized by a hyperchloremic metabolic acidosis and almost invariably by hypokalemia. However, in some forms (type IV), hyperkalemia may be present. In many patients, nephrocalcinosis and hypophosphatemia with osteomalacia may also occur.

The function of the kidneys in acid-base balance is to regulate the concentration of plasma bicarbonate ions. Normally, in the proximal renal tubules, approximately 85% to 90% of the bicarbonate ions that have been filtered by the glomeruli are reabsorbed, and hydrogen ions are excreted into the tubular urine in their place. In the distal renal tubules, the residual 10% to 15% of bicarbonate are absorbed. In addition, the distal tubules are responsible for the secretion of the daily load of nonvolatile acids (phosphoric, organic, etc.). This is accomplished by the secretion of hydrogen ions and by the secretion of NH_4^+.

In the distal (classic) type of RTA, there is a defect in hydrogen ion secretion. Since the daily acid load produced by metabolism cannot be excreted, a metabolic acidosis develops. The anions of these metabolic acids (phosphates, sulfates, etc.) are excreted as sodium salts, with resultant mild volume depletion due to sodium loss. This in turn stimulates marked sodium and chloride reabsorption. The net effect is a hyperchloremic acidosis. Excessive urinary loss of potassium ions is almost invariable and may be linked to the distal defects in hydrogen ion excretion and/or to hyperaldosteronism (which results from sodium depletion).

In the proximal type of RTA, there is reduction in the threshold of bicarbonate reabsorption, that is, when serum bicarbonate is less than 12 to 15 mEq/L, there is complete bicarbonate reabsorption. However, as serum bicarbonate concentration rises, the tubules show their inability to reabsorb bicarbonate ions so that large amounts of bicarbonate escape the proximal tubules, overwhelm the limited distal capacity for bicarbonate reabsorption, and appear in the urine. The result is a large loss of $NaHCO_3$, which results in a hyperchloremic metabolic acidosis. The distal tubules attempt to reclaim some of this $NaHCO_3$, which results in a large potassium loss. The urine of a patient with proximal RTA will be alkaline when efforts are made to maintain normal serum bicarbonate level. However, as the serum bicarbonate falls to the threshold value, bicarbonate reabsorption becomes complete, and the urine will have an acid pH.

It should be recognized that a great percentage of patients with RTA have defects of a mixed nature, with diminished distal acidification and mild bicarbonate wasting.

In type IV RTA, a mild to moderate hyperchloremic metabolic acidosis associated with a hyperkalemia occurs in patients with moderate renal insufficiency due to a variety of interstitial injuries. Defective distal tubular or collecting duct hydrogen ion and potassium excretion result from aldosterone deficiency or tubular resistance to aldosterone.

HYPOPHOSPHATEMIA

1. In proximal RTA, phosphate wasting may occur as a result of an associated defect in phosphate reabsorption.
2. In some instances, hypophosphatemia is a sign of the underlying cause of the RTA. For example, in vitamin D deficiency, hypocalcemia in-

duces secondary hyperparathyroidism, with resultant phosphate wasting.

3. In all patients with RTA, chronic acidosis causes hypercalciuria. This causes hypocalcemia with a resultant secondary hyperparathyroidism, which contributes to the hypophosphatemia.

NEPHROCALCINOSIS

Nephrocalcinosis or nephrolithiasis is seen primarily with distal RTA and results from several factors:

1. Hypercalciuria due to chronic acidosis
2. Chronically alkaline urine, in which calcium salts are less soluble
3. Hypocitraturia, which occurs in hypokalemia states (Citrate is an inhibitor of stone formation and its absence promotes stone formation.)

SYMPTOMS AND SIGNS

These depend on the age of the patient and on the electrolytes and other substances that are lost in the urine. Weakness may be present due to potassium loss. Disturbances in gait and bone pain are due to osteomalacia. X-ray examination will show signs of the rickets, osteomalacia or nephrocalcinosis, and pseudofractures, first described by Milkman, that are due to the osteomalacia. A Kussmaul type of hyperventilation may be present when the acidosis is severe.

LABORATORY FINDINGS

Blood

The findings vary greatly. However, the pH is low due to the acidosis and the serum chloride concentration is high (110 to 120 mEq/L). The serum bicarbonate concentration usually ranges from 20 to 12 mEq/L.

Hypophosphatemia is usually present. Occasionally, the serum phosphate concentration is normal. The serum calcium concentration is normal or slightly low. Hypokalemia is frequently present. Azotemia is either absent or minimal.

Urine

Patients with distal tubular acidosis characteristically show a urine with a high pH (6.0 to 7.0) regardless of the serum bicarbonate concentration. Patients with proximal renal tubular acidosis may show a urine with a normal pH (even less than 6.0) when the metabolic acidosis is severe and the serum bicarbonate concentration is low. (The reason is that reabsorption of bicarbonate ions in the proximal tubules may become complete in these patients when the serum bicarbonate concentration is low.)

In type IV RTA, the urine pH may be inappropriately high, but it can be low, particularly in those patients with aldosterone deficiency.

The specific gravity tends to become low and fixed. Hypercalciuria is often present. Glycosuria, ketonuria, or proteinuria may also be present.

Example: Patient with renal tubular acidosis.
pH 7.19
PCO_2 33 mm Hg
CO_2 content 14 mEq/L
Standard bicarbonate 14 mEq/L
Actual bicarbonate 13 mEq/L
Base excess -14 mEq/L

The pH is low. This indicates an acidosis. The negative base excess and the low standard bicarbonate indicate that a metabolic acidosis is present. The PCO_2 is within normal. This indicates respiratory balance. However, the actual bicarbonate is lower than the standard bicarbonate. This indicates that some degree of respiratory alkalosis is present. Therefore, a primary metabolic acidosis is present with a partially compensatory respiratory alkalosis.

Cation-Anion Balance:
Na 140   K 2.7 HCO_3 13   Cl 120
$$\begin{aligned} \text{Anion Gap} &= (Na + K) - (HCO_3 + Cl) \\ &= (140 + 2.7) - (13 + 120) \\ &= 142.7 - 133 \\ &= 9.7 \text{ mEq/L. This is normal.} \end{aligned}$$

DIAGNOSIS

Renal tubular acidosis can be suspected if a patient shows a hyperchloremic metabolic acidosis (serum chloride concentration 110 to 120 mEq/L) in association with nephrocalcinosis or sever hypokalemia or osteomalacia or pseudofractures.

Several methods have been described to differentiate distal from proximal renal tubular acidosis. The following tests are simple to perform:

1. In the patient with significant spontaneous acidosis (serum bicarbonate <18), the urine pH can be checked with a pH meter. In distal renal tubular acidosis, the urine pH will be consistently high (6.5 to 7.0), as has been pointed out above. A urine pH less than 6.0 excludes the possibility that distal renal tubular acidosis is present. (This rule does not

apply if a urinary tract infection, due to urease-producing bacteria, is present, because this will cause the urine pH to be higher than 7.0.)

2. In the patient who is not spontaneously acidotic, ammonium chloride is given orally by the method of Wrong and Davies (0.1 g per kg body weight, given over a period of 1 hour, and using either ammonium chloride solution or ammonium chloride in capsules). A fall of urine pH to less than 5.5 (in a period of 5 hours) indicates proximal tubular acidosis. (If the ammonium chloride loading test fails to produce a fall to less than 5.5, this suggests but does not necessarily indicate distal renal tubular acidosis.)

Recently, measurement of urinary pH during Na_2SO_4 loading, and measurement of urine-blood PCO_2 during $NaHCO_3$ loading have been used as sophisticated tools for assessing the precise nature of certain distal acidification defects.

The combination of nephrocalcinosis and osteomalacia, with pseudo-fractures, is nearly specific for distal renal tubular acidosis, when hypervitaminosis D is excluded by the patient's history (Courney and Pfister).

If ketonuria and glucosuria are present, this can simulate diabetes mellitus. However, in renal tubular acidosis, the blood sugar concentration is normal.

Renal tubular acidosis can be differentiated from renal rickets, because in renal rickets there is azotemia and an elevated serum phosphate concentration.

A metabolic acidosis similar to that found in renal tubular acidosis often occurs in the Fanconi syndrome. This usually is due to a genetic disturbance of renal tubular function for glucose, cystine and other amino acids, and phosphate. It is seen mostly in infants and children. The clinical picture is similar to that of renal tubular acidosis. However, the patient characteristically shows renal glycosuria, urinary excretion of cystine and other amino acids, and an increased urinary phosphate excretion. The blood shows normal serum glucose and amino acid concentrations, hypophosphatemia, normal serum calcium concentration, low serum bicarbonate and high chloride concentrations if acidosis is present, and a normal or slightly elevated blood urea nitrogen concentration. Nephrocalcinosis does not occur. In the later stages, glomerular function becomes decreased. This may cause retention of phosphate ions in the blood.

COURSE AND PROGNOSIS

Death may occur in children and young adults from progressive renal insufficiency. However, adults may show some of the electrolyte changes but no signs of renal insufficiency. Control of the metabolic abnormalities may help to avoid progressive renal insufficiency.

TREATMENT

The aim of treatment is to replace the bicarbonate ions that have been lost, and to stop the progress of the osteomalacia or rickets.

Patients with distal renal tubular acidosis can be treated with sodium bicarbonate orally in a dose of 4 to 6 g (48 to 72 mEq bicarbonate ions). However, if the serum bicarbonate concentration is approximately 22 mEq/L, sodium bicarbonate is not necessary.

Hypokalemia is generally improved by sodium bicarbonate supplementation; but in some patients potassium supplementation in the form of potassium citrate or bicarbonate is necessary.

Shohl's solution can be used in place of sodium bicarbonate. Each 1 mL contains approximately 1 mEq bicarbonate ions. Therefore, a daily dose of approximately 50 to 75 mL can be used.

Patients with proximal renal tubular acidosis will need larger doses of sodium bicarbonate or other alkaline salts and often require substantial potassium supplements.

Osteomalacia or rickets can be treated with a high-calcium diet and larger doses of vitamin D—20,000 to 100,000 units daily or 0.125 to 1.0 μg of 1.25 vitamin D_3—may be necessary. However, these doses may cause severe hypercalcemia with secondary renal failure. The serum calcium concentration should be checked every several weeks. If it rises above 10.5 mg/dL, the vitamin D therapy should be stopped.

Richards and his associates have reported the use of sodium bicarbonate alone in the treatment of osteomalacia of renal tubular acidosis.

In those patients who have RTA associated with hyperkalemia, potassium-binding resins, thiazide diuretics, furosemide, and sodium bicarbonate may help to correct the hyperkalemia and acidosis. Fludrocortisone is also useful in selected cases.

Bibliography

Albright, F, Burnett, CH, Parson, W, Reifenstein, EC, Jr, and Roos, A: Osteomalacia and late rickets: Various etiologies met in United States with emphasis on that resulting from specific form of renal acidosis: therapeutic indications for each etiological group and relationship between osteomalacia and Milkman's syndrome. Medicine 25:399, 1946.

Arruda, J, and Kurtzman, N: Metabolic acidosis and alkalosis. Clin Nephrol 7:201, 1977.

Courney, WR, and Pfister, RC: The radiographic findings in renal tubular acidosis. Radiology 105:497, 1972.

Davidman, M, and Schmitz, P: Renal tubular acidosis. A pathophysiologic approach. Hosp Pract, Jan 30, 1988, p 77.

DeFronzo, RA: Hyperkalemia and hyporeninemic hypoaldosteronism. Kidney Int 17:118, 1980.

Gennari, FJ, and Cohen JJ: Renal tubular acidosis. Ann Rev Med 29:521, 1978.

Gouttas, A, et al: Adult Fanconi syndrome. New York State J Med 65:295, 1965.

Harrington, TM, et al: Renal tubular acidosis. A new look at treatment of musculoskeletal and renal disease. Mayo Clin Proc 58:354, 1983.

Mason, AMS, and Golding, PL: Hyperglobulinemic renal tubular acidosis. BMJ 3:143, 1970.

Morris, RC, Jr: Renal tubular acidosis. Mechanisms, classification and implications. N Engl J Med 281:1405, 1969.

Morris, RC, Jr: Renal rubular acidosis, editorial. N Engl J Med 304:418, 1981.

Morris, RC, Jr, and Sebastian, A: Disorders of the renal tubule that cause disorders of fluid, acid-base, and electrolyte metabolism. In Maxwell, MH, and Kleeman, CR, (eds). *Clinical Disorders of Fluid and Electrolyte Metabolism.* 3rd ed. New York: McGraw-Hill, 1980.

Patterson, RM, and Ackerman, GL: Renal tubular acidosis due to amphotericin B nephrotoxicity. Arch Intern Med 127:241, 1971.

Pines, KI, and Mudge, GH: Renal tubular acidosis with osteomalacia. Am J Med 11:302, 1951.

Reynolds, TR: Renal tubular disorders. In Maxwell, MH, and Kleeman, CR (eds). *Clinical Disorders of Fluid and Electrolyte Metabolism.* 2nd ed. New York: McGraw-Hill, 1972.

Richards, P, et al: Treatment of osteomalacia of renal tubular acidosis by sodium bicarbonate alone. Lancet 2:994, 1972.

Sebastian, A, and Morris, R: Renal tubular acidosis. Clin Nephrol 7:216, 1977.

Sebastian, A, Schambelan, M, Lindenfeld, S, et al: Amelioration of metabolic acidosis with fludrocortisone therapy in hyporeninemic hypoaldosteronism. N Engl J Med 297:576, 1977.

Vander, AJ: *Renal Physiology,* 3rd ed. New York: McGraw-Hill, 1985.

Wilson, DR, and Siddiqui, AA: Renal tubular acidosis after kidney transplantation. Ann Intern Med 79:352, 1973.

Wrong, OM: Renal tubular acidosis. Letter. N Engl J Med 304:1548, 1981.

19

METABOLIC ACIDOSIS
SYNDROMES (Continued)

LACTIC ACIDOSIS

Lactic acidosis is a metabolic acidosis due to the accumulation of lactate ions above a concentration of 2 mEq/L in association with a decreased arterial pH.

Lactic acid is the end product of the anaerobic metabolism of glucose (dextrose). It is formed in nearly all tissues in the body, particularly in skeletal muscles and red blood cells. Glycogen is normally metabolized to pyruvic acid in the first stage of carbohydrate metabolism. If adequate oxygen is present, little lactic acid is formed because the pyruvic acid is metabolized to carbon dioxide. However, under anaerobic conditions, pyruvic acid is metabolized (reduced) to lactic acid in the cells. (This reaction occurs mainly in the liver.) Although this chemical reaction is reversible so that pyruvic acid can be formed from lactic acid, the kinetics of the reaction normally produces a lactate-pyruvate ratio of 10:1.

Lactic acid can accumulate in two ways:

1. By increased production of lactic acid. This occurs in lactic acidosis because there is an increased breakdown of glycogen in the liver. (An increased production of lactic acid also occurs with muscular exercise or hyperventilation, or when epinephrine, fructose, or glucagon is administered. However, these latter conditions do *not* produce a significant lactic acidosis.)
2. By decreased metabolism of lactic acid. Shock and hypoxia are the most common causes of this decreased metabolism of lactic acid.

ETIOLOGY

Lactic acidosis can occur from the following causes.

1. Shock. This is the most frequent cause of lactic acidosis, for reasons just mentioned. In addition, the arterial lactate concentration is a good prognosticator in shock. When the lactic acid concentration is below 4.3 mEq/L, almost all patients recover; when the concentration is between 4.4 and 8 mEq/L, there is only approximately a 33% chance of survival; when the lactic acid concentration rises above 8 mEq/L, there is only approximately a 10% chance of survival. However, when shock is treated appropriately and tissue perfusion improves, lactic acid will be flushed into the general circulation and its concentration in the blood will rise temporarily as the patient's condition improves.

2. Metabolic acidosis. Lactic acidosis also occurs when the pH falls to approximately 7.10 or less.

3. Diabetes mellitus. Lactic acidosis can occur in one of three ways in diabetic patients:

   a. If renal insufficiency due to shock, sepsis, pancreatitis, or any other cause, occurs, the diabetic patient is particularly susceptible to the development of lactic acidosis.

   b. Lactic acidosis can occur simultaneously with diabetic ketoacidosis. This combination can be suspected when a weakly positive Acetest (nitroprusside) reaction is found on the serum of a patient in diabetic ketoacidosis. The reason for this is that the Acetest is specific for aceto-acetate ketones, but does not measure beta-hydroxybutyrate and other ketones. (Measurement of beta-hydroxybutyrates and lactic acid should be made on such patients.)

   c. Phenformin (DBI) therapy of diabetes mellitus. (Phenformin has been withdrawn from general use, although it is still available as an investigational drug.)

4. Acute pulmonary edema due to left-sided congestive heart failure.

5. Generalized (grand mal) convulsive seizures.

6. Severe hypoxemia (PaO_2 below 35 mm Hg), or severe anemia (hemoglobin below 6 g/dL).

7. During cardiopulmonary bypass operations, especially if hypothermia is used during the bypass surgery.

8. Acute leukemia. An excessive amount of lactic acid is produced by the excessive numbers of white blood cells. In addition, tissue hypoxia occurs from sludging in small blood vessels. The situation is aggravated if leukemia infiltration of the liver occurs, producing impaired liver function.

9. AIDS. A number of cases of chronic lactic acidosis have been reported, presumably due to chronic viral or mycobacterial infection.

10. Excessive ethanol intake.

11. Spontaneous (idiopathic) causes. Lactic acidosis has been described in association with numerous infections or inflammatory conditions such as acute pyelonephritis, acute peritonitis, acute pancreatitis, subacute

bacterial endocarditis, acute poliomyelitis, and in noninfectious conditions such as gastrointestinal hemorrhage, acute myocardial infarction, and postoperatively. The mechanisms of lactic acidosis in these cases are not known. Shock or severe tissue hypoxia due to other causes is usually present, and is probably the precipitating factor producing the lactic acidosis.

SYMPTOMS AND SIGNS

Lactic acidosis usually develops acutely. Symptoms include weakness, fatigue, or moderate to marked dyspnea. Hyperventilation is a common finding. This may be slight cyanosis. Changes in consciousness may vary from mild lethargy to stupor and eventually to coma. Death usually occurs in hours or days.

These symptoms and signs are not specific for lactic acidosis and can occur with metabolic acidosis due to any cause.

LABORATORY FINDINGS

The normal arterial concentration of lactate is less than 1.5 mEq/L (approximately 10 mg/dL). A concentration greater than 2 mEq/L is abnormal. However, a rise in arterial lactate concentration to 2 to 3 mEq/L is usually associated with no change in pH, because buffers in the extracellular fluid can neutralize this increase in lactate ions. However, when the arterial lactate concentration rises above this, the pH begins to fall. When lactic acidosis is present, the arterial lactate concentration is usually higher than 7 mEq/L, and may rise as high as 30 mEq/L.

(*Lactate concentration in mEq/L can be converted to its concentration in mg/dL by* multiplying *by the factor 9. To convert lactate concentration in mg/dL to mEq/L,* divide *by this factor.*)

The normal arterial concentration of pyruvate is less than 0.15 mEq/L.

(*Pyruvate concentration in mEq/L can be converted to its concentration in mg/dL by* multiplying *by the factor 8.8. To convert pyruvate concentration in mg/dL to mEq/L,* divide *by this factor.*)

The Arterial Lactate-Pyruvate Ratio

Since the normal arterial lactate concentration is approximately 1.5 mEq/L, and the normal arterial pyruvate concentration is approximately 0.15 mEq/L or less, the arterial lactate-pyruvate ratio is normally approximately 10:1. When lactic acidosis is present, the lactate concentration rises much higher than the pyruvate concentration, so that the arterial lactate-pyruvate ratio may rise to 60:1.

Arterial blood should be used to determine lactate and pyruvate concentrations because contractions of the muscles of the arm occluded with a tourniquet will raise the lactate concentration in venous blood. (If venous blood is used, it should be drawn without stasis from a resting extremity. The venous lactate concentration exceeds the arterial lactate concentration by approximately 3 mEq/L.)

The pH is low and the anion gap is usually greater than 22 mEq/L.

Other Findings

Other laboratory findings include: leukocytosis and increased SGOT value, probably due to decreased blood flow through the liver. An increased serum phosphate concentration commonly occurs. Hypoglycemia in association with lactic acidosis has also been noted in some patients.

Example: Patient with lactic acidosis
pH 7.30 CO_2 content 9.0 mEq/L

Cation-Anion Balance:
Na 131   K 5   Cl 86 HCO_3 9 mEq/L
Anion Gap = $(Na + K) - (HCO_2 + Cl)$
$$= (131 + 5) - (9 + 86)$$
$$= 136 - 95$$
$$= 41 \text{ mEq/L. This is markedly abnormal.}$$

DIAGNOSIS

Lactate acidosis can be suspected when a metabolic acidosis occurs with an abnormal anion gap and diabetic ketoacidosis, azotemic acidosis, salicylate intoxication, ethylene glycol poisoning, paraldehyde or methanol intoxication can be ruled out. The presence of shock or severe hypoxia further suggests lactic acidosis. However, the diagnosis should be confirmed by measuring the arterial lactate concentration.

TREATMENT

1. Eliminate the source or sources of excessive lactate acid production. For example, if it is ethanol, stop it immediately.
2. Maintain an adequate peripheral perfusion of tissues and an adequate cardiac output. Correct hypoxia, if possible. If shock is present, vasoconstrictors such as dopamine (Intropin), or levarterenol (Levophed) should *not* be used, because they cause further vasoconstriction and may worsen the lactic acidosis. Instead, it is preferable to treat the patient with intravenous fluids, monitoring with CVP or with pulmonary-

wedge pressure measurements. Vasodilating drugs such as dopamine may also be helpful in association with intravenous fluids.

3. Correct the metabolic acidosis. Sodium bicarbonate is the drug of choice. It is given intravenously to raise the pH to approximately 7.30 (Chapter 38). Although there is no evidence that bicarbonate administration improves survival, it may provide extra time in which treatment of the cause of the lactic acidosis (e.g., antibiotics for sepsis) can be instituted.

   An alkalinizing solution such as lactated Ringer's solution (which contains lactate ions) should not be used. However, if a patient with unrecognized lactic acidosis is given sodium lactate, no harm will occur.

   When a patient in shock develops acute renal insufficiency and requires peritoneal dialysis, one should also remember that the commercially available peritoneal dialysis solutions contain 35 mEq/L lactate ions. Here again the lactate ions will not harm the patient, but they will not produce an alkalinizing effect until the peripheral perfusion of tissues improves and the lactate can be oxidized and bicarbonate ions formed.

4. If diabetic acidosis is also present, insulin and dextrose may also be of value (Freeman and Campbell).

5. Treat pulmonary edema due to left-sided congestive heart failure in the usual ways. (These patients do not need sodium bicarbonate to correct the lactic acidosis. This spontaneously disappears when the pulmonary edema disappears.)

Bibliography

Adrogué, HJ, et al: Assessing acid-base status in circulatory failure: Differences between arterial and central venous blood. N Engl J Med 320:1312, 1989.

Anderson, CT et al: Contribution of arterial blood lactate measurements to the care of critically ill patients. Am J Clin Path 68:63, 1977.

Bersin, RM, and Arieff, AI: Primary lactic alkalosis. Am J Med 85:868, 1988.

Chattha, G, Arieff, AI, Cummings, C, and Tierney, LM: Lactic acidosis complicating the acquired immunodeficiency syndrome. Ann Intern Med 118:37, 1993.

Cohen, RD: Lactic acidosis. Clinical considerations. Practical Cardiol 8:83, 1982.

Cohen, RD, and Woods, HF: *Clinical and Biochemical Aspects of Lactic Acidosis.* London: Blackwell Scientific, Baltimore: Williams & Wilkins, 1976.

Dahlquist, NR, et al: D-lactic acidosis and encephalopathy after jejunoileostomy. Mayo Clin Proc 59:141, 1984.

Fulop, M, et al: Lactic acidosis in pulmonary edema due to left ventricular failure. Ann Intern Med 79:180, 1973.

Fulop, M, and Hoberman, HD: Is lactic acidosis "spontaneous"? New York State J Med 77:24, 1977.

Goldberger, E: Cardiogenic shock. In *The Treatment of Cardiac Emergencies.* 4th ed. St. Louis: C.V. Mosby, 1984.

Humphrey, SH, and Nash, DA, Jr: Lactic acidosis complicating sodium nitroprusside therapy. Letter. Ann Intern Med 88:58, 1978.

Madias, NE: Lactic acidosis. Kidney Int 29:752, 1986.

Narins, RG, and Cohen, JJ: Bicarbonate therapy for organic acidosis: The case for its continued use. Ann Intern Med 196:615, 1987.

O'Connor, LR, Klein, KL, and Bethune, JE: Hyperphosphatemia in lactic acidosis. N Engl J Med 297:707, 1977.

Oliva, PB: Lactic acidosis. Am J Med 48:209, 1970.

Orringer, CE, et al: Natural history of lactic acidosis after grand-mal seizures. N Engl J Med 297:796, 1977.

Stackpoole, PW: Lactic acidosis: The case against bicarbonate therapy. Ann Intern Med 105:276, 1986.

Stackpoole, PW, et al: Treatment of lactic acidosis with dichloroacetate. N Engl J Med 309:390, 1983.

Stackpoole, PW, et al: Natural history and course of acquired lactic acidosis in adults. Am J Med 97:47, 1994.

Stackpoole, PW, Wright, EC: A controlled clinical trial of dichloracetate treatment in patients with lactic acidosis. N Engl J Med 327:1564, 1992.

Stolberg, L, et al: D-lactic acidosis due to abnormal gut flora. N Engl J Med 306:1344, 1982.

Weisfeld, ML, and Guerci, AD: Sodium bicarbonate in CPR. JAMA 266:2121, 1991.

20

METABOLIC ACIDOSIS SYNDROMES (Continued)

RENAL FAILURE: DIAGNOSTIC CONSIDERATIONS

The diagnosis of renal failure is generally established by simple laboratory measurement of the serum creatinine level, which provides an index of glomerular filtration rate (GFR). The term *renal failure* is somewhat arbitrary and will be discussed in the treatment chapters (21 and 22). As a guildeline, any substantive decline in renal function (>20% rise in serum creatinine) should be carefully scrutinized.

DEFINITIONS

The serum creatinine is a reasonably precise index of GFR, reflecting its relatively steady daily rate of endogenous production from muscle metabolism and its predominant excretion by glomerular filtration. However, several qualifying facts must be recognized:

1. The accuracy of estimating GFR from a serum determination depends on the relative stability of GFR. In acute renal failure (see below), the serum determination may be especially misleading; for example, moments after bilateral nephrectomy, despite a GFR of zero, serum creatinine will be normal. Over a period of many days, continued production of creatinine without excretion will result in retention and a progressive rise in serum creatinine. Thus, in patients with unstable GFR, the serum creatinine must be interpreted carefully and viewed as a potentially imprecise measure of GFR.
2. Even in stable patients, estimating GFR accurately from serum creatinine requires an understanding that the production rate of creatinine depends on muscle mass and will vary dramatically from one individ-

ual to another. The following frequently cited formula allows estimation of GFR based on serum creatinine, sex, age, and body weight.

$$\text{GFR (mL/min)} = \frac{(150 - \text{age}) \times \text{BW (kg)}}{72 \times \text{serum creatinine (mg/dL)}}$$

Thus, as a dramatic example, consider the following two patients with identical serum creatinine of 2.0 mg/dL.

a. 100-kg, 20-year-old man
b. 50 kg, 90-year-old woman

GFR for Patient a is 90 mL/min, while GFR for Patient b is 14 mL/min. Patient a has nearly normal GFR, while Patient b has marked insufficiency.

3. As GFR declines, creatinine becomes a less predictable marker because its tubular secretion may become substantial. Thus, in more advanced renal insufficiency, (GFR < 30 mL/min), the serum creatinine may provide a substantial overestimate of GFR.

Notwithstanding these caveats, the serum creatinine remains an excellent simple index for identifying marked reductions in GFR.

Although an abnormal serum creatinine is the most common way in which the physician discovers renal failure, a myriad of symptoms, signs, and laboratory abnormalities may be the presenting factor(s).

Symptoms
Generalized weakness
Sleep disturbance
Muscle cramps
Cognitive dysfunction
Anorexia, nausea, vomiting
Skeletal pain
Dyspnea on exertion
Paresthesias
Restless legs
Easy bruisability and/or bleeding

Signs
Pallor
Hypertension
Edema or other signs of circulatory overload
Ecchymoses
Pericardial rub

Laboratory Findings
Hyperkalemia
Acidosis

Hyperphosphatemia
Hypocalcemia
Anemia

ACUTE VS. CHRONIC RENAL FAILURE

The first step in diagnosis is establishing the acuity of the renal failure. Just as a prior chest x-ray is of critical value in evaluating a chest radiographic abnormality, previous serum creatinine determinations are the most objective means of assessing the timing of the development of reduced renal function. A concerted effort to obtain such important data may save substantial effort, inconvenience, cost, and discomfort. Without such data (obtained from history or old records), distinguishing acute from chronic renal insufficiency can be quite difficult, particularly since patients with underlying renal insufficiency are prone to episodes of acute renal failure. Thus, mixtures of acute and chronic renal failure in the same patient are not infrequent.

The history of symptoms may be helpful in establishing acuity; however, routine laboratory tests are frequently not helpful since electrolyte abnormalities may develop acutely. The presence of severe anemia (hemoglobin <8 g/dL) suggests chronic disease, but many patients with acute renal failure have complex associated problems that may have coincidentally resulted in severe anemia.

Two distinguishing features are most reliable.

1. The presence of radiographic evidence of renal osteodystrophy virtually ensures that renal disease is of longstanding duration. However, such features occur in only a small minority of patients presenting with chronic renal failure.
2. Small renal size (< 7 cm), best determined by ultrasonography (see below), is the most definitive evidence of chronic disease, as substantial renal shrinkage requires months to develop.

CHRONIC RENAL FAILURE

In the patient with definitive evidence of chronic advanced renal insufficiency, specific diagnostic evaluation may still be valuable. Although therapy directed at reversing the renal disease may not be possible, insight can be gained that may be prognostically useful for long-term planning (specifically for possible transplantation) or for family counseling.

A discussion of the differential diagnosis of chronic renal insufficiency is beyond the scope of this primer; however, the following data base is simply acquired:

HISTORY. Emphasizing family background, occupational or pharmaceutical exposures, hematuria, edema, any urologic symptoms, hypertension, and associated medical illness.

PHYSICAL EXAMINATION. Focusing on blood pressure, skin, and abdominal findings, including bruits.

LABORATORY FINDINGS. Urinalysis, sonogram, 24-hour urine collection for precise determination of creatinine clearance and urinary protein excretion.

The acquisition of this data base then allows a more specific approach to diagnosis. For example, the patient with heavy proteinuria would be evaluated for glomerular diseases, while the patient with severe hypertension, asymmetric kidneys, and an abdominal bruit might be evaluated for renovascular disease.

ACUTE RENAL FAILURE

The clinician should generally err on the side of assuming that renal failure is acute or may have an acute component. This strategy maximizes the opportunity to identify potentially reversible processes that may have contributed to a decline in GFR.

The same data base discussed above provides a framework for diagnostic decision making. However, an anatomical approach allows a complete analysis.

1. *Prerenal.* Although reduced renal perfusion may result from a variety of disturbances (see below), the pathophysiological consequences are uniform. As renal blood flow decreases, GFR is relatively preserved due to reflex adjustments in glomerular blood flow and resistance. In severe cases, however, the serum creatinine may exceed 5 mg/dL. BUN rises out of proportion, reflecting slow tubular flow and resultant urea reabsorption, with a high BUN/creatinine ratio (>20/1). This ratio, however, is frequently misleading, particularly in malnourished patients with low BUN production rates.

The hallmark diagnostic feature is avid tubular sodium reabsorption, which is most accurately assessed by determination of the fractional excretion of sodium (FE_{Na}) on a spot urine sample. FE_{Na} is the ratio of the clearance of sodium to the clearance of creatinine and is derived as follows:

$$FE_{Na} = \frac{Na \ clearance}{Creatinine \ clearance}$$

$$= \frac{Urine \ concentration \ (Na) \times Urine \ vol/S \ Na}{Urine \ concentration \ (creatinine) \times Urine \ vol/S \ creatinine}$$

This simplifies to

$$\frac{U \ Na/S \ Na}{U \ creatinine/S \ creatinine}$$

and accordingly requires only simultaneous measurement of urinary Na and creatinine, and serum Na and creatinine. Urine volume is mathematically unnecessary for the calculation.

FE_{Na} <.01 strongly suggests a prerenal component to a patient's acute renal insufficiency. Occasionally, a patient with true prerenal insufficiency may have a higher FE_{Na}, particularly in the setting of diuretic administration or metabolic alkalosis. Repeating the determination in 12 to 24 hours may resolve the former problem, whereas measuring the $FE_{Chloride}$ (rather than FE_{Na}) may resolve the latter dilemma.

An FE_{Na} < .01 also may occur with acute intrinsic renal failure, particularly in the setting of acute inflammatory processes such as acute glomerulonephritis or interstitial nephritis (see below).

The spectrum of prerenal failure includes:

- Low intravascular volume: Secondary extrinsic losses of salt and water (e.g., diarrhea, diuretics)
- Secondary intrinsic sequestration (e.g., pancreatitis, burns, severe hypoalbuminemia)
- Low cardiac output secondary to heart disease
- Hepatorenal syndrome, in which functional renal insufficiency develops despite anatomically normal kidneys, in the setting of severe liver failure.
- Vascular insufficiency: Aortic or renovascular disease may occasionally produce a prerenal pattern, although hypertension with normal renal function is the more characteristic clinical appearance of such patients.

As one proceeds with an anatomical approach, the diagnosis of acute renal failure (ARF) can be further classified as follows. (The reader is referred to other texts for specific discussion of each diagnostic category.)

2. Renal arterioles: Malignant hypertension, scleroderma, or vasculitis
3. Glomerulonephritis: Isolated or associated with systemic disease
4. Interstitial nephritis: Drug-induced, infectious, or idiopathic
5. Obstructive uropathy: Usually extrarenal but may include tubular obstruction secondary to uric acid crystallization
6. Renal venous obstruction (a rare phenomenon almost entirely limited to patients with underlying nephrotic syndrome)
7. Cortical necrosis: Occasionally, in clinical situations where hypotension is associated with disseminated intravascular coagulation, actual bilateral cortical necrosis may occur. This necrosis of the cortical areas of the kidney may be patchy and therefore compatible with life-sustaining renal function. However, when cortical necrosis is bilateral and extensive, recovery of renal function is virtually unprecedented. Disseminated intravascular coagulation or bilateral cortical necrosis can

occur as a result of intravascular coagulation and shock, as in burns, extensive trauma, transfusion reactions, gram-negative sepsis, acute pancreatitis, or obstetric complications such as premature separation of the placenta, pre-eclampsia, hypofibrinogenemia, and septic abortion.

8. Acute tubular necrosis: This entity is the most common variant, particularly in patients who develop renal insufficiency while hospitalized. A variety of insults may provoke this condition:

- Hypotension (of any cause)
- Toxic insults: drugs, contrast media
- Endogenous toxins: myoglobin, hemoglobin

The physiology involves a variable combination of profound renal vasoconstriction, tubular obstruction, and tubular injury resulting in backleak of filtered urine into the circulation.

Clinically, oliguria may be present, but when the acute tubular necrosis has a nephrotoxic cause, or when the patient has been treated with vigorous fluid replacement or renal vasodilators (e.g., dopamine infusion), it may not occur. The diagnosis is established by the clinical setting and an FE_{Na} that almost always exceeds .01. It may be confirmed by the presence of tubular cells, granular casts, and renal-tubular-cell casts.

ARF associated with predominant tubular obstruction and injury can be produced by antibiotics, such as amphotericin B, gentamicin, kanamycin, neomycin, polymyxin, or the urinary antiseptic phenazopyridine (Pyridium); by iodinated radiographic contrast agents; by heavy metals and their compounds, such as arsenic, bismuth, cadmium, and mercury, including the organic mercurial diuretics; by organic compounds such as carbon tetrachloride, chloroform, glycols, or methanol tetrachloroethylene; and by substances such as aniline dyes, carbon monoxide, chlordane, diesel fuel, Lysol and other phenols, quinacrine (Atabrine), and many others. Other causes of tubular injury include severe or extensive trauma, such as crush injuries or fractures; the release of hemoglobin into the circulation due to mismatched transfusions; sepsis, falciparum malaria (blackwater fever), mushroom poisoning, or venomous snake bites; and the release of myoglobin into the circulation, owing to burns, crush injuries, excessive muscular exercise, electric shock, heat stroke, severe depletion of potassium ions, cocaine ingestion, and a long list of acute infections. Predominant ischemic ARF is seen after major surgery or as a result of decreased circulating blood volume due to sodium and water loss, severe burns, acute myocardial infarction, or massive bleeding.

The course of ARF is often divided into an oliguric and a diuretic phase. However, many patients are never oliguric, especially when drugs are the cause of the ARF. Rarely, anuria may develop in the course of ARF, but it is more common with cortical necrosis. Obviously, the degree of renal failure is quite variable. Some patients will have only transient mild reductions in GFR, while others may develop prolonged periods of severely reduced GFR.

PROPHYLAXIS OF ACUTE RENAL FAILURE

During major surgery, the anesthetist should make certain that the patient has a urine output of at least 50 mL/hr (or even 75 to 100 mL/hr) (also see Chapter 37). In addition, patients with the nephrotic syndrome, multiple myeloma, or obstructive jaundice, or who are undergoing open heart, biliary, or gastrointestinal surgery are prone to ARF. Low-molecular-weight Dextran 40 must be used cautiously in elderly patients. Diagnostic radiography with a tri-iodinated dye also increases the likelihood of ARF.

Similarly, the clinician should avoid intravascular volume depletion and nephrotoxic drugs (especially aminoglycoside antibiotics and nonsteroidal anti-inflammatory drugs) in patients with underlying renal disease. Further, when aminoglycosides are used, blood levels must be carefully monitored in all patients. In clinical circumstances where oliguria develops in association with hypotension, the use of furosemide, mannitol, and low-dose intravenous dopamine may be of some value. Although these agents may not prevent the development of ARF, they do appear to convert oliguric ARF to nonoliguric ARF. This conversion often simplifies management from a fluid and electrolyte perspective.

Bibliography

Allon, M, Lopez, EJ, and Mink, W: Acute renal failure due to ciprofloxacin. Arch Intern Med 150:2187, 1990.
Anselo, J: Renal failure cured by chemical, foods, plants, animal serums and misuse of drugs. Arch Intern Med 150:505, 1990.
Badalamenti, S, Graziani, G, Salerno, F, and Ponticelli, G: Hepatorenal syndrome. Arch Intern Med 153:1957, 1993.
Bohle, A, Christensen, J, Vickot, F, et al: Acute renal failure in man: New aspects covering pathogenesis. Am J Nephrol 10:374, 1990.
Cameron, JS: Allergic interstitial nephritis: Clinical features and pathogenesis. Q J Med 66:97, 1988.
Conn, HF: Rational approach to the hepatorenal syndrome. Gastroenterology 65:321, 1973.
Diamond, JR, and Yoburn, DC: Nonoliguric acute renal failure. Arch Intern Med 142:1882, 1981.
Dossetor, JB: Creatinemia versus uremia. The relative significance of blood urea nitrogen and serum creatinine concentrations in azotemia. Ann Intern Med 65:1287, 1966.
Gault, MH, Longerich, LL, Hemett, JD, and Weslowski, C: Predicting glomerular function from adjusted serum creatinine. Nephron 62:2459, 1992.
Hilton, PJ, et al: Urinary osmolality in acute renal failure due to glomerulonephritis. Lancet 2:655, 1969.
Hollengang, NK, et al: Acute renal failure in man. Evidence for preferential renal cortical ischemia. Medicine 47:455, 1968.

Kassirer, JP: Clinical evaluation of kidney function-glomerular function. N Engl J Med 285:385, 1971.

Kim, KE, et al: Creatinine clearance in renal disease. A reappraisal. BMJ 4:11, 1969.

Lauler, DP, and Schreiner, GE: Bilateral renal cortical necrosis. Am J Med 24:519, 1958.

Lauler, DP, Schreiner, GE, and David, A: Renal medullary necrosis. Am J Med 29:132, 1960.

Levinsky, N: The interpretation of proteinuria and the urinary sediment. Disease-a-Month, March, 1967.

Levinsky, N: Pathophysiology of acute renal failure. N Engl J Med 296:1453, 1977.

Levy, M: Hepatorenal syndrome. Kidney Int 43:737, 1993.

Maher, JF: Nephrotoxicity of drugs and chemicals. Pharmacol Physicians 4:1, 1970.

Meyrier, A, Buchet, P, Simon, P, et al: Atheromatous renal disease. Am J Med 85:139, 1988.

Miller, T, Anderson, R, and Linas, S: Urinary diagnostic indices in acute renal failure. Ann Intern Med 89:47, 1978.

Moncrief, JW: Acute renal failure. Hints on how to avoid it. Consultant 13:76, 1973.

Montoreano, R, et al: Prevention of the initial oliguria of acute renal failure by the administration of furosemide. Postgrad Med 47:7, 1971.

Perlmutter, M, et al: Urine-serum urea nitrogen ratio. JAMA 170:1533, 1959.

Rimmer, JM, and Gennari, FJ: Atherosclerotic renovascular disease and progressive renal failure. Am J Med 1993, 118:712.

Sherman, RA, and Eisinger, RP: The use (and misuse) of urinary sodium and chloride measurements. JAMA 247:3121, 1982.

Villazon, A, et al: Polyuric syndromes in the critically ill patient. Crit Care Med 4:24, 1976.

21

ACUTE RENAL FAILURE:

MANAGEMENT CONSIDERATIONS

ARF results in a variety of potentially life-threatening complications. Despite remarkable advances in management, ARF remains a condition where in-hospital mortality rates may still exceed 50%. Although this very high rate often reflects the serious nature of the underlying conditions (sepsis, major vascular surgery, trauma, multiorgan failure), the metabolic burden of ARF certainly contributes to the poor prognosis. The consequences and management of ARF are reviewed below.

FLUID OVERLOAD

Judicious fluid management of the oliguric ARF patient may often avert serious overload. However, nutritional and medication requirements (antibiotics, pressors) often mandate substantial infusion volumes. In addition, hypoalbuminemia may contribute to sequestration of fluid. Significant central circulatory overload, manifest as pulmonary edema, requires direct management, whereas peripheral edema and ascites generally do not require therapy. Occasional patients may develop severe anasarca, which may threaten skin integrity.

Loop diuretic therapy (furosemide, bumetanide, ethacrynic acid) may be effective in those patients with less severe impairments of GFR. However, when pharmacological therapy fails, peritoneal dialysis or hemodialysis are highly effective means for removal of excess salt and water. Recently, the technique of continuous arteriovenous hemofiltration has been popularized, particularly for the management of overloaded ARF patients. The technique, which employs an extracorporeal filter placed between an indwelling arterial catheter and a venous return catheter, allows the removal of an ultrafiltrate of plasma at a rate of 10 to 20 mL/min.

HYPERKALEMIA

Urine flow tends to be the major determinant of serum potassium in ARF, with the serum potassium level reflecting the net balance between exogenous potassium input (diet, intravenous fluids, medications), catabolic rate (see below), and urine output. Despite very low GFR, nonoliguric patients may maintain normokalemia when potassium intake is meticulously restricted. Oliguric patients, however, particularly those who have had substantial tissue injury (e.g., surgery, rhabdomyolysis), will often require specific therapy.

A serum potassium level > 6.0 mEq/L must be assumed to be dangerous, whether or not concomitant electrocardiographic features are present (see Chapter 26). Patients with ARF tend to be more vulnerable to the electrophysiological effects of hyperkalemia than patients with chronic renal failure, who seem to develop a variable degree of adaptation to their chronic hyperkalemia. Nonetheless, a potassium level ≥ 6 mEq/L must always be approached with great care.

Nondialytic Management

The nondialytic management of hyperkalemia is discussed in Chapter 26. In hyperkalemic ARF patients, certain modifications should be noted. Although calcium infusion may still provide emergent electrical stabilization, and redistributive therapy with glucose/insulin or beta agonists may be transiently efficacious, bicarbonate therapy is not useful. Despite the usual concomitant acidosis, recent studies have shown no significant potassium-lowering effect of bicarbonate infusion. Potassium removal with cation resins remains useful, although generally such therapy will not be adequate to avoid dialysis in ARF patients. Beyond the inconvenience of resin therapy, an approximately 2 mEq sodium load accompanies the removal of each mEq of potassium. These factors are usually limiting, so that most oliguric ARF patients who develop hyperkalemia will require some form of dialysis.

Dialytic Removal

Potassium removal with any form of dialysis is dependent on the gradient between bloodstream and dialysate. Peritoneal dialysis (using a dialysate with zero potassium) can remove substantial amounts of potassium, but at a relatively slow rate. Even under optimal conditions, using 2-liter exchanges hourly, the maximal removal may be 10 to 15 mEq/hr. Hemodialysis, due to the rapid blood flow is far more efficient at potassium removal, with losses of 50 mEq/hr or more. Thus, for extreme hyperkalemia, hemodialysis is more rapidly effective. For maintenance therapy, however, peritoneal dialysis is quite effective because potassium removal proceeds continuously at a slow, steady rate—adequate to maintain normokalemia in most patients. Occasional patients with very high potassium production rates (usually ARF secondary to rhabdomyolysis) may require frequent hemodialysis for control.

METABOLIC ACIDOSIS

Complete cessation of renal acid excretion results in the retention of approximately 1 mEq/kg body weight of H^+ ion each day, which translates to a potential 2 mEq/L per day reduction in serum bicarbonate level. Thus, significant acidosis evolves predictably over a period of many days. A dramatic, sudden worsening should raise suspicion of a concomitant process such as lactic acidosis. Nonetheless, even in uncomplicated cases of ARF, serum HCO_3 levels may diminish to <10 mEq/L. Despite effective respiratory compensation, HCO_3 levels in this range are an indication for dialysis. Occasionally, HCO_3 supplementation may be appropriate in an effort to forestall dialysis, but patients with ARF so severe as to cause significant uremic acidosis generally have other strong indications for dialysis. Furthermore, HCO_3 administration (as $NaHCO_3$) is often contraindicated because the volume overload status of the patient may not permit further Na administration.

Peritoneal dialysis or hemodialysis are highly effective (details provided in Chapter 22).

HYPONATREMIA

Hyponatremia occurs frequently in ARF and generally reflects excessive iatrogenic administration of water. In oliguric ARF patients, a serum sodium level below 120 mEq/L constitutes an indication for dialysis, as diuretics and fluid restriction are generally futile. Any type of dialysis therapy will effectively normalize the serum sodium level.

CALCIUM AND PHOSPHORUS DISTURBANCES

Phosphorus retention may cause hypocalcemia, which is rarely of clinical significance. It is appropriate, however, to prevent hyperphosphatemia by avoiding phosphorus infusions and high-phosphorus nutrition, and by administering phosphorus-binding antacids. Since the latter can only bind ingested phosphorus, and since dialytic removal of phosphorus is poor, prevention is crucial. Severe hypocalcemia may produce seizures, with neuromuscular irritability (manifest as Chvostek's or Trousseau's signs) and electrophysiological disturbances (heralded by QT-interval prolongation), so that oral or intravenous calcium supplementation should be given when such features are present. However, in the absence of such clinical features, hypocalcemia does not necessarily warrant therapy, particularly since hyperphosphatemia is likely and may result in visceral precipitation of the administered calcium. Rhabdomyolytic ARF is particularly likely to produce extreme hyperphosphatemia and hypocalcemia, with actual precipitation of calcium salts in injured muscle tissue. If a decision is made to administer calcium, oral supplements are of little value, unless given with concomitant vitamin D supplementation (see below). Intravenous $CaCl_2$ (10 mL of 10% solution yielding approximately 10 mEq of calcium) must be given with great caution to avoid vascular extravasation, because it is extremely caustic. To avoid transient hypercalcemia, one ampoule should be given slowly, followed by a repeat serum calcium determination.

OTHER COMPLICATIONS

A variety of other complications may occur, although these are more frequently encountered in chronic renal failure (CRF). These complications, discussed more fully in Chapter 22, include the following.

Hypermagnesemia

Administering excessive magnesium to oliguric patients will cause hypermagnesemia. Magnesium levels as high as 5 mEq/L are generally well tolerated and are not commonly seen in ARF patients. Prevention, by avoidance of medications containing magnesium, is crucial; when extreme hypermagnesemia occurs, dialysis is the only effective therapy. As for potassium, hemodialysis is far more efficient than peritoneal dialysis in magnesium removal.

Bleeding

Uremia-associated platelet dysfunction may contribute to hemorrhage. In ARF patients with persistent bleeding (for example, postoperative or gastrointestinal) and marked azotemia, dialysis is indicated.

Pericarditis

Much more common in the course of CRF, pericarditis may nonetheless occur in ARF patients, reflecting an inflammatory serositis induced by uremic toxins. An asymptomatic pericardial friction rub is the usual presentation, but pain, fever, and tamponade may occur. Pericarditis is a strong indication for dialysis (any type).

Encephalopathy

The rapid accumulation of urea and other nitrogenous wastes may produce confusion, lethargy, coma, and seizures. Often these clinical features may be multifactorial, reflecting the serious underlying conditions that predispose to ARF, in addition to uremia itself. Electroencephalographic evidence of diffuse slowing may aid in distinguishing uremic encephalopathy, but it is generally unnecessary. Encephalopathy is also a strong indication for dialysis (any type).

Nutritional Deficiencies

Although a low protein intake may minimize BUN elevation, adequate provision of protein remains important in managing ARF patients who are critically ill. Patients who have undergone surgery or who have suffered burns, trauma, muscle injury, or sepsis are particularly likely to be highly catabolic, and sustain daily serious negative nitrogen balance. Adequate provision of protein—in the diet, in enteral alimentation, or in parenteral amino acid infusion—has been proven to improve survival, even though azotemia may be worsened and the need for dialysis increased. Generally, 1.5 g/kg per day of protein should be supplied to the critically ill patient. In addition, adequate provision of calories should not be overlooked, particularly in patients who are eating but are anorexic.

Bibliography

Abel, R, Beck, G, and Abbott, W: Improved survival of acute renal failure after therapy with intravenous essential L-amino acids and glucose. N Engl J Med 288:695, 1973.

Auger, RC, et al: Use of ethacrynic acid in mannitol-resistant oliguric renal failure. JAMA 206:891, 1968.

Baldwin, L, Henderson, A, and Hickman, P: Effect of low-dose dopamine on renal function after elective major vascular surgery. Ann Intern Med 120:744, 1994.

Barry, KG, and Berman, AR: Mannitol infusion. N Engl J Med, 264:1085, 1961.

Berlyne, GM, et al.: The dietary treatment of acute renal failure. Q J Med 36:59, 1967.

Betto, OS, and Stein, JH: Early management of shock and prophylaxis of acute renal failure in traumatic rhabdomyolysis. N Engl J Med 322:825, 1990.

Brown, JJ, et al: Renin and acute renal failure. BMJ 1:253, 1970.

Bullock, ML, and Shapiro, FL: Acute renal failure. Part 2. Hydration: first principle of prevention. Mod Med, April 29, 56, 1974.

Butkus, DE: Persistent high mortality in acute renal failure. Editorial. Arch Intern Med 143:209, 1983.

Cantarovich, R, et al: High dose furosemide in established acute renal failure. BMJ 4:449, 1973.

Conger, JD: Does hemodialysis delay recovery from acute renal failure? Semin Dial 3:3, 1990.

Finn, WF: Diagnosis and management of acute tubular necrosis. Med Clin North Am 74:4, 1990.

Kleinknecht, D, et al: Uremic and non-uremic complications in acute renal failure. Evaluation of early and frequent dialysis on prognosis. Kidney 1:190, 1972.

Lieberthal, W, and Levinsky, NG: Treatment of acute tubular necrosis. Semin Nephrol 10:571, 1990.

Myers, BD, Moran, SM: Hemodynamically mediated acute renal failure. N Engl J Med 314:a7, 1986.

Neilson, EG: Pathogenesis and therapy of interstitial nephritis. Kidney Dis 35:1257, 1989.

Rusell, JD, and Churchill, DN: Calcium antagonists and acute renal failure. Am J Med 87:306, 1989.

Siegler, RL, and Bloomer, A: Acute renal failure with prolonged oliguria. JAMA 225:133, 1973.

Smolens, P, and Stein, JH: Pathophysiology of acute renal failure. Am J Med 70:479, 1981.

Szerlip, HM: Renal dose dopamine: Fact and fiction. Ann Intern Med 115:153, 1991.

Turney, JH, Marshall, DH, Brownjohn, AM, et al: The evolution of acute renal failure. Q J Med 74:83, 1990.

Woods, J, Blythe, W, and Huffines, W: Management of malignant hypertension complicated by renal insufficiency. N Engl J Med 291:10, 1974.

22

CHRONIC RENAL FAILURE:

MANAGEMENT CONSIDERATIONS

Chronic renal failure (CRF) produces a myriad of multisystemic consequences. When therapy directed at improving renal function is futile or unsuccessful, each of these specific consequences must be addressed. Some may be managed only with dialysis; others may be controlled with more conservative approaches; still others do not respond to dialysis and require supplementary approaches.

ELECTROLYTE DISTURBANCES

Hyperkalemia

Those patients with disproportionate tubulointerstitial dysfunction may manifest hyperkalemia when GFR is quite well sustained. However, in general, hyperkalemia ($K \geq 6.0$ mEq/L) tends to occur late in the course of chronic renal disease and can often be avoided with judicious dietary restriction. A 2-g potassium diet, providing approximately 50 mEq of potassium, usually will prevent hyperkalemia. Occasionally, loop diuretic therapy may be useful in helping to control a tendency to hyperkalemia; but adequate sodium intake must be maintained. Cation exchange resins, because of their cost, distastefulness, and inconvenience, are not generally a mode of long-term treatment. Thus, the patient with CRF who manifests hyperkalemia despite satisfactory dietary restriction is generally best started on maintenance dialysis treatment (see below).

Metabolic Acidosis

As with hyperkalemia, severe acidosis generally occurs late in the course of chronic renal disease. However, tubulointerstitial damage may be associated with disproportionately severe acidosis relative to GFR. Generally, chronic hypobicarbonatemia of < 15 to 18 mEq/L is treated to prevent the potential (but unproven) acceleration of bone disease, which may result from the demands of chronic bone buffering of unexcreted acids of metabolism.

$NaHCO_3$ tablets (650 mg = 8 mEq), in a dose of 16 to 32 mEq per day, may empirically sustain serum HCO_3 levels; however, the sodium load is sometimes not tolerated or may necessitate increased doses of diuretics. Many patients experience gastrointestinal distress due to gastric CO_2 gas production. Sodium citrate in tablets or liquid (Shohl's solution) may be a more palatable alternative, where metabolism of each milliequivalent of citrate generates 1 mEq of HCO_3.

Notably, $CaCO_3$, which is often prescribed for its phosphorus-binding and/or calcium supplementary effects, is relatively poorly absorbed, so that it provides a minimal net HCO_3 dose.

Dialysis

Generally, the decision to dialyze is based on factors other than acidosis, but either peritoneal dialysis or hemodialysis is highly effective in reversing and controlling uremic acidosis. Peritoneal dialysis uses solutions with approximately 30 to 35 mEq/L of lactate, which is substantially absorbed through the peritoneal membrane. Although HCO_3 is actually lost from the bloodstream into the dialysate, the absorption of large quantities of lactate, which is metabolized to generate HCO_3, more than counterbalances these losses and corrects acidosis. Most patients receiving chronic peritoneal dialysis maintain serum HCO_3 levels of > 20 mEq/L.

Hemodialysis currently uses dialysate containing HCO_3. The dialysate HCO_3 concentration of approximately 30 mEq/L provides a high concentration gradient relative to the blood levels, which ensures a substantial HCO_3 infusion into the patient during each dialysis session. At the completion of a hemodialysis treatment, serum HCO_3 levels are generally 24 to 28 mEq/L. Over the ensuing two days, before the next treatment, daily acid retention may lower the level to 18 to 24 mEq/L, to be replenished at the next dialysis session. Historically, acetate was used as the principal dialysate source of HCO_3 (metabolized to HCO_3 by muscle and liver); however, most equipment designed after 1985 uses HCO_3 dialysate.

Hypermagnesemia

Although severe hypermagnesemia is unusual, it may occur in patients with acute or chronic renal failure who have inappropriately received high pharmacologic doses in the form of magnesium-containing antacids or laxatives. Magnesium levels > 5 mEq/L, which may be associated with altered mental status, weakness, and depressed neuromuscular responses, should be treated with dialysis. Most peritoneal dialysis and hemodialysis solutions contain approximately 1.5 mEq/L of magnesium to prevent hypomagnesemia in chronic dialysis patients. This normal level is nonetheless adequate to provide a sufficient gradient for substantial magnesium removal.

NEUROLOGIC MANIFESTATIONS

The development of either of the two major neurologic manifestations of uremia, encephalopathy or peripheral neuropathy, is a strong indication for dialysis.

Encephalopathy

Encephalopathy, with florid organic mental syndrome, asterixis, EEG changes, obtundation, or seizures, is a late uremic manifestation, which is more frequently observed today in the course of ARF. In the acute setting, severe encephalopathy may occur with BUN levels near 100 mg/dL, whereas in CRF, substantially higher levels of azotemia may be well tolerated. Subtle cognitive impairment may be demonstrable at much earlier stages, but rarely results in reported symptoms. The development of significant encephalopathy must be treated with dialysis. Conservative measures, such as protein restriction, which may lower the BUN level, are unlikely to reverse encephalopathy.

Peripheral Neuropathy

Peripheral neuropathy, most frequently manifest as symmetrical stocking-glove sensory disturbance, is a feature only of CRF, and is not seen in ARF. The sensation of "restless legs" is a common symptom and is of neuropathic origin. Rarely, motor function may also be affected. If the clinician is reasonably certain that uremia is responsible for a neuropathy, dialysis must be instituted. Frequently, concomitant diabetes, in the setting of renal insufficiency, may create substantial doubt about the specific etiology of the neuropathy.

Generally, peripheral neuropathy does not improve substantially even with dialysis, and stabilization is the best one can expect. Thus, early detection to institute dialysis before severe neuropathy has evolved is an important nephrologic strategy. A small percentage of CRF patients develop progressive uremic peripheral neuropathy, unresponsive to dialysis, where urgent renal transplantation becomes the preferred mode of therapy.

INFLAMMATORY MANIFESTATIONS

Inflammatory manifestations may include pericarditis, pleuritis, colitis, and gastritis. Of these, the first is the most frequent, most serious, and best documented. Uremic pericarditis is an inflammatory exudative process that is frequently associated with fever, pain, and leukocytosis. It may occur as a presenting manifestation of chronic or acute renal failure, but it also occurs commonly in the course of chronic dialysis patients. Uremic pericarditis constitutes an absolute indication for the initiation of dialysis, and often requires frequent and prolonged dialysis therapy. Refractory cases (particularly in the course of CRF) may require pericardial drainage.

Pleuritis, most often manifest as a left pleural effusion and associated with pericarditis, is a much less frequent uremic complication. The vast majority of pleural effusions seen in the setting of renal failure result from fluid overload (see below) or infection.

Gastritis and colitis are uremic complications seen only with extreme uremia. Such patients invariably have many strong indications for dialysis independent of the gastrointestinal features.

CARDIOVASCULAR COMPLICATIONS

Volume overload, manifest as edema, pleural effusion, and pulmonary vascular congestion, is a frequent expected complication of CRF. Underlying heart disease due to such disorders as longstanding hypertension or concomitant coronary artery disease often worsens the clinical problem.

Sodium restriction may successfully avert volume overload, particularly in CRF patients, and loop diuretics in high dosages may be efficacious. Generally, the development of substantial volume overload (particularly in the pulmonary circulation), if it is refractory to such conservative measures, constitutes a strong indication for dialysis.

One common clinical situation where volume overload may require early dialysis, despite the absence of other indications and despite a reasonably preserved GFR, is diabetic nephropathy. Here, the combined effects of hypertensive and arteriosclerotic heart disease with the nephrotic syndrome result in frequent severe overload states.

Patients receiving regular hemodialysis treatments are monitored carefully for evidence of fluid overload at each treatment session. The rate of fluid removal is based on the patient's weight gain since the previous dialysis. Fluid removal is specifically achieved by regulating the ultrafiltration rate across the dialyzing membrane. Most patients require three treatment sessions, each of 3 to 5 hours duration, weekly.

Chronic peritoneal dialysis is usually administered as a continuous process (CAPD—continuous ambulatory peritoneal dialysis). Some patients may be treated nightly for 8–12 hours. Fluid removal is achieved by instillation of hypertonic dialysate (1,500 mg/dL to 4,250 mg/dL glucose concentration) to withdraw excess salt and water along with urea and other waste products. Efficacy of fluid removal depends on the integrity and function of the peritoneal membrane. Some patients—particularly those who have had many episodes of peritonitis—become resistant to fluid removal and must be switched to hemodialysis.

BONE METABOLISM

The complex abnormalities of bone metabolism that characterize renal failure are beyond the scope of this text, but several therapeutic guidelines are presented here.

Phosphorus retention and deficiency of activated vitamin D are the two cornerstone pathological abnormalities that must be addressed. Successful therapy may control hyperparathyroidism and prevent osteodystrophy.

Early in the course of CRF, even subtle hyperparathyroidism should be prevented with low-phosphorus diet and appropriate phosphorus binders. Magnesium-based binders are relatively contraindicated due to potential hypermagnesemia. Aluminum-containing binders are generally avoided due to the proven hazard of aluminum accumulation, which may cause bone disease and potential encephalopathy. $CaCO_3$, which provides a modest calcium supplement, is a very effective phosphorus binder, and has been widely used. Recently, calcium acetate has been found to be a more efficient phosphorus binder relative to the absorbed calcium load. The chosen phosphorus binder (usually $CaCO_3$ or calcium acetate) should be administered 30–60 minutes after meals. Dosage must be titrated to control phosphorus levels and avoid hypercalcemia.

Vitamin D, administered as oral 1,25-dihydroxyvitamin D_3, is empirically given at a dosage of 0.25 to 0.5 µg/day, with caution to avoid hypercalcemia.

The reader is directed toward more specialized texts for details of the management of established renal osteodystrophy.

HORMONAL ABNORMALITIES

In addition to hyperparathyroidism (see above), numerous other endocrine disturbances occur. Insulin resistance (with paradoxical prolongation of the activity of administered exogenous insulin), hyperprolactinemia, and relative hypogonadism are among the disturbances. Specific therapeutic approaches occasionally are necessary.

HEMATOLOGIC COMPLICATIONS
Anemia

Anemia is frequently severe due to a combination of low erythropoietin levels, relative bone marrow suppression secondary to uremic toxins, shortened red blood cell survival, and excess external blood loss (blood drawing, epistaxis). As previously discussed, severe anemia may complicate ARF, particularly when concomitant serious illnesses are present.

As a general principle, dialysis will not substantially reverse the anemia of CRF, although some patients may achieve normal hemoglobin levels (particularly patients with preserved renal mass—for example, diabetic nephropathy, polycystic kidney disease). Synthetic erythropoietin has dramatically improved the well-being of chronic dialysis patients, but its effectiveness depends upon adequate control of uremia, reversal of deficiencies of iron or other nutrients, and the absence of serious acute concomitant illness. Accordingly, in the multisystemically ill ARF patient, erythropoietin administration is generally ineffective.

When clinically necessary, transfusion may be appropriate, but stable CRF patients frequently adapt to remarkably low hemoglobin levels, and may not be endangered by stable levels as low as 5 to 6 g/dL. Obviously, such levels are often incompatible with a vigorous, rehabilitated lifestyle, and represent a strong indication for erythropoietin administration.

Platelet Dysfunction and Uremic Bleeding

When BUN exceeds 80 mg/dL, platelet dysfunction is usually demonstrable by in vitro testing or bleeding-time determination. Clinical bleeding problems frequently develop in the course of CRF. Such patients often undergo surgery (vascular access, etc.) and GI hemorrhage is also a frequent complication, related to uremic colitis, a high frequency of peptic ulcer, and bowel angiodysplasia.

In patients at high risk of bleeding, vigorous dialysis to keep BUN below 80 is the first line of therapy; maintenance of the hemoglobin level above 8 to 9 g/dL also seems to reduce the bleeding tendency. Cryoprecipitate infusions, by providing von Willebrand's factor, are effective in lowering bleeding time in patients with serious bleeding. More recently, intravenous d DAVP, which has a similar mechanism of action, has been recommended in a dose of 0.4 μg/kg. Although effective for 12 to 36 hours, subsequent doses are ineffectual during a refractory period of several days when vascular stores of von Willebrand's factor are resynthesized.

High-dose estrogen therapy may also be used, particularly in angiodysplastic gastrointestinal hemorrhage.

IMPLICATIONS FOR DRUG ADMINISTRATION

A wide variety of pharmacological agents, or their toxic metabolites, are excreted by the kidneys. As a general rule, those agents with a narrow therapeutic window must be adjusted by measurement of blood levels. Dosage based on GFR and body weight must also be adjusted for dialytic removal. Numerous references provide guidelines. However, even some drugs that are predominantly handled by nonrenal metabolism may produce toxic effects idiosyncratically (e.g., benzodiazepines). Thus, general caution must always be exercised, particularly in the use of sedatives or relatively new agents.

Another notable pitfall is overestimation of GFR, based on serum creatinine level, particularly in patients with ARF (see Chapter 20). The reader is reminded that shortly after the development of severe ARF, the serum creatinine level will not yet have risen to its peak, despite a markedly low GFR. Dosage must be based on actual measured GFR or a projection based on the expected ultimate creatinine level.

SUMMARY

Numerous systemic problems are expected in CRF. Many can be ameliorated by dialysis. The decision to begin dialysis, however, is often subjective and requires interpretation of the risks of concomitant problems (e.g., heart disease), along with the traditional indications for dialytic therapy discussed above.

In the course of CRF, strategy is important. Efforts to prepare patients for the eventual need for dialysis or transplantation are important. Although the progression of chronic renal insufficiency is often unpredictable, timely creation of a fistula for vascular access is strongly advised. Meticulous interval history taking and examination are important in detecting subtle neuropathy, encephalopathy, and malnutrition. These complications must be avoided, as they may be incompletely reversed by dialysis.

Bibliography

Allon, M, Donlay, R, and Copkiney, G: Nebulized albuterol for acute hyperkalemia in patients on hemodialysis. Ann Intern Med 110:6, 1989.

Bailey, GL, and Sullivan, NR: Selected protein diet in terminal uremia. J Am Diet Assoc 52:125, 1968.

Bennett, WM, (ed): Drug prescribing in renal failure, 3rd ed. American College of Physicians, 1994.

Berger, EE, and Lowrig, EG: Mortality and the length of dialysis. JAMA 265:909, 1991.

Berl, T, Berns, A, Hyfer, W, et al: 1,25-Dihydroxycholecalciferol effects in chronic dialysis. Ann Intern Med 88:774, 1978.

Berlyne, GM, and Shaw, AB: Giordano-Giovannetti diet in terminal renal failure. Lancet 2:7, 1965.

Berlyne, GM: Red eyes in renal failure. Lancet 1:4, 1967.

Breslau N: Normal and abnormal regulation of 1,25 $(OH)_2$ D synthesis. Am J Med Sci 296:417, 1988.

David, DS, et al: Dietary management in renal failure. Lancet, 2:34, 1972. Also Am Heart J, 86:1, 1973.

Delmez, JA, Tindira, CA, Windus, DW, et al: Calcium acetate as a phosphorus binder in hemodialysis patients. J Am Soc Nephrol 3:96, 1992.

DeLuca, HF: The kidney as an endocrine organ. Production of 1,25-hydroxyvitamin D_3. N Engl J Med 289:359, 1973.

DeStrihou, CVY, and Frans, A: Pattern of respiratory compensation in chronic uremic acidosis. Nephron 7:37, 1970.

Donovitch, G, Bourgoignie, J, and Bricker, N: Sodium conservation in renal failure. N Engl J Med 296:14, 1977.

Eliahou, HE, et al: Acetate and bicarbonate in the correction of uremic acidosis. BMJ 4:399, 1970.

Eschbach, JW: Erythropoietin therapy for the anemia of chronic renal failure. *Kidney* 22:1, 1990.

Freeman, R: Treatment of chronic renal failure. An update. Editorial. N Engl J Med 312:577, 1985.

Gifford, JD, Rutsky, EA, Kirk, KA, and McDaniel, HG: Control of serum potassium during fasting in patients with end-stage renal disease. Kidney Int 35:90, 1989.

Giovannetti, S, and Maggiore, Q: A low nitrogen diet with proteins of high biological value for severe chronic uremia. Lancet 1:1000, 1964.

Ihle, BJ, Becker, GJ, Whitworth, JA, et al: The effect of protein restriction on the progress of renal insufficiency. N Engl J Med 321:1773, 1989.

Kurtin, P: Principles of nutritional support for patients with renal disease. Bull NY Acad Med 60:1002, 1984.

Lee, DBN, Goodman, WG, and Coburn, JW: Renal osteodystrophy: Some new questions on an old disorder. Am J Kidney Dis 11:365, 1988.

Lefebvre, A, de Vernejoul, MC, Gueris, J, et al: Optimal correction of acidosis changes progression of dialysis osteodystrophy. Kidney Int 36:1112, 1989.

Levin, DM, and Cade, R: Influence of dietary sodium on renal function in patients with chronic renal disease. Ann Intern Med 62:231, 1965.

Malluche, H, and Faugere, MC: Renal bone disease 1990: an unmet challenge for the nephrologist. Kidney Int 38:193, 1990.

Rose, WC, and Dekker, EE: Urea as a source of nitrogen for the biosynthesis of amino acids. J Biol Chem 223:107, 1956.

Salvesen, HA: Alkali treatment of renal acidosis. Acta Med Scand (suppl) 259:75, 1951.

Schiller, LR, Santa Ana, CA, Shiekh, MS, et al: Effects of the time of administration of calcium acetate on phosphorus binding. N Engl J Med 320:1110, 1989.

Tyler, HR: Neurologic disorders in renal failure. Am J Med 44:734, 1968.

23

ACUTE RENAL DISEASES AND ELECTROLYTE DISORDERS

Although acute renal diseases may produce ARF (reviewed in Chapters 20 and 21), they may also present with less dramatic reductions in GFR but with significant electrolyte and fluid implications. Those acute renal disorders that are particularly likely to produce such electrolyte manifestations are the focus of this chapter. A comprehensive discussion of acute renal diseases is beyond the scope of this primer and the reader is referred to a number of texts (see bibliography).

These disorders may be logically organized in an anatomic fashion:

- Prerenal (any condition characterized by reduced renal blood flow with normal intrinsic renal function)
- Disease of the renal vessels
- Glomerular disease
- Tubulointerstitial disease
- Postrenal (obstruction)

PRERENAL STATES

These conditions include

- Simple volume (water and electrolyte) depletion
- Low cardiac output
- Pericardial tamponade
- Cor pulmonale
- Cirrhosis
- Nephrotic syndrome
- Vena cava occlusion

Although an elevated BUN reading is the biochemical hallmark of renal hypoperfusion, the clinician must be aware that the BUN may be in normal range despite the presence of a prerenal state.

Although urinary urea excretion will always be quite low in such patients, concomitant low rates of urea production may keep the BUN in a normal range. Cirrhosis is the classic example of such a state, but patients with any of the above disorders often present with surprisingly normal BUN levels when protein intake has been low. Establishing the presence of a prerenal state thus depends on the presence of one of the above clinical disorders, along with low urinary sodium excretion (see below). If the BUN is normal, an elevated serum uric acid level will often provide confirmation (uric acid excretion is tightly correlated with sodium excretion). The serum creatinine is generally only modestly elevated, but more extreme elevations can occur (see Chapter 20).

Compensatory Responses to Hypoperfusion

The renal compensatory responses to hypoperfusion occur at three levels.

1. *Vascular.* The normal renal response to low flow (or low pressure) is vasoconstriction, which would further compromise renal perfusion. However, this is balanced by the release of local vasodilators, including endothelial relaxing factor (EDRF) and prostaglandins. These dilators support perfusion.
2. *Glomerular.* GFR is sustained by selective constriction of the efferent arteriole, mediated by release of renin (and production of angiotensin II).
3. *Tubular.* Compensation for reduced renal perfusion involves avid sodium retention throughout the nephron.

Biochemical Abnormalities

These compensatory mechanisms predispose to certain biochemical abnormalities:

HYPONATREMIA. Intense proximal sodium and chloride reabsorption limit the delivery of chloride to the ascending limb of the loop of Henle, where urinary dilution occurs. Furthermore, antidiuretic hormone (ADH) levels are frequently elevated in response to the basic hemodynamic prerenal disturbance. The net effect is an inability to excrete water, so that water ingestion in the setting of prerenal azotemia will result in hyponatremia.

HYPERKALEMIA. Although unusual, reduced sodium delivery and low tubular flow combine to limit potassium excretion. Even moderate potassium loads, which are normally easily excreted, may thus result in hyperkalemia.

Acid-Base Disturbances

Metabolic alkalosis often clinically accompanies volume-depleted states, usually as a result of diuretics or vomiting. However, in the absence of such factors, prerenal states may also be associated with a reduced renal H^+ excretory capacity. As described above, with regard to defective potassium excretion, reduced distal sodium delivery limits H^+ excretion so that an acidifying stimulus may not be appropriately matched by enhanced renal acid excretion. Diarrheal states such as cholera most commonly produce such a situation; HCO_3 loss in stool, accompanied by volume depletion, results in potentially severe hyperchloremic metabolic acidosis. Similarly, in cirrhosis, some patients may develop a functional type of "renal tubular acidosis" reflecting extreme tubular sodium reabsorption.

Therapeutic Implications

When NaCl depletion is the cause of the prerenal state, any of the aforementioned electrolyte abnormalities will be corrected by the administration of NaCl (usually as normal saline infusion). Hyponatremia will correct as restoration of arterial volume enhances distal sodium delivery and suppresses ADH levels. Hyperkalemia or acidosis will similarly correct with enhanced tubular urine flow (and distal sodium delivery), and metabolic alkalosis will correct as chloride administration allows renal HCO_3 excretion (see Chapter 29).

In other prerenal states, management should focus on correction of the fundamental problem (e.g., improving cardiac output, relieving tamponade, or treating proteinuria with immunosuppression). Frequently, the basic pathophysiology of the prerenal state cannot be corrected (e.g., cirrhosis or refractory congestive heart failure). Under these circumstances, hyponatremia must be managed by H_2O restriction. Hyperkalemia is generally mild, so that mild dietary potassium restriction generally suffices (see Chapter 26 for more detail). Acidosis, also generally mild, as seen in cirrhosis, requires no therapy. The approach to alkalosis in prerenal states is discussed in Chapter 29.

Vulnerability to Drugs

As a consequence of the renal compensation of prerenal states, agents that block prostaglandin formation will be especially poorly tolerated, with potentially dramatic reductions in renal blood flow, GFR, and potassium excretion.

Similarly, angiotensin converting enzyme (ACE) inhibitors have the potential to produce extreme declines in GFR and must be used with caution.

RENOVASCULAR DISEASE AND ATHEROSCLEROTIC DISEASE

Although the atherosclerotic and fibromuscular variants of renovascular disease are characterized by chronic hypertension with normal (or nearly normal) GFR, sudden events may occur to produce acute syndromes.

- *ARF* (see Chapter 2) in the setting of bilateral renal artery stenosis may be triggered by pharmacologic blood pressure reduction, particularly with ACE inhibitors.
- *Renal emboli* are seen principally with atherosclerotic renal involvement. The syndrome may be manifest with flank pain, gross hematuria or microhematuria, and variable reductions in GFR. Substantial elevation of LDH with modest increase in AST is characteristic, and isotopic scanning generally is confirmatory.
- *Hyponatremia* has been reported in a small number of patients with severe renal artery stenosis and concomitant renal hypoperfusion (as pathophysiologically described above).

GLOMERULONEPHRITIS (GN)

Acute glomerular inflammation can vary in severity from asymptomatic microhematuria to fulminant ARF, but the vast majority of cases are at the mild end of the spectrum. The causative factors include immune complex reactions to a variety of infections, and systemic disease (e.g., systemic lupus erythematosus, vasculitis). The reader is referred to standard texts for more detail.

Classic cases are characterized by glomerular inflammation, which is manifest clinically by sodium retention (with edema, hypertension, and occasionally pulmonary edema) out of proportion to the reduction in GFR. Examination of the urine sediment discloses moderate proteinuria (usually not in the nephrotic ranges) with hematuria, pyuria, red blood cell, and granular casts.

The intensity of sodium retention may contribute to hyperkalemia despite only modest reduction in GFR. The mechanism is presumed to be analogous to the hyperkalemia of prerenal states, although concomitant interstitial inflammation, which often histologically accompanies acute GN, may play a role.

Mild acute GN requires no intervention other than observation. However, on a general level, salt restriction and pharmacological control of blood pressure are usual therapeutic guidelines. In more severe cases, search for a specific diagnosis is critical to therapy. Even fulminant acute GN may fully resolve spontaneously (e.g., postinfectious GN), but other variants warrant specific treatment. In severe cases, recovery of renal function becomes unlikely when serum creatinine exceeds 5 mg/dL, so that rapid evaluation of acute GN is recommended even when impairment of GFR is not yet dramatic. Serological evaluation for SLE and other vasculitides and early renal biopsy usually provide a diagnosis. Specific treatment may include high-dose steroids and cyclophosphamide. A detailed description of the diagnostic and therapeutic approach to acute GN is beyond the scope of this primer.

ACUTE TUBULOINTERSTITIAL DISEASE

Acute tubulointerstitial diseases may acutely result in ARF (see Chapter 21), but many important syndromes may occur with only mild (or minimal) reduction in GFR. For a discussion of acute tubular necrosis, see Chapter 21.

Acute Interstitial Nephritis

Acute interstitial nephritis can rarely occur as an idiopathic syndrome (occasionally accompanied by uveitis). Viral or bacterial infections (Hanta virus, cytomegalovirus and adenovirus, leptospirosis, *Legionella*) may cause significant interstitial inflammation. Pyogenic bacteria rarely cause the syndrome of pyelonephritis. Drug-induced interstitial nephritis may be of an allergic type with concomitant rash and eosinophilia (most common with certain penicillins) or may be isolated to the kidneys with a lymphocytic process (as with nonsteroidal anti-inflammatory drugs).

In all of these conditions, clinical features of back pain and fever may be present, with inflammatory cells present in the urinalysis (granulocytes especially with bacterial pyelonephritis, eosinophils in allergic states, and lymphocytes in most others). Renal ultrasonography may confirm renal swelling or even focal inflammatory masses.

As noted above, GFR is usually only minimally impaired, as in bacterial pyelonephritis. Nonetheless, the tubulointerstitial inflammation may impair potassium and hydrogen ion excretion, with resultant hyperchloremic, hyperkalemic acidosis. Sodium retention may also occur, but is generally mild, and hypertension is unusual.

Treatment of life-threatening hyperkalemia should proceed along standard lines (Chapter 26); however, the generally mild hyperkalemia is usually manageable with dietary potassium restriction. Loop diuretics to enhance urine flow, which sometimes are helpful in chronic type IV renal tubular acidosis, may be of some value, as long as adequate sodium replacement is provided. Hyperchloremic acidosis is rarely severe enough to mandate specific therapy ($NaHCO_3$ orally or intravenously).

Metabolic Variants of Interstitial Nephritis

Hypercalcemia may produce a variable reduction in GFR with tubulointerstitial dysfunction, manifest as polyuria and polydipsia due to nephrogenic diabetes insipidus. Adequate water replacement and therapy of hypercalcemia should proceed concomitantly.

Under conditions of extreme *uric acid excretion* (particularly in the setting of chemotherapy for hematological malignancy), acute tubular uric acid sludging may occur. When severe, ARF may develop, but milder forms may be manifest as a tubulointerstitial nephritis. Prevention of massive uric acid excretion by allopurinol pretreatment before chemotherapy has virtually eliminated this entity. Diagnosis is established by high urinary uric acid excretion (urinary uric acid/creatinine ratio = 1) and crystalluria. Forced alkaline diuresis with $NaHCO_3$ infusion will treat mild cases by solubilizing the tubular uric acid.

OBSTRUCTION

Although severe obstruction will produce renal failure (see Chapter 20), milder obstruction frequently produces clinical or biochemical manifestations before the development of full-blown ARF. Most notably, azotemia out of proportion to the serum creatinine may occur, reflecting tubular urea reabsorption due to slow tubular flow. Similarly, potassium excretion may be limited, with resultant hyperkalemia; hyperchloremic acidosis may accompany the hyperkalemia. Although therapy is obviously addressed at relieving the mechanical obstruction, the important lesson is that the clinician should consider the possibility of obstruction when hyperkalemia, acidosis, and azotemia occur out of proportion to elevation of serum creatinine.

Bibliography

Badr, K, and Ichikawa, F: Prerenal failure: A deleterious shift from renal compensation to decompensation. N Engl J Med 319:623, 1988.

Choi, M, Fernandez, PC, Patnaik A, et al: Trimethoprim-induced hyperkalemia in a patient with AIDS. N Engl J Med 328:703, 1993.

Conte, G, Dal Canton, A, Imperatore, P, et al: Acute increase in plasma osmolality as a cause of hyperkalemia in patient with renal failure. Kidney Int 38:301, 1990.

Don, BR, Schambelan, M: Hyperkalemia in acute glomerulonephritis due to transient hyporeninemic hypoaldosteronism. Kidney Int 38:1159, 1990.

Hricik, DE: Captopril induced renal insufficiency and the role of sodium balance. Ann Intern Med 103:222, 1985.

Kamel, KS, Ethier, JH, Richardson, RMA, et al: Urine electrolytes and osmolality: When and how to use them. Am J Nephrol, 10:89, 1990.

Luscher, TF, Bock, HA, Yang, Z, and Diederich, D: Endothelium-derived relaxing and contrasting factors: Perspectives in nephrology. Kidney Int 39:575, 1991.

Packer, M, Lee, WH, Medina, N, et al: Functional renal insufficiency during long-term therapy with captopril and enalapril and enalapril in severe chronic heart failure. Ann Intern Med 106:346, 1987.

Patrono, C, and Dunn, MJ: The clinical significance of inhibition of renal prostaglandin synthesis. Kidney Int 32:1, 1987.

Relman, AS: The acidosis of renal disease. Am J Med 44:706, 1968.

Schrier, RW: Pathogenesis of sodium and water retention in high-output and low-output cardiac failure, nephrotic syndrome, cirrhosis, and pregnancy. N Engl J Med, 319:1065, 1988.

Schwartz, WB, and Relman, AS: Acidosis in renal disease. N Engl J Med 256:1184, 1957.

Whelton, A, Stout, RK, Spillman, PS, and Klassen, DK: Renal effects of ibuprofen, piroxicam, and sulindac in patients with asymptomatic renal failure: A prospective, randomized, crossover comparison. Ann Intern Med 112:568, 1990.

24

METABOLIC ACIDOSIS
SYNDROMES (Continued)

DIABETIC ACIDOSIS

The National Diabetic Data Group in 1979 described the following clinical classification of diabetes mellitus:

- Type I—insulin-dependent (formerly called juvenile-onset, or ketosis-prone) diabetes mellitus. The fasting plasma glucose concentration is more than 140 mg/dL. Insulin is needed to prevent ketosis.
- Type II—noninsulin-dependent (formerly called maturity-onset or ketosis-resistant) diabetes mellitus. The fasting plasma glucose concentration is more than 140 mg/dL. Insulin may be needed to control hyperglycemia. Ketosis does not develop unless the patient is subjected to stress of various kinds.
- Impaired glucose tolerance. The fasting plasma glucose concentration is less than 140 mg/dL.
- Gestational diabetes mellitus.
- Secondary diabetes mellitus, associated with certain conditions and syndromes, such as pancreatic disease, excessive glucocorticoid hormones (Cushing's syndrome), drug or chemically induced, and so on.

PATHOPHYSIOLOGY

The major sources of glucose (dextrose) in the body are food, liver glycogen, and glycogenesis from the metabolism of protein and fat. In the presence of insulin, a portion of the glucose is converted into glycogen in the liver. Part is oxidized to lactate and pyruvate, and then to carbon dioxide and water. A part of the glucose is also converted into acetate and then to amino acids and protein, or to fatty acids. Insulin also has a fat-sparing and protein-sparing effect, because it helps prevent the oxidation of fat and protein for energy.

The primary metabolic defect of a diabetic patient is a decreased ability to utilize glucose. This in turn is due either to a decreased secretion or a decreased effectiveness of insulin. The exact way in which insulin acts is not completely understood. It probably increases the passage of glucose into the cells through the cell membrane and stimulates carbohydrate metabolism in skeletal and cardiac muscles and in adipose tissues. It may also increase the conversion of glucose to glucose-6-phosphate. The glucose-6-phosphate can then be converted into glycogen or is further metabolized.

Diabetic ketoacidosis is characterized by the overproduction of glucose and ketone bodies in the liver, and by excessive mobilization of free fatty acids from adipose tissue. Recent studies by Unger and others indicate the pancreatic hormone glucagon is important in the pathogenesis of both diabetes mellitus and of diabetic ketoacidosis. For example, when a defect of insulin secretion is present, either an absolute excess or an excess of glucagon relative to the amount of available insulin can cause the liver to form glucose at a rate that exceeds the limited capacity of the diabetic patient to clear it from the bloodstream. McGarry and Foster have shown that insulin lack by itself will increase the supply of free fatty acids, but that glucagon is essential for the liver to produce ketone bodies in massive quantities. When the hyperglucagonemia of the diabetic patient is blocked, as by the administration of the hormone somatostatin, a lack of insulin results in a rise in the level of free fatty acids, but ketone production does not increase unless an excessive amount of glucagon is present.

When insulin is not secreted nor utilized, the following physiological and chemical disturbances occur:

1. Hyperglycemia develops because the insulin supply is inadequate. The concentration of glucose in the extracellular water and blood rises because glucose is not being utilized. When the renal circulation is normal, the plasma glucose concentration rarely rises higher than 400 mg/dL. However, when renal circulation is inadequate and water loss occurs, much higher blood glucose concentrations occur.

   The renal threshold for glucose is approximately 170 mg/dL. When this threshold is exceeded, glycosuria occurs. As a result large amounts of water and electrolytes are lost (osmotic diuresis) as well as glucose. And severe water loss can occur.

2. When the insulin supply is inadequate, the action of lipase is no longer inhibited. As a result, uncontrolled lipolysis occurs and the concentration of free fatty acids exceeds the capacity of the body to metabolize them. They are partially metabolized by the liver into ketones. The increased lipolysis also causes the fat content of the blood to rise greatly.

3. Hyperosmolality occurs because the high concentration of glucose in the blood increases the osmotic pressure of the extracellular water. This lowers the serum sodium concentration (Appendix IV).

When the plasma glucose concentration is more than 500 mg/dL, this suggests that significant hyperosmolality is present.

4. Metabolic acidosis and ketosis occur. Fat is metabolized at an excessive rate to supply energy. As a result large amounts of ketone acids (beta-hydroxybutyric acid and aceto-acetic acid) are formed. (This produces the metabolic acidosis with an abnormal large anion gap.)

   Acetone (formed from the aceto-acetic acid) also accumulates in the blood. It produces a characteristic fruity odor on the patient's breath, but it does not lower the pH.

   These metabolic and ketone acids react with the sodium bicarbonate of the blood, forming sodium ketone and metabolic acid salts, water, and carbon dioxide. The carbon dioxide is eliminated through the lungs. As a result, the bicarbonate–carbonic acid ratio and the pH fall, producing a metabolic acidosis.

5. Sodium and water loss occurs. This may be severe. This may be due to the osmotic diuresis. It may also be due to vomiting. One must remember that the low serum sodium concentration in patients with hyperglycemia may be more apparent than real (Appendix IV).

   The sodium and water loss is associated with hypotension and even with shock.

6. Hyperkalemia may occur because the metabolic acidosis and the absence of insulin cause a shift of potassium ions from the cells into the extracellular water. This movement of potassium ions out of the cells tends to produce an increased serum potassium concentration. Because potassium ions are continually lost with the osmotic diuresis, however, the serum potassium concentration may be high, normal, or low.

7. The triglyceride and cholesterol concentration of the blood increases owing to an increased synthesis of cholesterol in the absence of insulin.

8. Protein is metabolized at an excessive rate to supply glucose and energy. This increases the amount of nitrogenous wastes and acid metabolites in the blood.

9. The acidosis may cause a compensatory respiratory alkalosis, which may persist even after the pH has returned to normal. This is not unique to patients with diabetic acidosis, and occurs in all types of metabolic acidosis.

10. An acidosis associated with an excessive amount of lactic acid in the blood may develop with phenformin (DBI) treatment. (DBI is no longer marketed for general use, although it is still available as an investigational drug.) One should also remember that diabetic ketoacidosis and lactic acidosis may be present simultaneously.

11. A precipitating factor (or factors) must be sought in every patient who develops diabetic acidosis. Common precipitating factors include failure to take insulin and infections of any type. Other underlying factors include acute myocardial infarction, acute pancreatitis (the serum

amylase concentration may be elevated in diabetic acidosis in the absence of pancreatitis), endocrine disorders (hyperthyroidism, acromegaly, pheochromocytoma, Cushing's syndrome), rarely severe emotional stress, and occasionally drugs (for example, thiazide diuretics, furosemide, ethacrynic acid).

SYMPTOMS AND SIGNS

These have already been described in Chapter 17. The temperature is usually normal or subnormal. Therefore, even a slightly elevated temperature suggests that an infection may be present.

LABORATORY FINDINGS

Blood

The electrolyte concentrations vary greatly, and depend on the duration and degree of the acidosis and the presence of associated decreased renal function. A constant and characteristic finding is a low serum bicarbonate concentration. The anion gap is usually substantially increased. In occasional patients with mild, prolonged ketoacidosis, however, the anion gap may be only minimally increased. (The ketoacid anions are excreted in the urine with sodium and potassium, leaving behind hydrogen ions, which are balanced by enhanced chloride reabsorption.) Serum sodium level is usually low. This is due either to sodium loss or to the increased osmolality of the extracellular water, caused by the high glucose concentration in the blood (Chapter 11). If an excessive amount of water has been lost, the serum sodium concentration will be high.

Serum chloride concentration is usually normal. It may be low as a result of urinary excretion, or vomiting.

Serum potassium concentration is usually normal, or high, due to the acidosis. Even if the total potassium supply of the body is depleted, the serum potassium concentration may be normal or high. Occasionally, a low serum potassium concentration occurs. This may be due to a loss of potassium ions from vomiting or inadequate food intake because of anorexia. Breakdown of muscle tissue and failure of glycogen deposition in the liver also tend to deplete the body stores of potassium ions. (When excessive potassium and chloride ions are lost, a metabolic alkalosis may replace the diabetic metabolic acidosis.) A normal or low serum potassium concentration in the presence of acidosis is a presumptive sign of potassium loss.

The blood sugar level is characteristically high, and may reach or exceed 1500 mg/dL. Ketone acids are present in the blood and urine. A simple method of determining their presence is described below.

An elevated blood urea nitrogen (BUN) concentration is found in the majority of patients. This is a result of increased protein catabolism and prerenal azotemia, secondary to the loss of extracellular fluids.

The white blood count may be high, and values as high as 90,000/mm³ have been reported in uncomplicated diabetic patients with acidosis.

Serum amylase values may be abnormally high, even if acute pancreatitis is not present.

Urine

Ketonuria and glycosuria are present. Urinary ketone concentration may be high even when plasma ketone concentration is low. This is due to increased urinary excretion of the ketones, which results from the renal compensation for the metabolic acidosis.

Example: Moderate diabetic acidosis
  Blood sugar 450 mg/dL
  pH 7.34
  PCO_2 38 mm Hg
  Standard bicarbonate 20.3 mEq/L
  Actual bicarbonate 20 mEq/L
  Base excess -5 mEq/L
  CO_2 content 21 mEq/L

The pH is slightly low. This indicates a mild acidosis. The negative base excess and the low standard bicarbonate indicate that a metabolic acidosis is present. The PCO_2 is normal, indicating respiratory balance. However, the actual bicarbonate is slightly lower than the standard bicarbonate. This indicates that a respiratory alkalosis is present. Therefore, a mild metabolic acidosis is present with a compensatory respiratory alkalosis (see Chap. 15).

Cation-Anion Balance:
Na 135   K 5 HCO_3 20   Cl 92 mEq/L
Anion gap = $(Na + K) - (HCO_3 + Cl)$
      $= (135 + 5) - (20 + 92)$
      $= 140 - 112$
      = 28 mEq/L. This is abnormally high. It is due to the accumulation of keto acids.

Example: Patient with severe diabetic acidosis
  Blood sugar 950 mg/dL
  pH 7.2
  PCO_2 12.3 mm Hg
  Standard bicarbonate 8.3 mEq/L
  Actual bicarbonate 5 mEq/L
  Base excess $-$ 22.2 mEq/L

The pH is low, indicating a severe acidosis. The negative base excess and the low standard bicarbonate indicate that a metabolic acidosis is present. The low PCO_2 and the fact that the actual bicarbonate is lower than the standard bicarbonate indicate that a respiratory alkalosis is present. Therefore, a severe metabolic acidosis is present with a partially compensatory respiratory alkalosis (see Chapter 15).

Cation-Anion Balance:
Na 131   K 4.7 HCO_3 5   Cl 95 mEq/L
Anion gap = (Na + K) − (HCO_3 + Cl)
 = (131 + 4.7) − (5 + 95)
 = 135.7 − 100
 = 35.7 mEq/L. This is abnormally high. It is due to the accumulation of keto acids.

DIAGNOSIS

It has already been pointed out that patients with renal tubular acidosis may also show glycosuria and ketonuria. However, in these patients, the blood sugar concentration is normal, abnormal keto acids are not found in the blood, and the anion gap is normal. Acetone and reducing substances that give a false-positive test for glucose are also present in salicylate poisoning. In these patients, the blood sugar concentration is usually normal or slightly elevated. In addition, a positive ferric chloride test for salicylates in the urine is present (also see Chapter 25).

Ethyl alcohol ketoacidosis may simulate diabetic acidosis because the patient may be comatose and the blood glucose concentration may be slightly elevated (even higher than 300 mg/dL). However, if blood or urine tests for ketones are done with Acetest (Ames), a negative or minimally positive result may be obtained because the Acetest is sensitive only to aceto-acetate ketones, whereas there is an excessive amount of beta-hydroxybutyrate ketones in alcoholic ketoacidosis. Beta-hydroxybutyrate levels are not readily measurable. Thus, a high degree of suspicion and a mild positive blood Acetest reaction should strongly raise concern about this diagnosis.

The differential diagnosis of diabetic patients who develop coma is shown in Table 24–1.

COURSE AND PROGNOSIS

In spite of recent advances in therapy, a small percentage of patients with diabetic acidosis will die. However, many of these deaths are now due to associated pathological disturbances rather than to the diabetic acidosis.

TABLE 24–1
DIFFERENTIAL DIAGNOSIS OF COMA IN DIABETIC PATIENTS

Laboratory Tests	Diabetic Ketoacidosis	Hyperosmolal Hyperglycemic Nonketoacidosis	Hypoglycemia	Lactic Acidosis	Ethyl Alcohol Ketoacidosis
Plasma					
Glucose	High	Very high	Low	Normal, or high	Low, normal, or slightly high
Ketones	4 plus*	Absent	Absent	Absent	Slightly present‡
pH	Low	Normal	Normal	Low	Low
CO_2 content (or bicarbonate)	Low	Normal	Normal	Low	Low
Osmolality	High	Very high	Normal	Normal	High
Lactate	Normal	Normal or mildly elevated	Normal	Very high	Normal
BUN	Elevated	Elevated	Normal	Elevated	Normal or high
Urine					
Glucose	4 plus	4 plus	Absent†	Absent to 4 plus	Absent or present
Ketones	4 plus	Absent	Absent†	Absent	Absent‡

*4 plus or more in an undiluted sample.
†Urine that has been in the bladder for several hours may show glucose or ketones as a result of earlier hyperglycemia or ketonemia.
‡The Acetest reaction may be negative because the predominant ketone present is beta-hydroxybutyrate. A test for beta-hydroxybutyrate ketones will be positive.

PROPHYLAXIS

Every insulin-dependent diabetic patient should be taught to test his or her blood sugar. In addition, some brittle patients should also be taught to test the urine for acetone (ketone acids) and to report the presence of acetone to the physician immediately. The physician should also be aware that factors such as infection, trauma, surgical operation, irregular diet, inadequate insulin dosage, vomiting or diarrhea from any cause, pregnancy, thyrotoxicosis, or the acute onset of diabetes can precipitate diabetic acidosis.

TREATMENT

The treatment of diabetic acidosis is complicated because several independent disturbances may be present simultaneously. For example, in addition to a lack of insulin, sodium loss, water loss, potassium loss, shock, accumulation of keto acids producing a metabolic acidosis, a metabolic acidosis due to decreased renal function, even in the absence of previous renal disease, and a compensatory respiratory alkalosis that may persist even when the acidosis is corrected may be present.

The following plan of therapy can be used.

Emergency Treatment

A flowchart should be started (Table 24-2) to track the results of laboratory tests. In addition, notes should be made of the patient's vital signs and level of consciousness.

As soon as the patient is admitted to the hospital, the following tests should be done: blood sugar, plasma acetone, carbon dioxide content, pH, hematocrit and hemoglobin, blood urea nitrogen, potassium; urine sugar, acetone, and routine urine analysis; electrocardiogram; blood pressure and pulse. These tests can be repeated according to Table 24-2.

Treatment should include correction of the hyperglycemia and hyperosmolality, metabolic acidosis and ketosis, sodium loss, water loss, and potassium loss.

Use of Low-Dose Regular, Rapidly Acting Insulin

It has been found that large doses of intravenous (IV) or subcutaneous insulin used previously are not necessary. Regular insulin can be given IV or intramuscularly (IM). Then, when the acidosis is under control, the patient can receive insulin subcutaneously.

If the patient is hypotensive, insulin should be given IV rather than IM

TABLE 24–2

SCHEDULE OF LABORATORY TESTS THAT SHOULD BE DONE IN THE TREATMENT OF PATIENTS WITH DIABETIC ACIDOSIS

Hours of Treatment	0	1	2	3	4	5	6	7	8	9	10	11	12
Blood sugar	*				*				*				*
Ketones	*												
CO_2 content or bicarbonate	*				*				*				*
pH and P_{CO_2}	*				*				*				*
Hematocrit	*		*		*		*		*		*		*
Urea nitrogen	*												*
Potassium, sodium, chloride (magnesium)	*				*				*				*
Urine													
Sugar	*		*		*		*		*		*		*
Ketone	*				*				*				*
Analysis	*				*				*				*
Electrocardiogram	*				*				*				*
Blood pressure	*	*	*	*	*	*	*	*	*	*	*	*	*

*Indicates intervals at which the respective studies are usually performed.

because the intramuscular absorption from poorly perfused muscles may be erratic. When the blood pressure is stable, insulin can be given IV or IM.

A continuous infusion of regular insulin at a rate of 6 to 10 units per hours is usually adequate.

When insulin is given IV, some of it may bind to the glass container and to the plastic tubing. This can be counteracted by adding 100 units regular insulin to 1 liter full-strength (isotonic) saline solution and discarding the first 50 mL of the solution.

One milliliter per minute of this solution will deliver 6 units of insulin per hour. The solution should be given with an infusion pump if possible or with a pediatric microdrip bulb that delivers 1 mL with 60 drops.

100 units insulin in 1000 mL. (1 L) = 0.1 unit in 1 mL.

If 1 mL is delivered per min, 60 mL will be delivered in 1 hour. Therefore, $0.1 \times 60 = 6$ units of insulin will be delivered in 1 hour.

One must be careful not to lower the blood glucose concentration too fast. If this occurs, the plasma glucose concentration falls below the intracerebral glucose concentration because of the blood-brain barrier. This can lead to mental confusion and other neurological abnormalities.

The IV insulin is given at the rate described above until the blood glucose concentration falls to approximately 250 mg/dL. (With adequate insulin therapy, the blood glucose concentration should fall from 75 to 100 mg/dL per hour).

When the blood glucose concentration reaches 250 mg/dL and when the ketosis disappears, the IV insulin can be stopped and regular insulin subcutaneously should be started every 2 hours.

The dose of regular subcutaneous insulin can be determined from blood glucose concentrations, or from double-voided urine specimens (to make certain that one is not checking the glucose concentration of residual urine in the bladder).

Regular insulin can be given subcutaneously every 2 to 4 hours on the basis of blood sugar determinations.

Determining the Degree of Ketosis

The degree of ketosis can be determined in a general way, using the effect of plasma (or serum) on a crushed Acetest tablet. However, the test has several limitations:

1. It is inherently semi-quantitative.
2. It does not measure beta-hydroxybutyrate, which is often the predominant keto acid.
3. Shift from beta-hydroxybutyrate to acetoacetate often occurs during successful insulin therapy, so that increasingly positive Acetest reactions may be misleading.

Thus, sequential Acetest reactives are generally not valuable. Careful following of the sequential anion gap and HCO_3 levels are the best practical ways of monitoring clearance of ketoacidosis.

Insulin Resistance

If, after the first 2 hours of IV insulin therapy, the plasma glucose concentration is not decreasing and the arterial pH is not increasing, then the insulin dosage should be doubled every 2 hours until a significant response is observed (Schade and Eaton).

An alternate therapy to combat such insulin resistance is to give the patient 100 units of regular insulin IV. The dose may be doubled every 1 to 2 hours (100, 200, 400 units, etc.) if no response is obtained (Kleeman and Narins).

Use of Regular Insulin IM

Six to 10 units of regular insulin can be injected IM preferably into the arms rather than the buttocks, hourly. The same conditions described above for the use of IV insulin apply.

The blood sugar level should not be lowered too rapidly because, when severe hyperglycemia occurs, the glucose concentration of the interstitial spaces of the brain also rises, in spite of the blood-brain barrier. If the blood sugar concentration falls too rapidly with treatment, the osmotic pressure of the blood rapidly falls below that of the brain interstitial fluid. Therefore, water moves out of the blood and into the brain tissue and may cause cerebral edema and coma (Fulop, et al).

Sodium Loss

Most patients with diabetic acidosis show a loss of sodium ions as well as water. Therefore, intravenous fluids should be started with a sodium-containing solution such as isotonic saline (sodium chloride solution) (although some physicians prefer to start with half-strength sodium chloride solution). Two to 3 liters of isotonic sodium chloride solution can be given in the first 6 to 12 hours. The first 2 liters can be given at a rate of 500 to 1000 mL/hr. If more than 3000 mL of isotonic sodium chloride solution is given in the first 24 hours, a metabolic acidosis due to the high chloride content of the sodium chloride solution may be induced. Therefore, half-strength sodium chloride solution should be used after the first 3 to 4 liters of isotonic sodium chloride solution have been infused.

Patients may require as much as 6 liters or more of fluid to correct the water loss. If the patient is elderly or has organic heart disease, one should observe for signs of developing congestive heart failure such as increased respiratory rate, engorged liver, distended neck veins, and edema.

Shock

Sodium chloride solution may cause the shock to disappear. If this does not relieve the shock, dextran, plasma, or blood (if anemia is present) can be used.

Alkalinizing Solutions

There is a difference of opinion as to whether an alkalinizing solution should be used routinely in the treatment of diabetic acidosis. We believe that it is usually not necessary for the following reasons:

1. The basic cause of the acidosis is the lack of insulin and the accumulation of keto acids. Therefore, as insulin is given and the keto acids are metabolized, the acidosis disappears.
2. Sodium bicarbonate may paradoxically increase spinal fluid acidosis and may precipitate coma (Ohman, et al).
3. When diabetic acidosis is treated the usual way, rises in CO_2 content, serum bicarbonate concentration, and pH are associated with the elimination of keto acids from the blood. However, if sodium bicarbonate is given, it will cause only these values to rise and may obscure the persistence of a significant ketonemia.
4. When the CO_2 content or the serum bicarbonate concentration is raised too high with sodium bicarbonate therapy, a metabolic alkalosis may develop (Chapter 17).
5. Bicarbonate therapy may worsen tissue oxygen delivery by depleting red blood cell phosphates (2,3 DPG).

However, when the CO_2 content is below 10 mEq/L, or the serum bicarbonate concentration is below 9 mEq/L, or the pH is 7.1 or less, insulin is less effective. Therefore, sodium bicarbonate can be used. The dosage of sodium bicarbonate is described in Chapter 17.

Sugar Solutions

As was pointed out above, dextrose in water infusion is not needed until the blood glucose concentration falls to approximately 250 mg/dL. This may not occur for 4 hours or longer if the initial blood glucose concentration had been high.

When the blood glucose concentration has fallen to this level, there is danger that hypoglycemia may suddenly occur. If this occurs, neurological complications, described above, may develop. Hypoglycemia can be avoided by starting an infusion of 5% or 10% dextrose in water at this time. One should try to maintain the blood glucose concentration between 200 and 300 mg/dL for the first day of therapy. From 1 to 3 liters may be needed in the next 24 hours.

Potassium Salts

A marked urinary (or gastrointestinal) loss of potassium ions often occurs in patients with diabetic acidosis, and it has been estimated that such patients have a total potassium deficit of usually 3 to 10 mEq per kg body weight. However, it is not necessary to restore this loss in the first 24 hours of treatment. In addition, it may be dangerous to give potassium chloride while the patient is in shock and is passing only a small volume of urine. However, when the blood sugar concentration begins to fall, as after the sixth hour of treatment, or when the urine output increases, or when the serum potassium concentration falls to 4 mEq/L or lower, or when the electrocardiogram begins to show signs of hypokalemia, potassium ions may be needed to prevent serious hypokalemia.

Approximately 40 mEq/L of potassium ions (3 g of potassium chloride) can be given intravenously in the saline or dextrose solution being infused. It is sometimes necessary to give as much as 200 to 300 mEq of potassium ions during the first 24 hours of treatment.

The electrocardiogram or preferably serum potassium concentrations can be used to determine the amount of potassium chloride needed and to prevent hypokalemia.

Phosphate and Magnesium Salts

It has been shown that patients with diabetic acidosis lose phosphate and magnesium ions during therapy. However, the addition of these ions does not seem to increase the rate of recovery.

If desired, potassium phosphate can be given at a rate of 2.5 mM per hour. Potassium phosphate is available in 1-mm vials (for dilution and intravenous use) that contain 3 mM phosphate and approximately 4.5 mEq potassium.

Magnesium sulfate can be given IV as 500 mL of a 2% solution, given over a period of 4 to 6 hours.

Other Therapy

Gastric aspiration with a Levin tube is indicated only if there is severe vomiting or gastric dilatation. Lavage of the stomach is not necessary, nor is the instillation of either a saline or sodium bicarbonate solution.

It is not necessary to catheterize the bladder routinely. This should be done only if the patient does not produce a urine sample after 3 or 4 hours of treatment, or is comatose.

Bibliography

Alberti, KGMM, Hockaday, TDR, and Turner, RC: Small doses of intramuscular insulin in the treatment of diabetic "coma." Lancet 2:515, 1973.

Andrué, HJ, Barrero, J, and Eknoyan, G: Salutary effects of modest fluid replacement in the treatment of adults with diabetic ketoacidosis: Use in patients without extreme fluid deficit. JAMA 262:2108, 1989.

Andrué, HJ, et al: Plasma acid-base patterns in diabetic ketoacidosis. N Engl J Med 307:1603, 1982.

Assal, JP, et al: Metabolic effects of sodium bicarbonate in management of diabetic ketoacidosis. Diabetes 23:405, 1974.

Bendezu, R, et al: Experience with low-dose insulin infusion in diabetic ketoacidosis and diabetic hyperosmolarity. JAMA 138:60, 1978.

Bolli, GB, and Gerich, JE: The "dawn" phenomenon. A common occurrence in both non–insulin-dependent and insulin-dependent diabetes mellitus. N Engl J Med 310:746, 1984.

Carroll, P, and Matz, R: Uncontrolled diabetes mellitus in adults. Diabetes Care 6:579, 1981.

Cobble, SP: Insulin: not recommended in infusions. JAMA 230:468, 1974.

Connors, JM: Insulin therapy in diabetic ketoacidosis, comments. Ann Intern Med 86:109, 1977.

Cooperman, MT, et al: Clinical studies of alcoholic ketoacidosis. Diabetes 23:433, 1974.

Farah, D, et al: Paracetamol interference with blood glucose analysis. A potentially fatal phenomenon. BMJ 285:172, 1982.

Felig, P: Diabetic acidosis. N Engl J Med 290:1360, 1974.

Felts, PW: Ketoacidosis. Med Clin North Am 67:831, July 1983.

Fisher, JN, Shahshahani, MN, and Kitabchi, AE: Diabetic ketoacidosis. Low-dose insuline therapy by various routes. N Engl J Med 297:238, 1977.

Foster, DW, and McGarry, JD: The metabolic derangements and treatment of diabetic ketoacidosis. N Engl J Med 309:159, 1983.

Fulop, M, et al: Ketotic hyperosmolar coma. Lancet 2:635, 1973.

Gerich, JE, et al: Prevention of human diabetic ketoacidosis by somatostatin. Evidence for an essential role of glucagon. N Engl J Med 292:985, 1975.

Glasgow, AM: Hyperglycemic response to massive doses of commercial insulin. Diabetes, 19:28, 1970.

Jenkins, DW, Eckel, RE, and Craig, JW: Alcoholic ketoacidosis. JAMA 217:177, 1971.

Jimenez, JA, et al: Metabolic alkalosis in diabetic ketosis. JAMA 233:1193, 1975.

Kleeman, CR, and Narins, RG: Diabetic acidosis and coma. In Maxwell, MH and Kleeman, CR (ed.): *Clinical Disorders of Fluid and Electrolyte Metabolism,* 3rd ed. New York, McGraw-Hill, 1980.

Kreisberg, RA: Diabetic ketoacidosis. New concepts and trends in pathogenesis and treatment. Ann Intern Med 88:695, 1978.

Lucas, CP, Grant, N, Daly, WJ, and Reaven, GM: Diabetic coma without ketoacidosis. Lancet 1:75, 1963.

Matz, R: Diabetic coma. Guidelines in therapy. NY State J Med 74:642, 1974.

Matz, R: Diabetic acidosis. Rationale for not using bicarbonate. NY State J Med 76:1299, 1976.

Metzter, AL, and Rubenstein, AH: Reversible cerebral edema complicating diabetic ketoacidosis. Br Heart J 3:746, 1970.

Mishbin, RI: Insulin resistance in ketoacidosis, correspondence. N Engl J Med 297:893, 1977.

Molnar, GD, and Service, FJ: Low-dosage continuous insulin infusion for diabetic coma. Editorial notes. Ann Intern Med 81:853, 1974.

Munro, JF, et al: Euglycemic diabetic ketoacidosis. BMJ 2:578, 1973.

National Diabetes Data Group: Classification and diagnosis of diabetes mellitus and other categories of glucose intolerance. Diabetes 28:1039, 1979.

Oh, MS, Carroll, HJ, and Uribarri, J: Mechanism of normochloremic and hyperchloremic acidemia in diabetic ketoacidosis. Nephron 54:1, 1990.

Ohman, JL, Jr, et al: The cerebrospinal fluid in diabetic ketoacidosis. N Engl J Med 284:283, 1971.

Page, M, McB, et al: Treatment of diabetic coma with continuous low-dose infusion of insulin. BMJ 2:687, 1974.

Pagliara, AS: Managing ketoacidosis in diabetic patients. Consultant, p. 121, March 1981.

Peterson, L, et al: Insulin absorbance ot polyvinylchloride surfaces with implications for constant infusion therapy. Diabetes 25:72, 1976.

Podolsky, S: Nonketotic diabetic coma in the cardiac patient. Cardiovasc Rev Reports 4:201, 1983.

Roggin, GM, et al: Ketosis and metabolic alkalosis in a patient with diabetes. JAMA 221:296, 1970.

Schade, DS, and Eaton, RP: Diabetic ketoacidosis. Pathogenesis, prevention, and therapy. Clin Endocrinol Metab 12:321, 1983.

Sherwin, RS, and Felig, P: Hyperglucagonemia in diabetes, letter. N Engl J Med 299:1366, 1978.

Siegel, AJ, Steinke, J, and Bell, WR: Insulin-resistant diabetic coma. Arch Intern Med 134:562, 1974.

Taylor, AL: Diabetic ketoacidosis. Postgrad Med 66:161, 1980.

Warren, SE: False-positive urine ketone test with captopril, letter. N Engl J Med 303:1003, 1980.

Zileli, MS, et al: Oxazepam intoxication simulating non-ketoacidotic diabetic coma. JAMA 215:1986, 1971.

25

METABOLIC ACIDOSIS SYNDROMES (Continued)

SALICYLATE POISONING

Salicylate poisoning is commonly observed in infants and children under the age of 1 year. However, it also occurs in adults. It can be produced by the oral ingestion of acetylsalicylic acid (aspirin), methyl salicylate (oil of wintergreen), salicylic acid, sodium salicylate, or even by the use of salicylic acid ointments.

PATHOPHYSIOLOGY

Salicylates cause two types of acid-base disturbances. First, a primary stimulation of the respiratory center of the brain occurs. This produces a marked hyperventilation and a primary respiratory alkalosis. Within 3 to 24 hours usually, sometimes within 1 hour, the salicylate disturbs carbohydrate metabolism and causes a depletion of liver glycogen. As a result, ketone and particularly lactic and pyruvic acids accumulate in the body. This causes a primary metabolic acidosis. Hyperglycemia may also develop. The salicylates also interfere with prothrombin and fibrinogen formation in the liver.

When the respiratory alkalosis develops, the renal compensatory mechanisms cause an excretion of bicarbonate and other basic salts. This tends to produce a compensatory metabolic acidosis superimposed on the lactic acidosis. The respiratory alkalosis can also produce hypokalemia, which may be severe and may persist even after the metabolic acidosis has developed.

(Eichenholz has shown that if the respiratory alkalosis is prevented, by having subjects who have received an excessive amount of salicylates inhale a mixture high in carbon dioxide, the metabolic acidosis does not develop.)

The toxicity of salicylates is related more to their blood level than to

233

the amount ingested. Ordinarily, the toxic blood salicylate level is 30 mg/dL. However, severe intoxication can occur at a lower blood concentration. Conversely, no toxicity may occur in other patients with a much higher blood salicylate concentration.

SYMPTOMS AND SIGNS

These vary with the age of the patient. In adults, the classic symptoms of salicylism occur—vertigo, tinnitus, impaired hearing, and visual blurring. Anorexia, nausea, vomiting, sweating, pallor, flushing, cyanosis, and tetany may also occur. In addition, pulmonary edema may develop, either as a direct lung injury or due to iatrogenic fluid overload.

Numbness and tingling of the face, lips and extremities may occur as a result of the hyperventilation. Fever is usually present. Bleeding may also develop. Later erythema, scarlatinal, or desquamative rashes may appear.

Signs of central nervous toxicity are also common—hyperventilation, mental confusion, excitement or hyperactivity, disorientation, or delirium (salicylate "jag"). Muscle twitchings or convulsions can also occur, and may be followed by progressive central nervous system depression with lethargy, stupor, coma, and death (terminal respiratory acidosis). (This is probably due to an abnormally low glucose concentration in brain cells, produced by the salicylates.) Acute renal failure or injury to the liver may also develop.

LABORATORY FINDINGS

Blood

The blood findings depend on the presence of respiratory alkalosis, or metabolic acidosis, and on the occurrence of vomiting or other losses of water and electrolytes. Water loss and hypernatremia are common. Hyperglycemia or hypoglycemia may be present. The white blood count may be elevated.

Urine

Oliguria may be present, with albumin, red blood cells, and casts. Positive tests for glucose or ketone acids and acetone may be present but may be false positives. However, salicylate poisoning can cause a true diabetes-like condition to develop temporarily.

Salicylic acid can be detected in the urine by means of the ferric chloride test. A sample of urine is boiled to vaporize acetone and ketone substances. Then a 10% solution of ferric chloride is added. This causes a strong purple color in the presence of salicylic acid.

Example: An adult who has taken an excessive amount of acetylsalicylic acid (aspirin).

    Blood salicylate concentration 60 mg/dL

    pH 7.4

    P_{CO_2} 18.4 mm Hg

    CO_2 content 11.6 mEq/L

    Standard bicarbonate 16.3 mEq/L

    Actual bicarbonate 11 mEq/L

    Base excess − 10.5 mEq/L

The pH is normal. However, the P_{CO_2} is low. This indicates that a respiratory alkalosis is present. Similarly, the actual bicarbonate is lower than the standard bicarbonate, because of the respiratory alkalosis.

The low standard bicarbonate and the negative base excess indicate that a metabolic acidosis is also present. Therefore, a respiratory alkalosis and a metabolic acidosis are present (Chapter 15).

Cation-Anion Balance:

Na 140   K 4.0 HCO_3 11   Cl 106 mEq/L

Anion gap = (Na + K) − (HCO_3 + Cl)

           = (140 + 4) − (11 + 106)

           = 144 − 117

           = 27 mEq/L. This is abnormally high and is due to the accumulation of lactic and other metabolic acids.

DIAGNOSIS

Salicylate poisoning can be confused with diabetic acidosis and coma because both conditions may show hyperpnea, hyperglycemia, ketonemia, glycosuria, and ketonuria. The urinary test for salicylic acid has been described above. One should also remember that a true diabetic-like state can be produced by salicylate poisoning.

The best way to make a diagnosis of salicylate poisoning is to obtain a history of salicylate ingestion and to find a high blood salicylate concentration.

COURSE AND PROGNOSIS

Salicylate poisoning is a serious condition because death often occurs in spite of vigorous treatment. Death is probably due to a toxic encephalopathy.

PROPHYLAXIS

Salicylate toxicity does not usually occur in adults until a daily dose of aspirin, for example, exceeds 5 g (15 five-grain tablets). There is no direct correlation between salicylate dosage and the appearance of even mild toxic symptoms, such as tinnitus.

Salicylate dosage must be carefully regulated, especially in elderly patients. In addition, changes in the urine pH (due to changes in diet, medication, and so on) directly affect blood salicylate levels—the lower the urinary pH, the higher the blood salicylate level.

TREATMENT

Serum salicylate concentration should be determined. If it is higher than 70 mg/dL, this is an indication for hemodialysis. (Peritoneal dialysis is relatively ineffective in removing salicylates.)

If the patient is seen early after the ingestion of salicylates, gastric lavage with isotonic saline solution, using a wide-bore Jacques, 30-gauge French tube, can be done (although the value of this has been questioned). Sodium bicarbonate should *not* be used for stomach lavage, because it increases the absorption of salicylates from the gastrointestinal tract.

Oral administration of an aqueous suspension of activated charcoal in an amount up to 10 times the amount of salicylates that have been ingested may also reduce the salicylate absorption. This should be done preferably within 30 minutes (or within several hours) after the salicylates have been ingested. Vomiting can be induced, using syrup of ipecac, if the patient is awake and alert. (Activated charcoal should not be given prior to the administration of ipecac, because it inactivates ipecac.)

During the stage of respiratory alkalosis, dextrose in water should be given intravenously to enhance renal excretion of the salicylates. The dextrose also prevents excessive lowering of the glucose content of the brain cells. The water counteracts the water loss produced by hyperventilation and/or fever.

When metabolic acidosis develops, particularly when the pH is low, sodium bicarbonate should be given intravenously because the metabolic acidosis is associated with increased ionization of the salicylate ions and their increased movement out of the blood and into cells. This increases the salicylate toxicity, even though the serum salicylate level falls when this happens.

The amount of sodium bicarbonate should be determined from changes in pH. However, because the respiratory alkalosis may persist longer than the metabolic acidosis, the pH should be raised to only 7.30—but not higher—to prevent the development of severe alkalosis (respiratory and metabolic). Excessive sodium bicarbonate must be avoided because of the potential for pulmonary edema.

Potassium chloride should be given intravenously in conjunction with the sodium bicarbonate. Large doses may be needed, particularly if hypokalemia develops.

Calcium gluconate or chloride can be given for tetany. Vitamin K_1 oxide can be given if bleeding occurs. Fever is treated symptomatically.

Bibliography

American Hospital Formulary Service: Salicylates. Category 28:08.

Anderson, RI, et al: Unrecognized adult salicylate intoxication. Ann Intern Med 85:745, 1976.

Arena, FP, et al: Salicylate-induced hypoglycemia and ketoacidosis in a nondiabetic adult. Arch Intern Med 138:1153, 1978.

Cohen, AS: Differential diagnosis of salicylate intoxication and diabetic acidosis. N Engl J Med 254:457, 1956.

Eichenholz, A: Respiratory alkalosis. Arch Intern Med 116:699, 1965.

Eichenholz, A, Mulhausen, RO, and Redleaf, PS: Nature of acid-base disturbance in salicylate intoxication. Metabolism 12:164, 1963.

Ferguson, RK, and Boutros, AR: Death following self-poisoning with aspirin. JAMA 213:1186, 1970. Also JAMA 15:298, 1971.

Gabow, PA: How to avoid overlooking salicylate intoxication. J Crit Illness 1:77, 1986.

Hill, JB: Salicylate intoxication. N Engl J Med 288:1110, 1973.

Knochel, JP: The paradox in salicylate poisoning. J Crit Illness 1:3, 1986.

Koppes, GM, and Arnett, FC: Salicylate hepatotoxicity. Postgrad Med 56:193, 1974.

Levy, RI: Overwhelming salicylate intoxication in an adult. Acid-base changes during recovery with hemodialysis. Arch Intern Med 119:399, 1967.

Matthew, H: Gastric aspiration and lavage. Clin Toxicol 3:179, 1970.

Mongan, E, et al: Tinnitus as an indication of therapeutic serum salicylate levels. JAMA 226:142, 1973.

Rupp, DJ, et al: Acute polyuric renal failure after aspirin intoxication. Arch Intern Med 143:1237, 1983.

Singer, RB: Acid-base disturbance in salicylate intoxication. Medicine 33:1, 1954.

Temple, AR: Acute and chronic effects of aspirin toxicity and their treatment. Arch Intern Med 141:364, 1981.

Vivian, AS, and Goldberg, IB: Recognizing chronic salicylate intoxication in the elderly. Geriatrics 37:91, 1982.

Zimmerman, HJ: Effects of aspirin and acetaminophen on the liver. Arch Intern Med 141:333, 1981.

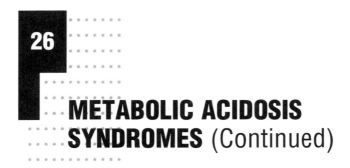

METABOLIC ACIDOSIS
SYNDROMES (Continued)

HYPERKALEMIA

Hyperkalemia is present when the serum potassium concentration is higher than 5.5 mEq/L.

Although it is possible to measure the total exchangeable body potassium experimentally, such measurements are not available for clinical purposes. Therefore, most physicians use the terms *hyperkalemia* (hyperpotassemia) and *hypokalemia* (hypopotassemia), which merely describe the serum potassium concentration, to indicate potassium excess and potassium loss. Unfortunately, a change in serum potassium concentration does not always correspond to a similar change in total exchangeable body potassium. For example, a low, normal, or high serum potassium concentration may exist with a low or normal total exchangeable body potassium level. However, it has been shown that an excess of total exchangeable body potassium may not occur in a patient with azotemic acidosis, for example, even though hyperkalemia may be present and even though the patient may die from the toxic effects of potassium.

One of the serious difficulties in studying potassium excess or potassium loss is that the potassium is essentially an intracellular ion. Measurement of serum potassium concentration merely indicates the extracellular concentration of the ion. For this reason, the electrocardiographic patterns of hyperkalemia and hypokalemia have been used instead of the serum potassium concentrations to determine whether hyperkalemia or hypokalemia is present. However, even this method is not completely accurate, as will be pointed out in this chapter and in Chapter 30.

Potassium balance is normally maintained by a daily dietary intake and excretion of about 50 to 100 mEq. This is equivalent to 3.73 to 7.46 g of potassium chloride. This is associated with a normal serum potassium concentration between 3.5 to 5.0 mEq/L.

PATHOPHYSIOLOGY

Both respiratory and metabolic acidosis (including diabetic and azotemic acidosis) are associated with hyperkalemia, which probably occurs as a compensatory mechanism. When the acidosis develops, the hydrogen ion concentration of the extracellular water increases. This causes potassium ions to move out of the cells into the extracellular water, and causes hydrogen and sodium ions to move into the cells. Conversely, the rapid infusion of a potassium salt, such as potassium chloride, will produce a metabolic acidosis.

The relations of potassium disturbances to muscle paralysis can be better understood by means of the following brief outline of the physiology of muscle contraction: The transmission of a nerve impulse from nerve endings to the motor end plate of muscle is due to the release of acetylcholine. Further conduction of the stimulus along the muscle fiber is related to electrical currents produced by potassium. This occurs because there is a potential difference of 90 millivolts between the inner (negative) and outer (positive) surface of the muscle fiber membrane. In other words, the membrane of the muscle fiber is polarized. The polarization is due to the difference in the concentration of potassium inside and outside the cells. The potassium concentration in the cell is very high, approximately 150 mEq/L, whereas the extracellular potassium concentration is low, approximately 4 mEq/L. When the muscle is stimulated, potassium moves out of the cell, depolarizes the cell membrane, and causes a stimulus to spread along the length of the muscle fiber.

The importance of this polarized state of the muscle cell membrane is that a persistent increased or decreased polarization can block the spread of the stimulus along the muscle fiber. It can therefore cause either muscle weakness or paralysis.

Hypopolarization occurs when the concentration of potassium outside the cell is decreased, due to hypokalemia (or the concentration of potassium within the cell is increased). When the muscle is now stimulated, the degree of depolarization produced by acetylcholine is not sufficient to start the spread of the stimulus along the muscle fiber.

Hyperpolarization occurs with hyperkalemia (or when the potassium concentration within the muscle cell falls). When this occurs, the transmission of a stimulus along the muscle is also prevented.

Although potassium disturbances inside or outside the cell can cause muscle weakness or paralysis, measurements of potassium concentrations inside the cell cannot be done clinically. Therefore, muscle paralysis due to potassium disturbances is usually described in relation to hypokalemia or hyperkalemia.

The most serious effect of hyperkalemia is on the heart. Intraventricular conduction disturbance occurs with or without atrioventricular (AV) dissociation. Finally, ventricular fibrillation and cardiac arrest develop. Hyperkalemia also effects the peripheral nerves. Potassium is capable of stimulating pain receptors. This is the reason for the paresthesias that may develop.

ETIOLOGY

It has already been mentioned that an excess of total body potassium may not occur, in contrast to the retention and accumulation of sodium ions. Hyperkalemia may occur, however, in the following situations:

1. Spurious or artifactual causes. Artifactual hyperkalemia may occur if the blood sample hemolyzes, if there is venous stasis and muscular exercise of the extremity during a venipuncture, or if the venipuncture is done near the site of an intravenous infusion of potassium chloride. (A severe and dangerous hyperkalemia may occur if a bolus of potassium chloride solution is injected into the side arm of an intravenous infusion bottle and if the bottle is not inverted and agitated to disperse the potassium chloride throughout the bottle.)

   Hyperkalemia has been noted in vitro in patients with an abnormal elevation of the blood platelet count. Extreme leukocytosis in leukemia may also spuriously elevate the serum potassium level. These patients show no clinical or electrocardiographic signs of hyperkalemia.
2. Primary renal disease (acute or chronic renal failure). Hyperkalemia does not occur until the creatinine clearance decreases to approximately 10 mL/min or less. However, in patients with renal diseases that disproportionately interfere with tubular function (for example, obstructive uropathy, interstitial nephritis), hyperkalemia may occur with creatinine clearance only moderately reduced. Some of these patients may have renin deficiency (see No. 5 below).
3. Acidosis (metabolic or respiratory). Acidosis is associated with a rise in serum potassium concentration, even to a hyperkalemic level. Hyperchloremic metabolic acidosis is the most likely to produce this effect. This is not associated with clinical signs in most patients, but ventricular fibrillation and death due to hyperkalemia have been described in patients who develop acute respiratory acidosis, or in severely burned patients.
4. Adrenocortical insufficiency (Addison's disease). Most of these patients show neither clinical nor electrocardiographic signs of hyperkalemia. Rarely, severe and even fatal hyperkalemia may occur.
5. Hyperkalemia due to renin deficiency occurs with total adrenal insufficiency, the progressive loss of sodium ions and water and the decreased plasma volume stimulate renin release. However, in isolated hypoaldosteronism, renin activity is low. The primary disturbance is a defect in renin secretion. The hypoaldosteronism is secondary to this.

The defect in renin secretion is due to damage to the juxtoglomerular apparatus of the kidneys. Pathologically it is associated with pyelonephritis, nephrosclerosis, hyperparathyroidism, diabetes, gout. It can also be produced by nonsteroidal anti-inflammatory drugs, such as indomethacin.

6. Drugs. Hyperkalemia can also occur as a result of potassium-sparing diuretics, such as triamterene (Dyrenium) or spironolactone (Aldactone), and from other drugs (succinylcholine) when given to patients with neuromuscular disease; arginine, when given to patients with renal failure; aminocaproic acid, if renal function is decreased; antineoplastic drugs, probably as a result of destruction of neoplastic cells; arginine infusion if used in an azotemic patient; isoniazid (INH), if excessive doses are given; cephaloridine (Loridine); or penicillin G, potassium. (Each million units for intravenous use contains 1.7 mEq potassium ions.) Beta blockers, particularly those of the noncardioselective type, may also contribute to hyperkalemia by blocking $beta_2$-receptor-mediated cellular potassium uptake. Also, heparin may occasionally induce hyperkalemia by interfering with aldosterone biosynthesis.

7. Exogenous sources.
   a. Diet. When foods containing an excessive amount of potassium salts are ingested, hyperkalemia may develop. Normally, potassium balance is regulated by the urinary excretion of potassium ions. About 80% of ingested potassium salts is excreted in the urine, and approximately 20% in the stool. A normal person can take a single oral dose of 10 g potassium chloride without toxic effects. The dose will be excreted in approximately 4 to 8 hours. Even when the urinary elimination of potassium ions is impaired, as in patients with renal failure, signs of hyperkalemia do not usually appear. However, when the urinary output falls below 400 or 500 mL a day, the ingestion of a diet that contains a normal amount of potassium ions can cause hyperkalemia.
   b. Excessive intravenous administration of potassium chloride (or any potassium salt). The concentrations of potassium chloride that can be safely given intravenously to patients are described in Chapter 30. However, if the potassium chloride is infused too rapidly, or if renal insufficiency, inadequate urinary output, or acidosis is present, hyperkalemia may develop from the infusion of a small concentration of potassium chloride.

      One should remember that salt substitutes contain potassium chloride as a major ingredient. A salt substitute will not cause hyperkalemia in a patient with normal renal function, but hyperkalemia can occur if the salt substitute is given to a patient with renal failure.

c. A rapid transfusion of a large volume of bank blood (which may contain 20 mEq/L potassium ions or more, particularly if the blood is more than 10 days old). However, recent data have suggested that frank hyperkalemia is quite unlikely.

8. Endogenous sources. Tissue trauma liberates intracellular potassium ions. For example, hyperkalemia has been noted in the *crush syndrome*. However, the hyperkalemia in these patients is probably due mostly to the acute renal tubular failure that is present.

Hyperkalemia can also be classified according to pathophysiology, according to the presence of decreased and renal failure, decreased aldosterone secretion, potassium-sparing diuretics, and so on, or the presence of excessive exogenous potassium ions (diet, intravenous potassium salts, bank blood, and so on), or the presence of endogenous release of potassium ions (tissue trauma, succinylcholine, acidosis, and so on).

One should remember that hyperkalemia is frequently the result of numerous factors simultaneously present. For example, a patient with acute failure may also develop hyperkalemia due to acidosis, dietary excess of potassium salts, and tissue destruction.

SYMPTOMS AND SIGNS

Vague muscle weakness is usually the first symptom of hyperkalemia. Muscle paralysis develops over a period of several days. It is usually first noticed in the legs, then in the trunk and in the arms. The facial and respiratory muscles are affected last. The paralysis usually spares the muscles supplied by the cranial nerves.

The paralysis is flaccid, like what occurs with hypokalemia. Paresthesias of the face, tongue, feet, and hands may occur. Later, anesthesia may occur. In addition, the muscles are irritable and will respond to tapping or squeezing. Vibratory and position senses may be decreased or absent.

In spite of the muscle paralysis, the patient usually remains alert and apprehensive, and consciousness may persist until cardiac arrest and death occur. The heart rate may be slow and regular. In other patients, a slow or rapid irregular rate may be present.

There is no direct relation between the degree of muscle weakness or paralysis and the serum potassium concentration. However, when it reaches 10 to 12 mEq/L, ventricular fibrillation, cardiac arrest, and death usually occur.

A rare hereditary type of periodic muscle paralysis is associated with hyperkalemia, *adynamia episodica hereditaria*. Attacks can be precipitated by the ingestion of potassium chloride, and can be relieved by intravenous calcium gluconate, or by glucagon (30 µg per kg of body weight) intravenously, or epinephrine (0.25 to 0.4 mL of a 1:1000 dilution) subcutaneously. Dextroamphetamine sulfate in a daily dose of 10 to 15 mg (in the form of Dexedrine Spansules, S.K.F.) has been found helpful in preventing attacks. The way in which this drug causes a fall of serum potassium concentration is not known. Carbonic anhydrase inhibitors and other diuretics that promote the excretion of potassium have also been found helpful.

ELECTROCARDIOGRAM

The electrocardiographic changes that occur with hyperkalemia (Fig. 26–1) can be related in a general way to the serum potassium concentration:

- At a concentration of approximately 6 to 7 mEq/L, tall peaked T waves with a narrow base and a normal or decreased QT occur *(A)*.
- At approximately 8 mEq/L, the P waves disappear or wander in and out of the QRS *(B)*.
- At approximately 10 mEq/L, wide, aberrant QRS complexes appear *(C)*.
- At approximately 11 mEq/L, biphasic deflections, caused by a fusion of the QRS complex, ST segment, and the T wave, appear *(D)*.
- At 12 mEq/L (or even at a lower concentration of 10 mEq/L), ventricular fibrillation and cardiac standstill and death may occur *(E)*.

With the onset of the wide aberrant QRS complexes and the loss of the P waves, an idioventricular rhythm develops that is similar to what occurs in complete AV block. The ventricular rate may be regular, irregular, slow, or rapid, and the tracing may even resemble a ventricular tachycardia. In addition, the shape of the abnormal QRS complexes may vary from beat to beat.

Marked hyperkalemia is sometimes associated with transient electrocardiographic patterns that simulate myocardial infarction. Elevation of ST segments, coved or inverted T waves, and even transient Q waves may ap-

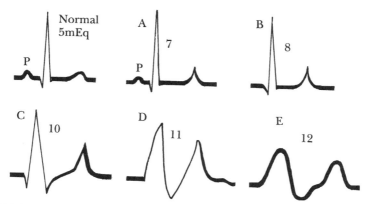

FIGURE 26–1. Electrocardiographic patterns of kyperkalemia.

pear. These pseudoinfarct patterns should disappear when the serum potassium concentration is lowered.

These electrocardiographic findings may not occur in patients with Addison's disease and with adrenocortical insufficiency in spite of the hyperkalemia that is present. The electrocardiogram may be normal, or the T waves may be flat or their direction reversed. In addition, when such patients are treated with desoxycorticosterone (DOCA) and the serum potassium concentration falls, the T waves may become large and normal again, in spite of the lowering of the serum potassium concentration. Alternatively, as in many patients with Addison's disease, the T-wave abnormalities may become more marked in spite of clinical improvement.

The presence of peaked T waves is not itself a pathognomonic sign of hyperkalemia, because such T waves may occur normally, or with myocardial infarction, intracranial hemorrhage, cardiac rupture, hemopericardium and so on.

LABORATORY FINDINGS

The serum potassium concentration is elevated to 5.5 mEq/L, or higher. The serum sodium concentration is often decreased. Serum calcium concentration may be normal or decreased. Other laboratory findings indicative of respiratory or metabolic acidosis are present.

If pseudohyperkalemia due to an increased platelet count is suspected, the potassium concentration of *plasma*, rather than serum, should be measured, because the potassium ions are released during clotting.

DIAGNOSIS

Hyperkalemia can be suspected in a patient with oliguria, anuria, or renal disease, or in a patient who is receiving potassium salts therapeutically who begins to complain of paresthesias. The serum potassium concentration will be 6 mEq/L, or higher. The electrocardiogram will show signs of hyperkalemia (except in patients with Addison's disease).

COURSE AND PROGNOSIS

The development of hyperkalemia is serious in patients with oliguria or anuria. Similarly, the cause of death in acute respiratory acidosis is probably the hyperkalemia that develops and causes ventricular fibrillation.

PROPHYLAXIS

Potassium should not be given to any patient with oliguria or anuria. In addition, even if a potassium deficit exists, as in a patient with diabetic acidosis, potassium should not be administered until the severity of the acidosis has decreased greatly, and the urinary output has increased.

One should also remember that the use of a low-sodium diet, such as the rice diet for a hypertensive patient who also has renal impairment, can cause a decrease in renal blood flow and a marked hyperkalemia. The hyperkalemia can be corrected in such patients by increasing the sodium content of the diet.

TREATMENT

Emergency Treatment

When the serum potassium concentration is 7.0 mEq/L or higher, or if the electrocardiogram shows serious changes such as disappearance of P waves or widening of the QRS complex, the following emergency treatment can be done:

1. Hypertonic 25% dextrose can be given intravenously into a large vein such as the superior vena cava with 1 unit of regular insulin per 4 or 5 g dextrose (1 unit insulin per 10 g dextrose if renal failure is present) (also see page 227). In a period of one-half hour 200 to 300 mL can be given. The serum potassium concentration will begin to fall in about one-half to 1 hour and will remain lowered for approximately 4 to 6 hours.

   An infusion of hypertonic dextrose causes the secretion of endogenous insulin. If the infusion is stopped suddenly, hypoglycemia may develop. This may be severe, if insulin had been added to the infusion bottle. For this reason, it is advisable to follow an infusion of hypertonic dextrose with an infusion of 250 to 500 ml of 5% dextrose in water.

2. Calcium gluconate or chloride can be given intravenously in a dose of 50 to 100 mL at a rate of 2 mL. Chamberlain has given as much as 90 mL of a 10% calcium chloride solution intravenously in a period of 5 minutes to treat hyperkalemia. When this is done, the patient should be monitored with an electrocardiograph, and the injection stopped as soon as electrocardiographic signs of hyperkalemia disappear. (The serum potassium concentration remains unchanged.) If necessary, the patient can then be given a daily dose of 100 mg of a 10% solution of calcium gluconate, as a prophylactic measure, if there is a possibility that the hyperkalemia will recur.

   The use of calcium salts to counteract hyperkalemia is contraindicated if the patient is receiving digitalis.

3. Hypertonic (7.5%) sodium bicarbonate solution given intravenously (Chapter 38) can lower the serum potassium concentration. It is most likely to be useful in patients with metabolic acidosis, but often is of little value, particularly in patients with chronic failure.

4. Beta agonists, such as terbutaline, are also effective.
5. Hemodialysis or peritoneal dialysis is also effective in lowering the serum potassium concentration. Hemodialysis, which is far more rapid in removing potassium, is the preferred modality in extreme cases.
6. Repeated electrocardiograms or serum potassium determinations should be used to check the therapy. However, the electrocardiogram cannot be used as a guide to the treatment of hyperkalemia in patients with Addison's disease.

Nonemergency Treatment

The following can also be done to lower the serum potassium concentration when a dangerous level of hyperkalemia is not present:

1. Low-potassium, high-carbohydrate diet can be prescribed. A low-potassium diet contains 40 mEq potassium ions or less daily. This is equivalent to approximately 3 g of potassium chloride daily. Table 26–1 lists foods high in potassium which should be avoided, foods low in potassium which can be used as desired, and the potassium content of other foods.
2. A sodium polystyrene sulfonate (Kayexalate) resin can also be used to remove potassium ions from the colon. The sodium ions of the resin are partially released and replaced by potassium ions. The potassium-containing resin is then excreted in the stool. Each gram of resin binds approximately 1 mEq potassium ions. This can cause a significant decrease in serum potassium concentration. However, an effect may not be apparent for several hours; therefore, the resin cannot be used for the emergency treatment of hyperkalemia.

The average adult dose of the resin is 15 g (approximately 4 heaping teaspoonfuls) orally, 1 to 4 times daily. The resin can be suspended in 150 to 200 mL of water, flavored with syrup. It can also be given by nasogastric tube. Twenty milliliters of a 70% sorbitol syrup is often given with each dose of resin. The sorbitol can even be given every 2 hours. Its purpose is to produce a mild diarrhea and in this way to prevent fecal impaction.

The resin can also be given rectally, once or twice daily, in a dose of 30 g suspended in 200 mL of water, or in equal amounts of water and 2% methylcellulose suspension, or in 10% dextrose solution. The enema should be at body temperature and should be retained for 4 to 10 hours, if possible. It should be followed by a cleansing enema. Rectal administration is not as effective as oral administration.

When the resin is used in a patient with acute renal failure, the amount of water given with the resin should be measured. In this way, excessive administration of water will be prevented.

Serum potassium concentrations should be determined daily during

TABLE 26–1
POTASSIUM CONTENT OF FOODS*

Minimal Potassium Content: butter or margarine, carbonated water, cranberry juice or sauce, ginger ale, gumdrops or jelly beans, lollypops or Charms, root beer, salad oil, sugar or honey, water ices or popsicles. Also spices (allspice, anise, basil, bay leaf, caraway, celery flakes, celery salt, chili powder, cinnamon, cream of tarter, curry, garlic, garlic powder, ginger, horseradish, mace, marjoram, mint leaves, dry mustard, nutmeg, onion powder, paprika, pepper, poppy seeds, rosemary, sage, sesame seeds, tarragon, thyme, turmeric, vanilla extract).

High Potassium Content: chocolate, coffee, cocoa, tea, dried fruits, dried peas or beans, ice cream or sherbet, milk desserts, molasses, whole grain breads and cereals, wild rice (also see Table 30–1).

The potassium content of other foods is as follows:

Dairy Products: 2 mEq potassium ions supplied by milk or cream, 1/2 cup, or sour cream, 1/4 cup. 1.75 mEq potassium ions supplied by cottage cheese, 1/2 cup, or cream or processed cheese, 1 oz.

Breads and Cereals: 1.25 mEq potassium ions supplied by: bread, 1 slice; cooked cereal (cornmeal, farina, cream of wheat, hominy grits, oatmeal), 1/2 cup; dry cereal (corn flakes, puffed rice, puffed wheat, shredded wheat), 1/4 cup; cooked macaroni, noodles, spaghetti, or rice, 1/2 cup; dry cereals (corn flakes, puffed rice, puffed wheat, shredded wheat), 3/4 cup.

Fruits: 2.5 mEq potassium ions supplied by: apple, 1 small; apple juice, 1/2 cup; applesauce, 1/3 cup; blueberries, fresh, 1 cup; orange, 1/2 small; peaches, canned, 1/2 cup; pears, canned, 1/2 cup; pineapple, canned, 1/2 cup (or 1 slice). 3.5 mEq potassium ions supplied by: fruit cocktail, 1/2 cup; grapes, seedless, 1/2 cup; grape juice, 1/2 cup; grapefruit, 1/2 medium; grapefruit juice, 1/2 cup; peach, fresh, 1 small: pineapple juice, 1/2 cup; pear, fresh, 1/2 small; strawberries, fresh, 10 large; strawberries, frozen, slices, 1/2 cup; tangerine, 1; watermelon, 1/2 cup.

Eggs: 1.75 mEq potassium ions supplied by: 1 egg, medium, prepared any way.

Meat and Poultry: 3 mEq potassium ions supplied by: 1 ounce of beef, lamb, liver, veal, chicken, or turkey.

Seafood: 1.75 mEq potassium ions supplied by: lobster, fresh, 1 ounce; oysters, fresh, 4; shrimp, fresh 1 ounce. 3 mEq potassium ions supplied by: 1 ounce cod, halibut, haddock, or salmon

Vegetables: 3 mEq potassium ions supplied by: beans, green or waxed, canned, 1/2 cup; beets, canned, 1/4 cup; carrots, canned, 1/4 cup; cucumber, 4 slices; corn, canned, 1/2 cup; lettuce, 2 large leaves; onions, cooked, 1/2 cup; peas, canned, 1/2 cup; summer squash, 1/2 cup; turnips, 1/2 cup. 6 mEq potassium supplied by: asparagus, frozen, 6 spears; broccoli, frozen, 1 stalk (or 1/2 cup); cabbage, raw, 1 cup; cabbage, cooked, 1/2 cup; cauliflower, cooked, 1 cup; corn, fresh, 1 4-inch ear; eggplant, cooked, 1/2 cup; okra, 1/2 cup; potato, boiled without skin, 1/4 cup; potato, candied sweet, 2 halves; potato, baked sweet, 1/2 small; pumpkin, canned, 1/2 cup; rutabagas, cooked, 1/2 cup; winter squash, frozen, 1/2 cup; tomato, 1 small; tomato juice, 1/2 cup.

---

*A low-potassium diet contains 40 mEq potassium ions or less daily. This is equivalent to approximately 3 g of potassium chloride daily.

resin therapy, and the resin should be stopped when the serum potassium concentration falls to 4 or 5 mEq/L. (The resin should be stopped when the serum potassium concentration falls to a level that is slightly higher than desired. The reason for this is that the resin that is already present in the gastrointestinal tract continues to remove potassium ions until it is eliminated in the stool.)

Adverse effects of the resin include anorexia, nausea, vomiting, hypokalemia, hypokalcemia, severe constipation, and even fecal impaction. Because hypokalemia may occur, the resin must be used cautiously in patients receiving digitalis preparations to avoid digitalis toxicity (which can be precipitated by hypokalemia). Similarly, when the resin is used for more than several days, it can cause a marked loss of calcium (and magnesium) ions. This can be prevented by determining the serum calcium concentration. If it begins to fall, calcium chloride or gluconate can be given intravenously.

Since sodium ions are released into the large intestine by the resin, they may be absorbed into the body. Therefore, the resin should be used cautiously if congestive heart failure is present.

Bibliography

Bellet, S, and Wasserman, F: The effects of molar sodium lactate in reversing the cardiotoxic effect of hyperpotassemia. Arch Intern Med 100:565, 1957.

Blumberg, A, Weidmann, P, and Gnadinger, M: Effect of various therapeutic approaches on plasma potassium and major regulating factors in terminal renal failure. Am J Med 85:507, 1988.

Bostic, O, and Duvernoy, WFC: Hyperkalemic cardiac arrest during transfusion of stored blood. J Electrocardiol 5:407, 1972.

Brown, MJ, Brown, DC, and Murphy, MB: Hypokalemia from beta$_2$ receptor stimulation by circulating epinephrine. N Engl J Med 309:1414, 1983.

Brown, RS: Extrarenal potassium homeostasis. Kidney Int 30:116, 1986.

Bushinsky, DA, and Gennari, FJ: Life-threatening hyperkalemia induced by arginine. Ann Intern Med 89:632, 1978.

Chamberlain, MJ: Emergency treatment of hyperkalemia. Lancet 1:464, 1964.

Cooperman, LH: Succinylcholine-induced hyperkalemia in neuromuscular disease. JAMA 213:1867, 1970.

Don, BR, Sebastian, A, Cheitlin, M, et al: Pseudohyperkalemia caused by fist clenching during phlebotomy. N Engl J Med 322:1290, 1990.

Egan, TJ, and Klein, R: Hyperkalemic familial periodic paralysis. Pediatrics 24:761, 1959.

Ethier, JH, Kamel, KS, Magner, PO, et al: The trans-tubular potassium concentration in patients with hyperkalemia. Am J Kidney Dis 15:309, 1990.

Fenech, FF, and Solar, NG: Hyperkalemic periodic paralysis starting at age of 48. BMJ 2:472, 1968.

Goldfarb, S, et al: Acute hyperkalemia induced by hyperglycemia. Ann Intern Med 84:426, 1976.

Graber, M, Subramani, K, Copish, D, and Schwab, A: Thrombocytosis elevates serum potassium. Am J Kidney Dis 12:116, 1988.

Haddad, A, and Strong, E: Potassium in salt substitutes, letter. N Engl J Med 292:1082, 1975.

Herz, P, and Richardson, JA: Arginine-induced hyperkalemia in renal failure patients. Arch Intern Med 130:778, 1972.

Howard, JA, and Kosowsky, BD: Electrocardiographic diagnosis of hyperkalemia in the presence of ventricular pacing and atrial fibrillation. Chest 78:491, 1980.

Hultgren, HN, Swenson, R, and Wettach, G: Cardiac arrest due to oral potassium administration. Am J Med 58:139, 1975.

Kurtzman, NA, Gonzalez, J, DeFronzo, RA, and Giebish, G: A patient with hyperkalemia and metabolic acidosis. Am J Kidney Dis 15:333, 1990.

McArdle, B: Adynamia episodica hereditaria and its treatment. Brain 85:(I), 121, 1962.

Magner, PO, Robinson, L, Halperin, RM, et al: The plasma potassium concentration in metabolic acidosis: A re-evaluation. Am J Kidney Dis 11:220, 1988.

Nicolis, GL, et al: Glucose-induced hyperkalemia in diabetic subjects. Arch Intern Med 141:49, 1981.

Perez, G, Siegel, L, and Schreiner, GE: Selective hypoaldosteronism with hyperkalemia. Ann Intern Med 76:757, 1972.

Pollen, RH, and Williams, RH: Hyperkalemia neuromyopathy in Addison's disease. N Engl J Med 263:273, 1960.

Pongpaew, C, Na Songkhla, R, and Kozam, RL: Hyperkalemic cardiac arrhythmia secondary to spironolactone. Chest 63:1023, 1973.

Popovtzer, MM, et al: Hyperkalemia in salt-wasting nephropathy. Arch Intern Med 132:203, 1973.

Rabelink, TJ, Koomas, HA, Henlaae, RJ, Dorhout Mees, EJ: Early and late adjustment to potassium loading in humans. Kidney Int 38:942, 1990.

Rimmer, JM, Horn JF, Gennari FJ: Hyperkalemia as a complication of drug therapy. Arch Intern Med 147:876, 1987.

Salem, MM, Rosa, RM, Batlle, DC: Extrarenal potassium tolerance in chronic renal failure: Implications for the treatment of acute hyperkalemia. Am J Kidney Dis 18:421, 1991.

Schambelan, M, et al: Isolated hypoaldosteronism in adults. A renin-deficiency syndrome. N Engl J Med 287:576, 1972.

Thomson, RL: Potassium penicillin G. N Engl J Med 271:1218, 1964.

Van Dellen, RG, and Purnell, DC: Hyerkalemic paralysis in Addison's disease. Mayo Clin Proc 44:904, 1969.

Walker, BR, et al: Hyperkalemia after triamterene in diabetic patients. Clin Pharmacol Ther 13:643, 1972.

Williams, FA, Jr, et al: Acquired primary hypoaldosteronism due to an isolated zona glomerulosa defect. N Engl J Med 309:1623, 1983.

Williams, ME, and Rosa, RM: Hyperkalemia: Disorders of internal and external potassium balance. J Intensive Care Med 3:63, 1988.

Williams, RHP: Potassium overdosage. A potential hazard of nonrigid parenteral fluid containers. BMJ 1:714, 1973.

27

ALCOHOLIC KETOACIDOSIS

Chronic alcoholics frequently develop high-anion-gap acidosis in the setting of binge drinking and poor nutrition. Beta-hydroxybutyric acid is the predominant acid, but acetoacetic and lactic acid may contribute. Starvation-induced insulin deficiency and hyperglucoagonemia promote the release of free fatty acids. The associated liver glycogen depletion sets the stage for accumulation of ketoacids, which are synthesized from the free fatty acids. Stress and extravascular volume depletion worsen the state by inducing increased levels of growth hormone, cortisol, and catecholamines—which all antagonize insulin action.

CLINICAL FEATURES

Alcoholic ketoacidosis (AKA) occurs in chronic alcoholics who stop eating but continue to consume large quantities of alcohol. In the vast majority of patients, symptoms include anorexia, nausea, vomiting, and abdominal discomfort. Tachycardia and tachypnea are regular features. Abdominal tenderness may be present, but not abdominal distention, rebound tenderness, or decreased bowel sounds. When present, the latter signs indicate a complication such as pancreatitits, hepatitis, or pneumonia. Hypothermia may be present (particularly when there is concomitant hypoglycemia). Fever is unusual unless there is a complicating process. Altered mental status is infrequent, unless there is an associated metabolic or structural brain problem.

LABORATORY TESTS

Leukocytosis may be present due to stress. Anemia is common. The BUN level may be elevated. Liver function tests may be abnormal. Levels of pancreatic enzymes such as amylase or lipase may be elevated, but do not necessarily indicate that pancreatitis is present.

A high-anion-gap acidosis results from the accumulation of beta-hydroxybutyrate and acetoacetate. Occasionally a lactic acidosis will also appear. As beta-hydroxybutyrate determination is not clinically available, the nitroprusside (Acetest) reaction is the most useful diagnostic test. Performed on serum, the reaction is almost always positive in AKA. As it is a semiquantitative assay for acetoacetate, its degree of reactivity provides no insight into severity. Blood pH, HCO_3 level, and the size of the anion gap provide such quantitative information. In less than 5% of AKA patients, the Acetest reaction may be totally negative. In such cases, the clinical diagnosis is supported by a normal lactate level, exclusion of any toxic ingestion, and a suggestive clinical presentation.

Serum sodium is mildly low in approximately one third of patients, usually reflecting salt depletion. Severe hyponatremia is unusual and suggests some concomitant condition. Serum potassium and magnesium levels are often low due to the effects of vomiting and chronic alcoholism.

The serum glucose level is usually normal or slightly elevated. Hypoglycemia occurs in approximately 10% of patients.

A test for ethanol is usually positive, although a substantial number of patients will have undetectable levels.

In addition to the wide anion gap acidosis, other acid-base abnormalities may be present. Metabolic alkalosis due to vomiting may be present and can be inferred when the pH and HCO_3 levels are not especially low and the anion gap is quite wide. Respiratory alkalosis, which may be acute or chronic, may further complicate the picture. Such a disturbance would be suggested by a PCO_2 substantially lower (and a pH substantially closer to normal) than would be expected for the degree of hypobicarbonatemia.

Hypophosphatemia and hypomagnesemia are common.

PROGNOSIS

The prognosis is generally good unless acute pancreatitis or sepsis is present. The acidosis generally clears in 12 to 24 hours with appropriate therapy.

TREATMENT

The decreased intravascular volume must be replenished with normal saline. Dextrose should be administered to hypoglycemic patients. Hypokalemia, hypophosphatemia, and hypomagnesemia should be treated as indicated. Improvement is noted within 12 to 24 hours in virtually all patients. Refractory acidosis strongly suggests some concomitant problem. Intravenous bicarbonate is rarely indicated, unless the pH is 7.10 or less. Insulin is rarely needed.

Bibliography

Hamburger, SA, Rush, DR, and Bosker, G: Endocrine and Metabolic Emergencies. Bowie, MD: Robert J. Brady, 1984.

Hamburger, SA, and Soloffi, A: Alcholic ketoacidosis—A review of 30 cases. J Women's Med Assoc 37:106, 1982.

Wrenn, KD, et al: The syndrome of alcoholic ketoacidosis. Am J Med 91:19, 1991.

Halperin, ML, et al: Metabolic acidosis in the alcoholic. Metabolism 32:308, 1983.

Androgue, HJ, et al: Salutary effects of moderate fluid replacement in the treatment of alcoholic ketoacidosis. JAMA 262:210, 1989.

28

RESPIRATORY ALKALOSIS

Primary respiratory alkalosis occurs as a result of a decreased partial pressure of carbon dioxide in the alveolar air, due to hyperventilation. It is the least common type of acid-base disturbance.

A compensatory respiratory alkalosis can also occur as a result of a metabolic acidosis. In such patients, the respiratory alkalosis may continue even though the metabolic acidosis is corrected (see Chapter 17).

Synonyms: Carbonic acid deficit, hypocapnia.

PATHOPHYSIOLOGY

Respiratory alkalosis occurs as a result of hyperventilation. This should not be confused with an increased respiratory rate (tachypnea), which may or may not be associated with hyperventilation. Conversely, hyperventilation can occur with a normal respiratory rate. The characteristic findings of hyperventilation are an increased tidal volume and increased alveolar ventilation.

When hyperventilation occurs, a large amount of carbon dioxide is eliminated from the body. This causes the bicarbonate–carbonic acid ratio and the pH to rise.

Compensatory mechanisms occur to restore the pH. The normal excretion of an acid urine by the kidneys decreases. Instead, the kidneys suppress hydrogen ion formation, suppress ammonia formation, suppress chloride ion excretion, and no longer conserve bicarbonate ions (see Chapter 12). In addition, potassium ions move from the extracellular water into the cells, and hydrogen and sodium ions move from the cells into the extracellar waters. As a result of all of these changes, a compensatory metabolic acidosis develops.

Respiratory alkalosis is also associated with an accumulation of lactate ions, which can lead to a metabolic acidosis independent of the usual compensatory metabolic acidosis.

ETIOLOGY

Respiratory alkalosis occurs as a result of stimulation of the respiratory center. The most common cause is the functional hyperventilation due to anxiety (hyperventilation syndrome). Other causes include central nervous system lesions involving the respiratory center of the medulla, such as encephalitis, brain tumor, or intracranial surgery; hypermetabolic conditions due to fever, especially gram-negative sepsis, hyperthyroidism, alcoholic intoxication (delirium tremens), or exercise; salicylate or paraldehyde intoxication or disulfiram plus alcohol; conditions associated with increased cardiac output, such as anemia, beriberi, or cirrhosis of the liver; assisted respiration with either a pressure-cycled or volume-cycled respirator; hypoxia due to congestive heart failure, congenital heart disease with a right-to-left shunt, pulmonary atelectasis, high altitude residence, or pulmonary fibrosis (alveolar capillary block). In addition, the condition may occur in patients with serious abdominal disease such as peritonitis, ascites, or metastatic neoplasms. It also may occur after the administration of progestational drugs.

Acute respiratory alkalosis can also occur as a compensatory reaction in respiratory acidosis patients who have received a tracheotomy due to the sudden increase in alveolar ventilation.

SYMPTOMS AND SIGNS

The most characteristic clinical picture occurs in the *hyperventilation syndrome*. The patient may complain of dizziness, which is not true vertigo but lightheadedness; circumoral paresthesias; numbness and tingling of the fingers and toes; sweating; palpitation; tinnitus; and tremulousness. Additional symptoms include dyspnea and air hunger; profuse sweating with a feeling of intense fear or panic or a feeling of unreality; muscle cramps; severe precordial chest pain including a sensation of tightness around the chest; or epigastric or lower abdominal pain with nausea, vomiting, or diarrhea; blurred vision; and loss of voice.

(Pitts and McClure have shown that the clinical picture of the hyperventilation syndrome can be experimentally produced in normal subjects by an intravenous infusion of sodium [DL] lacate.)

Signs include the hyperventilation and signs of tetany such as carpopedal spasm. Chvostek's and Trousseau's signs can also be elicited.

Atrial or ventricular tachyarrhythmias may also develop. These may be due to the alkalosis and/or the associated hypokalemia.

Convulsive tendencies are exaggerated by hyperventilation, and grand mal or focal convulsions can be provoked. The electroencephalogram shows paroxysmal or continuous slow waves with high voltage. However, these changes cannot be correlated with the arterial pH.

Mental and neurological symptoms and signs are likely to occur when the pH rises to 7.54 or higher (Kilburn).

When acute respiratory alkalosis occurs as a result of tracheotomy, the patient may develop shock or arrhythmias, including ventricular fibrillation.

LABORATORY FINDINGS

The P_{CO_2} is characteristically low, the pH is high, and CO_2 content and the actual bicarbonate are low. However, the standard bicarbonate level remains normal unless a compensatory metabolic acidosis occurs (Chapter 15).

It must be noted that acute respiratory alkalosis is associated with only modest metabolic compensation, i.e., the serum bicarbonate is expected to diminish by 2.5 mEq for each 10 mm Hg drop in P_{CO_2}. As respiratory alkalosis persists, progressive compensation occurs so that the serum bicarbonate is expected to diminish by 5 mEq for each 10 mm Hg drop in P_{CO_2}. Thus, the pH will be substantially more alkalotic in the patient with acute hyperventilation.

The bicarbonate concentration is low and the chloride concentration is reciprocally elevated. The serum sodium concentration may be normal or low due to a slightly increased sodium excretion by the kidneys. The serum potassium concentration is characteristically normal. A variable elevation of the arterial lactate concentration occurs. The serum phosphate concentration falls, but the serum calcium concentration remains normal.

The electrocardiogram of respiratory and metabolic alkalosis is similar (Chapter 29).

Example: Prolonged respiratory alkalosis due to encephalitis
P_{CO_2} 18 mm Hg
pH 7.5
CO_2 content 14.5 mEq/L
Standard bicarbonate 20.5 mEq/L
Actual bicarbonate 14 mEq/L
Base excess -4.5 mEq/L

The pH is high. This indicates an alkalosis. The P_{CO_2} is low. This indicates that a respiratory alkalosis is present. This is further indicated by the fact that the actual bicarbonate level is lower than the standard bicarbonate level. The negative base excess and the low standard bicarbonate value indicate that a metabolic acidosis is present. Therefore, a primary respiratory alkalosis is present with a partially compensatory metabolic acidosis.

Cation-Anion Balance:

Na 136   K 4 HCO_3 14   Cl 109 mEq/L

$$
\begin{aligned}
\text{Anion gap} &= (\text{Na} + \text{K}) - (HCO_3 + \text{Cl}) \\
&= (136 + 4) - (14 + 109) \\
&= 140 - 123 \\
&= 17 \text{ mEq/L. This is normal.}
\end{aligned}
$$

DIAGNOSIS

The hyperventilation of primary respiratory alkalosis can be confused with the hyperventilation resulting from a compensatory metabolic acidosis. However, tetany does not occur with the compensatory hyperventilation of a metabolic acidosis.

The pH is crucial in differential diagnosis. For example, a high pH in association with the low PCO_2 suggests a primary respiratory alkalosis with (or without) a compensatory metabolic acidosis. A normal pH in association with the low PCO_2 suggests a simultaneous primary respiratory alkalosis and a primary metabolic acidosis. A low pH in association with the low PCO_2 suggests a primary metabolic acidosis and a compensatory respiratory alkalosis.

COURSE AND PROGNOSIS

The condition is usually self-limited. In severe cases, catatonia and coma may occur.

TREATMENT

Treatment of the hyperventilation syndrome is difficult. The physician can make the patient aware of the cause of the symptoms by having him or her hyperventilate and precipitate symptoms. Then the patient should breathe into a paper bag (not a plastic bag) held closed around the nose and mouth to make the symptoms disappear.

A 5% carbon dioxide mixture with 95% oxygen has been used to treat patients with respiratory alkalosis. However, this can be dangerous because the respiratory center of patients with respiratory alkalosis is sensitive to carbon dioxide. Therefore, the inhalation of carbon dioxide may cause an increased hyperventilation. Patients with cerebral lesions can breathe a mixture of 5% carbon dioxide and 95% oxygen until clinical signs disappear.

If the PCO_2 is quickly restored to normal, the compensatory metabolic acidosis that is present may lower the pH to a dangerous level. It is therefore preferable to decrease the hyperventilation by using sedatives. In addition, it may be necessary to replace the bicarbonate ions that have been lost.

Bibliography

Ackerman, SH, and Sachar, EJ: The lactate theory of anxiety. A review and reevaluation. Psychosom Med 36:69, 1974.

Eichenholz, A, et al: Primary hypocapnia. A cause of metabolic acidosis. J Appl Physiol 17:283, 1962.

Eichenholz, A: Respiratory alkalosis. Arch Intern Med 116:689, 1965.

Gambino, SR: Acid-base balance in tetanus. JAMA 187:307, 1964.

Greene, NM: Fatal cardiovascular and respiratory failure associated with tracheotomy. N Engl J Med 261:846, 1959.

Halsam, MT: The relationship between the effect of lactate infusion on anxiety states and their amelioration by carbon dioxide inhalation. Br J Psychiat 125:88, 1974.

Kiely, JM: Organic disease presenting as hyperventilation syndrome. Psychosomatics 11:326, 1970.

Kilburn, KH: Shock, seizures and coma with alkalosis during mechanical ventilation. Ann Intern Med 65:977, 1966.

Krapf, R, Beeler, I, Hertner, D, and Hulter, HN: Chronic respiratory alkalosis—The effect of sustained hyperventilation on renal regulation of acid-base equilibrium. N Engl J Med 324:1394, 1991.

Krapf, R, Caduff, P, Wagdi, P, Staubli, M, and Hulter, HN: Plasma potassium response to acute respiratory alkalosis. Kidney Int 47:217–224, 1995.

Lane, DJ, Rout, MW, and Williamson, DH: Mechanism of hyperventilation in acute cerebrovascular accidents. BMJ 3:9, 1971.

Pitts, FN, Jr, and McClure, JN, Jr: Lactate metabolism in anxiety neurosis. N Engl J Med 277:1329, 1967.

Wilson, RF, et al: Severe alkalosis in critically ill surgical patients. Arch Surg 105:197, 1972.

29

METABOLIC ALKALOSIS SYNDROMES

Metabolic alkalosis is an alkalosis that results from a loss of hydrogen (and chloride) ions, or an excess of base (bicarbonate ions).

PATHOPHYSIOLOGY

When hydrogen ions are lost, or bicarbonate ions are retained in the body, the bicarbonate–carbonic acid ratio increases and the pH rises. As a result of this, the kidneys compensate for the rise in pH, just as in respiratory alkalosis (Chapter 28). In addition, breathing becomes more shallow and the PCO_2 rises, so that a respiratory acidosis develops to compensate for the metabolic alkalosis. In the past, it has been assumed that the compensatory respiratory acidosis was minimal, because respiratory acidosis might produce decreased oxygen saturation of the blood; in addition, the retention of carbon dioxide would serve as a stimulus for hyperventilation, which would reduce the PCO_2. However, studies have shown that the compensatory respiratory acidosis that develops in a patient with a primary metabolic alkalosis may be so severe that the PCO_2 may rise above a value of 55 mm Hg (Tuller and Mehdi; Lifschitz, et al and other researchers). (A PCO_2 value above 55 mm Hg has been considered a sign of primary respiratory acidosis, but this criterion is no longer valid.)

The electrolyte disturbances that occur in metabolic alkalosis are described below.

ETIOLOGY

Metabolic alkalosis can occur in the following situations:

1. When hydrochloric acid is lost from the body due to vomiting, gastric suction, or villous adenoma of the sigmoid colon.

Normally, the parietal cells of the stomach form carbonic acid from carbon dioxide and water by means of the enzyme carbonic anhydrase. The carbonic acid dissociates into hydrogen and bicarbonate ions. The hydrogen ions enter the lumen of the stomach along with chloride ions to form hydrochloric acid. The bicarbonate enters the bloodstream, producing the transient "alkaline tide" noted after meals.

In the alkaline medium of the intestines, the intestinal epithelial cells also form carbonic acid from carbon dioxide and water by means of carbonic anhydrase. However, the hydrogen ions pass back into the circulation through the lumen of the gut. This restores the neutrality of the blood, because the hydrogen ions that enter the blood from the intestinal cells neutralize the bicarbonate that had passed into the blood from the stomach.

When hydrogen ions are lost from the gastrointestinal tract, as in vomiting, the bicarbonate that passes into the blood from the stomach is not neutralized. This causes the bicarbonate–carbonic acid ratio and the pH to rise, producing a metabolic alkalosis. In addition, the vomiting also causes a loss of chloride and potassium ions that aggravate the alkalosis.

Alkalosis due to vomiting can occur in an otherwise normal patient. In addition, vomiting can occasionally cause an alkalosis in a patient with chronic renal disease. It is comparatively uncommon, because there is a high incidence of achlorhydria in these patients. Therefore, even if vomiting occurs, little hydrochloric acid is lost.

The excessive use of milk and an antacid, such as sodium bicarbonate or particularly calcium carbonate, in the treatment of a patient with peptic ulcer can produce not only a metabolic alkalosis but also severe hypercalcemia with renal insufficiency and azotemia *(milk-alkali syndrome)*.

2. When excessive sodium bicarbonate, or other alkaline salts such as sodium or potassium acetate, lactate, or citrate, are given orally or parenterally.

When sodium bicarbonate, for example, is ingested, the bicarbonate ions combine with the hydrochloric acid of the gastric juice, the hydrogen ions are neutralized, and carbon dioxide is formed and eliminated, namely,

$$NaHCO_3 + HCl \rightarrow H_2CO_3 + NaCl + CO_2 \uparrow$$

3. When excessive potassium ions are lost as a result of diarrhea, vomiting, cirrhosis of the liver, or any other condition (Chapter 31).

4. When hydrogen and chloride ions are lost from the body from excessive use of the thiazide diuretics, or from the use of the "loop" diuretics, furosemide (Lasix), or ethacrynic acid (Edecrin). (A metabolic alkalosis may also develop because of a loss of potassium ions in the urine [see Chapter 30].)

The thiazides inhibit the reabsorption of sodium ions in the distal renal tubule, and in this way increase the excretion of sodium and chloride ions in the urine (see Chapter 10). However, more chloride than sodium ions are excreted. Potassium and ammonium ions are also excreted with the excess chloride ions.

When the patient becomes refractory to the thiazide diuretics due to a low sodium intake or decreased renal blood flow, or when excessive amounts of the diuretics are given, the excretion of chloride ions continues. However, a large amount of potassium or ammonium ions, instead of sodium ions, is excreted along with the chloride ions. The mechanism by which the loss of potassium ions produces a metabolic alkalosis is discussed in Chapter 30. The excretion of each ammonium ion is associated with a loss of a hydrogen ion.

Furosemide and ethacrynic acid act by inhibiting active chloride reabsorption in the ascending limb of the loop of Henle. They are associated with an excretion of sodium and potassium ions. A large amount of water is also excreted from the kidneys.

When a large amount of water is excreted as a result of the action of either furosemide or ethacrynic acid, the bicarbonate–carbonic acid ratio may become higher because of the increased concentration of extracellular water. This is called a *contraction alkalosis.*

5. When prolonged hypercalcemia is associated with a metabolic alkalosis. This is probably due to loss of potassium ions in the urine resulting from disturbed renal tubular function produced by the hypercalcemia.

6. When metabolic alkalosis occurs during the diuretic phase of acute renal failure. This is also due to an excessive loss of potassium ions in the urine.

7. When metabolic alkalosis is due to the effects of aldosterone or a similar mineralocorticoid steroid, as in primary aldosteronism, Cushing's syndrome, malignant hypertension, renal artery stenosis, and so on (see Chapter 31).

Most metabolic alkalosis patients can be treated with chloride ions in the form of sodium chloride (*saline-responsive* metabolic alkalosis) rather than potassium chloride (which is preferable). This is due to the fact that these patients have a decreased (arterial) blood volume, from vomiting, for example. This stimulates the secretion of aldosterone, which causes an increased urinary loss of potassium ions. In addition, a decreased blood volume is associated with an increased reabsorption of bicarbonate ions from the tubular urine. When a large amount of sodium chloride is given to such a patient, either intravenously or even orally, chloride ions are supplied, the blood volume rises, the excessive secretion of aldosterone stops, the excessive urinary loss of potassium ions stops, and the excessive reabsorption of bicarbonate ions from the kidney tubules stops. As a result, metabolic balance reappears.

However, when the metabolic alkalosis is due to the effects of excessive aldosterone or another mineralocorticoid steroid, as in primary aldosteronism, the patient will not respond to sodium chloride and requires potassium chloride. This is known as a *saline-resistant* metabolic alkalosis. (A *saline-resistant* metabolic alkalosis can also occur when metabolic alkalosis is due to depletion of potassium ions and the serum potassium concentration is less than 2 mEq/L.)

Table 29–1 shows the different causes of saline-responsive and saline-resistant metabolic alkalosis.

The usual *saline-responsive* metabolic alkalosis can be differentiated from a *saline-resistant* metabolic alkalosis by means of the urinary chloride concentration, because in a *saline-responsive* metabolic alkalosis there are only minimal chloride ions in the urine (less than approximately 10 mEq/L unless the patient is receiving diuretics). However, when a *saline-resistant* metabolic alkalosis is present (and the patient is not receiving diuretics), the chloride concentration of the urine is more than approximately 10 mEq/L.

(The relative absence of chloride ions in patients with metabolic alkalosis due to the usual causes [loss of hydrogen and chloride ions resulting from a loss of gastric secretions, or from diuretic therapy] is as follows: When sodium ions are reabsorbed from the tubular filtrate into the blood, chloride ions are also usually reabsorbed, to preserve electroneutrality. However, when a metabolic alkalosis occurs due to a continued gastrointestinal loss of chloride ions, most if not all of the chloride ions that reach the tubular filtrate are reabsorbed, so that little or none appears in the urine.)

8. Bartter's syndrome (see Chapter 31).

9. With *overcompensatory metabolic alkalosis (posthypercapnic metabolic alkalosis)*. Chronic respiratory acidosis is associated with a compensatory metabolic alkalosis, with a loss of hydrogen and chloride ions in the urine and a retention of bicarbonate ions, so that hypochloremia and an elevated serum bicarbonate concentration develop. If the cause of

TABLE 29–1
CAUSES OF SALINE-RESPONSIVE AND SALINE-RESISTANT METABOLIC ALKALOSIS

Saline-Responsive	Saline-Resistant
Loss of HCl by vomiting, etc.	Primary aldosteronism
Diuretics associated with loss of	Bartter's syndrome
Cl⁻ ions through kidneys*	Cushing's syndrome
Abrupt relief of chronic hypercapnia	Licorice ingestion
Villous adenoma of colon	Severe K⁺ depletion

*These include thiazides and loop diuretics.

the respiratory acidosis is suddenly removed and the P_{CO_2} suddenly decreases, a severe metabolic alkalosis may develop because of the elevated serum bicarbonate concentration. This will persist until the patient is given chloride ions (either in the form of sodium or potassium chloride or an acidifying salt such as ammonium chloride, 1-lysine monohydrochloride, or dilute hydrochloric acid).

Overcompensatory metabolic alkalosis usually occurs in patients with chronic pulmonary disease and congestive heart failure who are treated with a low-sodium diet and diuretics.

10. With *contraction alkalosis.* If the volume of extracellular water decreases rapidly, for example, as the result of the diuretic ethacrynic acid or furosemide, the concentration of extracellular bicarbonate will increase. Theoretically, the concentration of dissolved carbon dioxide should also similarly increase and the pH should remain unchanged. However, the increased concentration of dissolved carbon dioxide will raise the carbon dioxide pressure of the blood and increase the diffusion of carbon dioxide into the alveolar air, where it is removed during respiration. As a result, the bicarbonate–carbonic acid ratio and the pH rise. The metabolic alkalosis produced in this way has been called a *contraction alkalosis.* It is the reverse of a *dilution acidosis* (Chapter 17).

SYMPTOMS AND SIGNS

It is difficult to separate the clinical symptoms and signs of patients with metabolic alkalosis from those of their associated disease processes, and especially from the symptoms and signs of hypokalemia (Chapter 30). A characteristic clinical picture of metabolic alkalosis occurs after a large amount of absorbable antacid medication is taken over a long time. Anorexia, nausea, and painless vomiting may occur. The patient may become confused and mentally unreliable. These patients have been described as being "difficult." This stage may be followed by drowsiness and coma. Tetany is another common sign of either metabolic or respiratory alkalosis.

Tetany

Tetany can be caused by either an increased pH or a decreased serum calcium concentration. If the serum pH is normal, tetany may occur when the serum calcium concentration decreases to 7.5 to 7 mg/dL or lower (4.25 to 3.5 mEq/L or lower). However, a low pH decreases the tendency to tetany. This is the reason tetany does not appear in metabolic acidosis due to chronic renal disease, where the serum calcium concentration is low. When both the serum calcium and potassium concentrations are low, tetany is also inhibited. However, tetany will appear when the serum potassium concentration is elevated and the serum calcium concentration remains low. A high serum potassium concentration does not induce tetany when the serum calcium concentration is normal.

Tetany can therefore be corrected by either lowering the pH or raising the serum calcium concentration, if the pH is normal. If the low serum calcium is due to an increased serum phosphate concentration, the serum calcium concentration can be raised only by lowering the serum phosphate concentration.

In addition, when a patient is treated for hypokalemia, the serum calcium concentration should be checked. If hypocalcemia is also present, it should be treated along with the hypokalemia.

Electrocardiogram

Patients with metabolic and respiratory alkalosis may show a characteristic electrocardiographic pattern that results from sinus tachycardia and a relative prolongation of the QT interval. The pattern consists of a T (or U) wave that approaches or actually merges with the P wave that follows (TP phenomenon).

Electroencephalogram

Gross slowing or rhythmic activity may be present.

LABORATORY FINDINGS
Blood

In a patient with uncomplicated metabolic alkalosis, the pH is high, indicating the alkalosis. The PCO_2 is normal or elevated.

The bicarbonate concentration is high and the chloride concentration is reciprocally low. Serum sodium concentration is normal or high. Serum potassium concentration may be normal or low.

Urine

The urine is usually alkaline, due to renal compensatory changes. However, if the alkalosis is due to potassium loss, the urine may be acid.

Example: Patient with metabolic alkalosis due to excessive vomiting
pH 7.56
PCO_2 46 mm Hg
CO_2 content 41.4 mEq/L
Standard bicarbonate 39 mEq/L
Actual bicarbonate 40 mEq/L
Base excess +16.2 mEq/L

The pH is high. This indicates an alkalosis. The positive base excess and the high standard bicarbonate indicate that a metabolic alkalosis is present. The PCO_2 shows a high normal value. Therefore, respiratory balance is present. However, the actual bicarbonate is higher than the standard bicarbonate. This indicates that some degree of respiratory acidosis is present. Therefore, a primary metabolic alkalosis is present with a partially compensatory respiratory acidosis (see Chapter 15).

Cation-Anion Balance:
Na 137   K 3.5 HCO_3 40   Cl 88 mEq/L
Anion gap = (Na + K) − (HCO_3 + Cl)
    = (137 + 3.5) − (40 + 88)
    = 140.5 − 128
    = 12.5 mEq/L. This is normal.

DIAGNOSIS

A metabolic alkalosis should be suspected in any patient who has vomited, who has received large amounts of absorbable alkaline salts, who has lost potassium, who shows electrocardiographic signs of hypokalemia, or who shows hypoventilation or tetany. The diagnosis is confirmed by finding a high CO_2 content and a high pH.

COURSE AND PROGNOSIS

The course and prognosis depend on the cause of the metabolic alkalosis.

PROPHYLAXIS

Absorbable alkali should be given cautiously to patients. This applies not only to those with peptic ulcer, for example, but also to those with metabolic acidosis who are being treated with alkalizing solutions. In addition, electrolytes should be replaced in patients who vomit or who are being treated with gastric suction. Patients with intractable vomiting should receive histamine-2-receptor blockers (cimetidine, ranitidine, etc.) to prevent further gastric hydrochloric acid loss.

Patients with congestive heart failure who receive daily doses of a diuretic, such as a thiazide, furosemide, or ethacrynic acid, should receive prophylactic potassium chloride to prevent a metabolic alkalosis. A carbonic anhydrase inhibitor (see page 267) can also be used to prevent the development of a metabolic alkalosis, because it increases the concentration of chloride ions in the body and enhances renal bicarbonate excretion.

Potassium chloride can be given in a daily dose up to 5 to 10 g. Numerous stock potassium chloride solutions are now available (Chapter 30). Potassium chloride can also be used as a salt substitute for sprinkling on food. The only contraindications to its use are severe renal disease and acidosis, because if the potassium ions are not excreted, muscular and nerve paralysis and death may occur. When potassium salts are used for patients with congestive heart failure, the serum potassium concentration in the body should be periodically checked.

TREATMENT

The aim of treatment is to correct the disturbance that has produced the metabolic alkalosis. For example, if vomiting or gastric suction is the cause, solutions containing saline and potassium chloride should be infused in a volume approximate to the volume of gastric juice that has been lost. If potassium deficiency is present due to any other cause, the patient should also receive potassium in the form of potassium *chloride.*

Ammonium Chloride

Ammonium chloride has been used in the treatment of metabolic alkalosis due to vomiting or gastric suction. However, in these patients, potassium loss is also present. For this reason, solutions containing sodium chloride and potassium chloride are preferable.

Ammonium chloride can also be used to treat metabolic alkalosis due to diuretics such as the thiazides. (It is rarely used now for this purpose but may be valuable in patients with concomitant congestive heart failure.) Uncoated tablets of ammonium chloride are prescribed orally in a daily dose of 6 to 12 g. (Enteric coated tablets should not be used. They may not dissolve in the intestines.) The ammonium chloride should be used for only 3 days each week, because the ammonium ions are metabolized to urea by the liver. The chloride ions are excreted along with sodium ions and water by the kidneys. The loss of sodium ions causes a diuresis and a loss of edema fluid. If the ammonium chloride is given for more than 3 days at a time, ammonia is produced by the kidneys and chloride ions are excreted along with the ammonia. As a result, sodium ions are not eliminated and no diuresis occurs. In addition, the ammonium chloride may be retained in the body, causing a metabolic acidosis.

If the patient cannot tolerate the ammonium chloride orally, it can be given intravenously in the form of a 2.14% solution. One should not attempt to raise the serum chloride concentration above 95 mEq/L with the intravenous solution. In addition, the serum chloride concentration should not be raised more than 15 mEq/L in one infusion in this way.

Either solution can be given at a rate up to 120 mL/hr.

Example: Man weighting 70 kg. Serum chloride concentration 75 mEq/L. It is desired to raise serum chloride concentration to 90 mEq/L.

Extracellular water is 20% of body weight.

$70 \times .2 = 14$ liters extracellular water.

Unit chloride deficit is 90 mEq/L $-$ 75 mEq/L = 15 mEq/L.

Total chloride deficit is $14 \times 15 = 210$ mEq/L.

Each liter of the 2.14% ammonium chloride solution contains 399.5 mEq chloride.

Therefore, 210/399.5 liter or approximately 526 mL is needed.

The following rule, based on the above calculations, can also be used:

0.50 mL of the 2.14% ammonium chloride solutions per kg of body weight will raise the serum chloride concentration 1mEq/L.

Thus, in the above example of a 70-kg man with a chloride deficit of 15 mEq/L, the amount of 2.14% ammonium chloride solution needed is $70 \times 15 \times 0.50 = 525$ mL.

Dilute Hydrochloric Acid (U.S.P., 10%)

This is a satisfactory substitute for ammonium chloride. It can be conveniently given by mouth. The dose is 20 mL daily. The patient sips 5 mL of the acid in a full glass of water, 4 times a day, through a glass tube to protect the teeth. The 20 mL of hydrochloric acid has a chloride content equivalent to about 3 g of ammonium chloride.

The duration of therapy with chloride salts depends on the degree of chloride depletion. It may take several days to a week or more. The patient usually responds within 2 to 3 days.

Intravenous Hydrochloric Acid

Hydrochloric acid can also be given intravenously when extreme metabolic alkalosis is present, and the patient has not responded to the usual treatment.

Intravenous hydrochloric acid can be given as a 0.05 normal (N) to 0.2 N solution. A 0.15 N solution in water (150 mEq HCl per liter of H_2O) is approximately isotonic. The 0.15 N solution can also be given in a 5% dextrose in water solution.

A 0.15 N solution is prepared by adding 150 mL of 1.0 N hydrochloric acid to 850 mL of sterile water, or by diluting 12.5 mL of reagent grade hydrochloric acid (35 to 38%) to a total volume of 1000 mL with sterile water.

The 0.15 N solution can be given at a rate of up to 125 mL/hr. A glass container should be used because hydrochloric acid may react with a plastic container.

The hydrochloric acid must be given through a central venous catheter. If it is given into a peripheral vein, it will cause sloughing of the surrounding tissues. Supplemental potassium chloride is given as needed to correct any associated hypokalemia.

Knutson has suggested that hydrochloric acid can be given into a periphral vein if it is buffered in an amino acid solution and infused with a fat emulsion.

The dose of IV hydrochloric acid can be calculated in several ways:

1. From the plasma bicarbonate level:
   mEq HCl needed = $(HCO_3$ observed $- 24) \times 0.5 \times$ body weight (kg)
2. From the plasma chloride concentration:
   mEq HCl needed = $(100 - Cl$ observed$) \times 0.2 \times$ body weight (kg)

About one half to two thirds of the calculated deficit should be given during the first 24 hours to prevent overcorrection.

When loss of hydrochloric acid is severe, as in postoperative patients or in the Zollinger-Ellison syndrome, a patient can lose a massive amount of gastric juice with a high hydrochloric content. Abouna et al. have given as much as 600 mEq IV hydrochloric acid per 24 hours.

Excessive ammonium chloride or hydrochloric acid can cause a severe acidosis, disorientation, confusion, and coma. It is also dangerous to give these agents to patients with a primary respiratory acidosis who develop a high CO_2 content as a result of a compensatory metabolic alkalosis. If the metabolic alkalosis is eliminated by the ammonium chloride, the patient may die from the respiratory acidosis. Ammonium chloride is also contraindicated in cirrhosis of the liver, or in patients with right-sided heart failure and liver damage, because it can precipitate hepatic coma.

Sodium Chloride

Sodium chloride, in the form of oral table salt or saline solution given intravenously, can be used to correct a metabolic alkalosis, unless sodium ions are contraindicated because of congestive heart failure, edema, ascites, or a *saline-resistant* metabolic alkalosis.

Carbonic Anhydrase Inhibitors

Patients with severe congestive heart failure may develop a metabolic alkalosis due to thiazide or other diuretic therapy, and may become refractory to the action of the diuretic. A carbonic anhydrase inhibitor such as acetazolamide (Diamox) may be effective in decreasing the alkalosis and in restoring the sensitivity of the patient to the diuretic. The following schedule may be beneficial:

Diamox, 250 mg 2 or 3 times a day for 3 days
Ammonium chloride, 6 to 9 g a day for 3 days, simultaneously

The diuretic can then be resumed on the fifth day.

The carbonic anhydrase inhibitors can produce drowsiness or paresthesias as side reactions. Disorientation has also been observed in edematous patients with impaired liver function. In addition, drug fever and rashes may occur, probably due to the sulfonamide structure of the carbonic anhydrase inhibitors.

Other Acidifying Agents

L-Lysine monohydrochloride has also been used to produce a mild metabolic acidosis in order to increase the effect of diuretics in patients with heart failure. It increases the serum chloride concentration, which may be lowered as a result of the diuretics.

L-Lysine monohydrochloride can be given in a dose of 10 to 40 g a day, for 3 to 5 days. Each gram yields 5 mEq chloride ions. Forty grams is equivalent to 11 g of ammonium chloride, or 12 g of calcium chloride. It can be given as a 40% solution in cold fruit juice or in regular or low-sodium milk. Therefore, 1 teaspoonful (5 mL) contains 2 g. It may cause side effects such as abdominal cramps or transient diarrhea.

Treatment of Metabolic Alkalosis Complicated by Severe Respiratory Acidosis

Mechanical ventilation using a respirator should be avoided. Instead, the primary metabolic alkalosis should be corrected.

Bibliography

Abouna, GM, et al: Intravenous infusion of hydrochloric acid for treatment of severe metabolic alkalosis. Surgery 75:194, 1974.
Alexander, CS: T-P phenomenon. An electrocardiographic clue to unsuspected alkalosis. Arch Intern Med 116:220, 1965.
Cannon, PJ, et al: "Contraction" alkalosis after diuresis of edematous patients with ethacrynic acid. Ann Intern Med 62:979, 1965.
Clark, RG, and Norman, JN: Metabolic alkalosis in pyloric stenosis. Lancet I:1244, 1964.
Coe, FL: Metabolic alkalosis. JAMA 238:2288, 1977.
Fulop, M: Hypercapnia in metabolic alkalosis. New York State J Med 76:19, 1976.
Galla, JH, Bonduris, DN, and Luke, RG: Effects of chloride and extracellular fluid volume on bicarbonate re-absorption along the nephron in metabolic alkalosis in the rate. Reassessment of the classic hypothesis on the pathogenesis of metabolic alkalosis. J Clin Invest 8:41, 1987.
Galla, JH, Gifford, JD, Luke, RG, and Rome, L: Adaptions to chloride-depletion alkalosis. Am J Physiol 261:R771, 1991.
Garella, S, Chazan, JA, and Cohen, JJ: Saline-resistant metabolic alkalosis or "chloride-wasting nephropathy." Report of four patients with severe potassium depletion. Ann Intern Med 73:31, 1970.

Javaheri, S, et al: Compensatory hypoventilation in metabolic alkalosis. Chest 81:296, 1982.

Javaheri, S, and Kazemi, H: Metabolic alkalosis and hypoventilation in humans. Am Rev Respir Dis 136:1011, 1987.

Kassirer, JP, and Schwartz, WB: Correction of metabolic alkalosis in man without repair of potassium deficiency. Re-evaluation of the role of potassium. Am J Med 40:19, 1966.

Kassirer, J, Berkman, P, Lawrenz, D, and Schwartz, W: Critical role of chloride in correction of hypokalemic alkalosis in man. Am J Med 38:172, 1965.

Knutsen, OH: New method for administration of hydrochloric acid in metabolic alkalosis. Lancet 1:953, 1983.

Kraft, AR, Tompkins, RK, and Zollinger, RM: Recognition and management of the diarrheal syndrome caused by nonbeta islet cell tumors of the pancreas. Am J Surg 119:163, 1970.

Kurtzman, NA: Metabolic alkalosis. The Kidney, 9: no. 6, November, 1976.

Kurtzman, NA, White, MG, and Rogers, PW: Pathophysiology of metabolic alkalosis. Arch Intern Med 131:702, 1973.

Lifschitz, MD, Brasch, R, Cuomo, AJ, and Menn, SJ: Marked hypercapnia secondary to severe metabolic alkalosis. Ann Intern Med 77:405, 1972.

Miller, PD, and Berns, AS: Acute metabolic alkalosis perpetuating hypercarbia. A role for acetazolamide in chronic obstructive pulmonary disease. JAMA 238:2400, 1977.

Mulhausen, R, Eichenholz, A, and Blumentals, AS: Acid-base disturbances in patients with cirrhosis of the liver. Medicine 46:85, 1967.

Oliva, PB: Severe alveolar hypoventilation in a patient with metabolic alkalosis. Am J Med 52:817, 1972.

Roggin, GM, et al: Ketosis and metabolic alkalosis in a patient with diabetes. JAMA 211:296, 1970.

Rosen, RA, Julian, BA, Dubovsky, EV, et al: On the mechanism by which chloride corrects metabolic alkalosis in man. Am J Med 84:449, 1988.

Rubin, AL, et al: Use of L-lysine monohydrochloride in combination with mercurial diuretics in treatment of refractory fluid retention. Circulation 21:332, 1960.

Seldin, DW, and Rector, FC, Jr: The generation and maintenance of metabolic alkalosis. Kidney Int 1:306, 1972.

Tuller, MT, and Mehdi, F: Compensatory hypoventilation and hypercapnia in primary metabolic alkalosis. Am J Med 50:290, 1971.

Wesson, DE: Augmented bicarbonate re-absorption by both the proximal and distal nephron maintains chloride-deplete metabolic alkalosis in rates. J Clin Invest 84:1460, 1989.

Wesson, DE: Depressed distal tubule acidification corrects chloride-deplete metabolic alkalosis. Am J Physiol 259:F636, 1990.

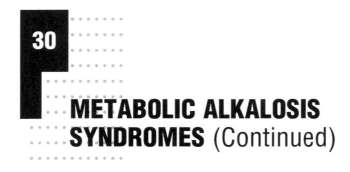

METABOLIC ALKALOSIS SYNDROMES (Continued)

HYPOKALEMIA

Hypokalemia (hypopotassemia) is present when the serum potassium concentration is lower than 3.5 mEq/L.

Serum potassium concentrations can be misleading because a loss of total body potassium can be present with a normal serum potassium concentration. This can occur in several different ways:

1. Hemoconcentration is present, due to either water loss or sodium loss.
2. When acidosis is present, there is a shift of potassium from the cells into the extracellular water. Therefore, serum potassium concentration may be normal or even high in the presence of potassium loss. This occurs, for example, during diabetic acidosis. Conversely, alkalosis causes potassium to move from the extracellular water into the cells. Therefore, the serum potassium concentration may appear to be low without loss of potassium from the body.

The average daily intake of the potassium ion ranges from 50 to 75 mEq. This is equivalent to 3.73 to 5.6 g of potassium chloride, and is adequate for the normal needs of the body.

PATHOPHYSIOLOGY

In Chapter 26 it was pointed out that a loss of total exchangeable body potassium is not necessarily associated with hypokalemia, and that the serum potassium concentration in such patients may be low, normal, or even high, depending on the associated presence of water loss or acidosis.

It can be stated as a general rule that potassium loss promotes a metabolic alkalosis, and, conversely, that a metabolic or respiratory alkalosis promotes hypokalemia.

Potassium loss promotes metabolic alkalosis in the following way: When potassium ions are lost from the cells, sodium and hydrogen ions move from the extracellular water into the cells to replace the potassium. However, for every 3 potassium ions lost from the cell, only 2 sodium ions enter the cell. The remaining potassium ion is replaced by a hydrogen ion. This causes a decreased hydrogen ion concentration of the extracellular water, and a metabolic alkalosis. A similar loss of potassium ions occurs through the kidneys. Normally, potassium ions are completely filtered by the glomeruli. Then they are completely reabsorbed in the proximal tubules. Finally, approximately 10% of the potassium ions that had been originally filtered are actively secreted by the distal tubular cells into the urine, and are excreted.

The secretion of potassium ions from the distal tubular cells into the urine occurs in association with a reabsorption of sodium ions from the tubular urine into the tubular cells (and into the blood), although these two processes do not occur at the same anatomical site. If the number of potassium ions available for exchange with sodium ions is decreased, hydrogen ions, instead of potassium ions, will be excreted into the tubular urine, while sodium ions are reabsorbed. The urinary loss of hydrogen ions also causes a metabolic alkalosis. In addition, the hydrogen ions in the urine cause the urine to show an acid pH even in the presence of a metabolic alkalosis. This is a characteristic finding of metabolic alkalosis associated with potassium loss.

Alkalosis, conversely, causes hypokalemia. Potassium ions move from the extracellular water into the cells, and hydrogen ions move from the cells into the extracellular water, in an attempt to raise the hydrogen ion concentration and lower the pH of the extracellular water toward normal.

The relation of hypokalemia to muscle paralysis is discussed in Chapter 26.

Hypokalemia causes an important abnormality of renal function, namely, an inability of the kidneys to concentrate urine normally. As a result, the osmolality of the urine falls to a value only slightly above that of the plasma *(hyposthenuria)*. The urinary specific gravity also becomes low. (The hyposthenuria is characteristically resistant to the action of vasopressin.) As a result, nocturia, polyuria, thirst and polydipsia may occur.

Insulin is necessary for potassium ions to enter cells. Therefore, patients with diabetes mellitus may not be able to tolerate large doses of potassium salts. If renal insufficiency is present, a potassium-sparing diuretic such as traimterere may easily induce hyperkalemia.

The pathophysiological mechanisms by which the hypokalemia occurs in other clinical conditions are discussed below.

ETIOLOGY

The following conditions tend to decrease the serum potassium concentration and to cause hypokalemia. A loss of total exchangeable potassium may or may not be present.

1. Hypokalemia due to a loss of potassium ions from the body. This can occur in at least three ways:
   a. Loss of potassium ions from the gastrointestinal tract. This can cause two patterns of hypokalemia:
      i. Hypokalemia associated with a loss of gastric juices *(upper GI syndrome)*. This occurs with persistent vomiting, particularly with pyloric obstruction. The hypokalemia is associated with a metabolic alkalosis due to the loss of hydrogen ions from the gastric juice.
      ii. Hypokalemia associated with a loss of lower intestinal fluids. This can occur with diarrhea due to any cause, with intestinal fistulas, or with a *villous adenoma of the colon* (or from long-term surreptitious use of laxatives or excessive enemas). A large number of chloride ions are lost, in addition to the potassium (and sodium) ions, so that the hypokalemia is associated with a metabolic alkalosis.

      Patients with *nonbeta islet cell tumor of the pancreas* often show a profuse watery diarrhea ("pancreatic cholera"), hypokalemia, and characteristic achlorhydria (WDHA syndrome).

      Hypokalemia may also occur in patients with the Zollinger-Ellison syndrome (nonbeta islet cell adenomas of the pancreas; excessive hydrochloric acid secretion by the stomach with peptic ulcers of esophagus, stomach, duodenum, or jejunum, chronic diarrhea, and hypokalemia. Some of these patients also have hyperparathyroidism).

      Hypokalemia due to diarrhea has also been reported in *medullary carcinoma of the thyroid*. The carcinoma cells secrete prostaglandins, which stimulate intestinal secretions and produce the diarrhea. The syndrome may be a variant of the Zollinger-Ellison syndrome (see above). However, peptic ulcers are not present.

      Another factor in producing hypokalemia with lower intestinal losses is that feces contain an appreciable amount of potassium ions. (From 8 to 15 mEq potassium ions are normally excreted in the feces daily. A much greater loss occurs with diarrhea.)

      In patients with hypokalemia due to gastrointestinal losses, the actual serum potassium concentration may be misleading because severe water loss, sodium loss, or acidosis may be present. Therefore, the serum potassium concentration may be normal (or high) in spite of a loss of total exchangeable body potassium and a low potassium concentration in the cells.

      The electrocardiogram will reflect the serum potassium concentration. In cholera, for example, where there may be a high serum potassium concentration due to the associated metabolic acidosis, the electrocardiogram may show signs of hyper-kalemia. Conversely, patients with hypokalemia secondary to gastric losses may show the classic electrocardiographic patterns of hypokalemia.

b. Loss of potassium ions through the urine. This can occur in several ways:

   i. Diuretics, such as the thiazides, ethacrynic acid, or furosemide. An important action of these diuretics is the excretion of chloride ions in the urine. The chloride is usually excreted with sodium, ammonium, or potassium ions. Potassium loss this way may be severe, especially in patients who are on a low-sodium diet and receive a large amount of the diuretics. (Surreptitious diuretic use is occasionally a cause of hypokalemia.)

   ii. Excessive administration of bicarbonate or other alkaline salts. In these patients, the potassium loss is due to its urinary excretion in association with the urinary excretion of excess bicarbonate ions.

   iii. Decreased intake of potassium ions (orally or parenterally). Malnourished or semistarved patients have a low intake of potassium salts, but a continued excretion of potassium ions occurs. Apparently, the kidneys have an incomplete homeostatic mechanism for the conservation of potassium ions, and as much as 20 mEq can be excreted in the urine daily for a long time, even if a person is on a potassium-free diet.

     When a patient is given a large volume of potassium-free fluids parenterally, the hypokalemia that occurs is partly due to dilution of the blood with the intravenous fluids. In addition, a large number of potassium ions is excreted in the urine, for reasons just mentioned.

   iv. The effect of aldosterone or other mineralocorticoid hormones (see Chapter 31). Postoperative potassium loss and the potassium loss that occurs in Cushing's syndrome have the same mechanism. Large doses of corticosteroids can also cause a severe potassium loss.

   v. Renal tubular dysfunction. Potassium loss can occur in patients with renal tubular acidosis (Chapter 18) and in patients with uretero-enterostomy.

   vi. Diuretic phase of acute renal failure.

   vii. Massive doses of sodium penicillin G (100 million units a day) may be associated with potassium loss through the kidneys. Apparently, penicillin promotes the urinary excretion of potassium ions by interfering with distal tubular cation transport. Amphotericin B, gentamicin, and carbenicillin may also cause potassium loss through the kidneys. The hypokalemia that often occurs in patients with acute myeloid leukemia is also partly due to loss of potassium ions through the kidneys.

   c. Loss of potassium ions through the skin. Excessive sweating, particularly in persons acclimatized to tropical climates (where the potassium loss in sweat may equal or exceed the sodium loss).

2. Intracellular shifts of potassium ions. This can occur in the following conditions:

   a. Hypokalemia due to the transfer of potassium ions from the blood into the liver and muscle cells. Potassium is needed by the liver to convert glucose to glycogen. The ingestion of food, particularly carbohydrates, causes the secretion of insulin, which stimulates the liver cells. As a result, the concentration of potassium in the blood falls. A similar lowering of serum potassium concentration occurs after the parenteral injection of insulin.

   b. Hypokalemic periodic paralysis. The fall in serum potassium concentration, by the mechanism described above, is probably the direct cause of attacks of familial periodic paralysis. This type of hypokalemia is not associated with a decreased total exchangeable body potassium. However, patients who experience attacks of periodic paralysis show a lowered muscle potassium concentration, even during periods between attacks. This suggests that chronic potassium loss is present in these patients.

   c. The action of an anabolic hormone, such as testosterone. Potassium ions enter the muscle cells, where they are utilized to build muscle protein. However, in these patients, the electrocardiogram does not show signs of hypokalemia. The reason for this is not known.

   d. Alkalosis, either respiratory (Chapter 28) or metabolic (Chapter 29). The low serum potassium concentration may or may not indicate a loss of potassium from the body.

   e. Treatment of megaloblastic anemia. When hematopoiesis starts, a large number of potassium ions enter the young red blood cells, and serious hypokalemia may result.

   f. Beta-2 agonist. These agents cause potassium movement into cells. Their administration is responsible for the mild hypokalemia seen in treated asthma patients.

3. Combination factors. Numerous factors producing hypokalemia may be present simultaneously or in sequence. For example, hypokalemia may occur in uncomplicated cirrhosis of the liver, if diarrhea is present. Renal tubular acidosis may also be a factor in the potassium loss. When cirrhosis is associated with ascites, hypokalemia may be due to secondary aldosteronism, or to the effect of diuretics.

4. Pseudohypokalemia. This can occur with leukemia, where metabolically active white blood cells may take up potassium from the plasma in vitro after blood drawing. Prompt laboratory processing of plasma will avoid this phenomenon.

PATHOLOGY

When potassium loss occurs for a long time, it may cause hydropic and degenerative changes in the convoluted tubules of the kidneys, without significant glomerular or vascular changes. These renal changes are associated with a hyposthenuria that is resistant to vasopressin (ADH).

Potassium loss can also cause degeneration of the myocardium. Loss of striation of the cells occurs. This is followed by poor staining of the cytoplasm and finally by karyorrhexis and karyolysis. In addition, infiltration of the myocardium by neutrophilic polymorphonuclear leukocytes and large mononuclear cells occurs. Later, fibrosis occurs.

SYMPTOMS AND SIGNS

The clinical symptoms and signs of hypokalemia are mostly nonspecific and may occur in seriously ill patients who do not show hypokalemia. They include: anorexia, nausea and vomiting, abdominal distention, decreased bowel sounds, paralytic ileus, muscle weakness, absent or diminished deep tendon reflexes, and a depressed mental state. Thirst and polyuria may also occur.

Neuromuscular symptoms and signs do not usually appear until the serum potassium concentration falls to approximately 2.5 mEq/L, and may not even be present when it reaches 2 mEq/L. Muscle weakness first develops, then paralysis. Paresthesias or severe pain the muscles may also be present. The muscle weakness is most prominent in the legs, especially in the quadriceps muscles. Later, the respiratory muscles become weakened. The diaphragm becomes paralyzed before the intercostal muscles and the accessory muscles of respiration. As a result, a characteristic "fish-mouth" type of breathing, characterized by pursing of the lips, occurs. The muscles innervated by the cranial nerves are almost never affected. Instead of muscle weakness due to actual muscle atrophy. In spite of the muscle weakness, deep tendon reflexes and the abdominal and cremasteric reflexes remain normal. The electroencephalogram also is normal.

Central nervous symptoms may include lethargy, drowsiness, irritability, confusion. Rarely coma, delirium, and hallucinations occur.

Occasionally, tetany may occur when hypokalemia has been corrected. This is due to a concomitant hypocalcemia whose effects have been inhibited by the hypokalemia.

Postural hypotension is common.

Nocturia, polyuria, and polydipsia may occur because the kidneys lose their capacity to concentrate urine normally. The resultant loss of water through the urine also produces thirst.

The most characteristic signs of muscle paralysis associated with hypokalemia are seen in *familial periodic paralysis*. The attacks can occur spontaneously, or can be precipitated by substances such as epinephrine, desoxycorticosterone acetate, corticotropin (ACTH), insulin, dextrose, or a large carbohydrate meal, which reduce the serum potassium concentration. The attacks can occur when the serum potassium concentration is at a low normal level, such as 3.5 mEq/L, which would have no effect on the normal person. (Hyperthyroidism may also induce attacks.)

ELECTROCARDIOGRAM

Assuming that there are no local alterations of the potassium content of heart muscle (due to muscle injury or ventricular strain) the electrocardiographic changes which occur in hypokalemia can be correlated in a general way with the level of potassium in the serum.

Figure 30–1 shows some of the common changes seen, which include:

1. Lowering and broadening of the T wave *(A)*. The QT interval is also slightly prolonged. Such a pattern may occur when the serum potassium is merely at a low normal level, for example, 3.5 mEq/L.

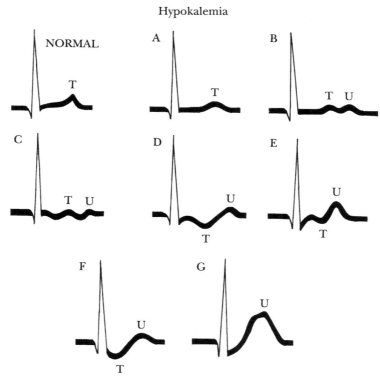

FIGURE 30–1. Electrocardiographic patterns of hypokalemia.

2. Low, broad T waves with a double summit, due to superimposition of the U wave on the T *(B)*. The QT interval may appear markedly prolonged in such cases. However, the prolongation may be more apparent than real because it may be difficult to determine where the T ends and the U begins. As a consequence, the QU interval, rather than the QT interval, is often measured.

3. Depression of the ST segment and slight lengthening of the QT interval *(D,E.)*. The ST may be slightly depressed, or may show several small undulations *(C)*. D, E, F, G, show more marked ST deviations. These ST segments have a sagging appearance, characteristic of hypokalemia.

4. Downward T waves and prominent U waves *(D,E,F)*. Such a pattern is best seen in precordial leads such as V_1 through V_4, which overlie the right ventricle and thus have an rS or RS pattern.

5. Increase in P wave amplitudes and widening of the QRS interval.

6. Numerous arrhythmias, including sinus bradycardia, prolonged PR interval, Wenckebach type of AV block, paroxysmal supraventricular tachycardia with AV block. Arrhythmias due to digitalis toxicity may be precipitated or worsened.

Although *A* through *G* show the progressive changes that can occur as hypokalemia becomes more marked, these progressive changes do not always occur, and it may be impossible to determine the exact degree of hypokalemia from the electrocardigram.

LABORATORY FINDINGS
Blood

The normal serum potassium concentration varies from 3.5 to 5.0 mEq/L (13.7 to 19.5 mg/dL). Signs of hypokalemia are usually associated with serum concentrations of 3 mEq/L (12 mg/dL) or less. The serum calcium concentration may be normal, low, or high in association with the hypokalemia. (Serum potassium concentration should always be determined in hypocalcemic tetany. If the hypokalemia alone is corrected, tetany may be precipitated.)

With severe hypokalemia, laboratory findings of a metabolic alkalosis, including a high bicarbonate concentration and a high CO_2 content, are present (Chapter 29).

One should remember that if an acidosis is present, the serum potassium concentration tends to be high, regardless of the total exchangeable body potassium. A normal or low serum potassium concentration in an acidotic patient therefore indicates a severe potassium loss. Conversely, in alkalosis, the serum potassium concentration tends to be low, even when the total exchangeable body potassium is normal. Significant potassium loss should be suspected in an alkalotic patient when the serum potassium concentration is below 2.5 mEq/L.

Potassium loss may cause decreased carbohydrate tolerance, so that an elevated fasting blood sugar level and a diabetic glucose tolerance test response may develop. (If this happens when a patient is receiving diuretics, it can be corrected by also giving potassium chloride in conjunction with the diuretic.)

Urine

Hypokalemia is associated with a decreased ability of the kidneys to concentrate urine normally. Therefore, when the hypokalemia is severe, the urine osmolality decreases to approximately that of the serum. The urine shows an acid pH, but it is rare for the urinary pH to decrease to 5.0 or lower.

The urinary potassium excretion is low (less than 30 mEq a day), in association with the hypokalemia. However, if the hypokalemia is due to diuretics, to renal tubular acidosis, or to the diuretic phase of acute renal failure, the urinary potassium excretion will be high (more than 40 mEq a day).

DIAGNOSIS

The sudden development of marked muscle weakness or paralysis, or loss of deep tendon reflexes, or paralytic ileus, is suspicious of potassium loss. The electrocardiogram will usually show signs of hypokalemia in these patients, even if the serum potassium concentration appears normal.

Hypokalemia due to aldosterone and other mineralocorticoid hormones is discussed in the next chapter.

COURSE AND PROGNOSIS

Severe potassium loss can cause death. This is probably one of the reasons that some diabetic patients with acidosis have died in the past, even though the acidosis was apparently corrected.

Hypokalemia may worsen the clinical status of a patient with cirrhosis of the liver, owing to the concomitant alkalosis, which promotes ammonia trapping in brain cells. Therefore, hepatic insufficiency and coma may be precipitated if such a patient is treated vigorously with diuretics, such as the thiazides, furosemide, or ethacrynic acid, which cause an increased urinary excretion of potassium ions.

PROPHYLAXIS

Potassium loss should be anticipated. If the patient has severe losses of gastrointestinal fluids, or is receiving intravenous fluids, the serum potassium concentration should be determined and potassium chloride given as indicated (also see below).

One of the most common causes of potassium loss is the use of long-term diuretics without supplemental potassium chloride. If potassium chloride is contraindicated, potassium loss can be prevented in these patients by the concomitant use of a potassium-sparing diuretic, such as spironolactone (Aldactone) or triamterene (Dyrenium). Supplemental potassium chloride may also be necessary for patients who are receiving long-term corticosteroid treatment.

TREATMENT

Potassium loss must be treated with potassium salts. Potassium chloride is the salt of choice, although potassium phosphate or other potassium salts can be used if there is no serum chloride deficit. If an acidosis is present along with the hypokalemia, an alkalinizing potassium salt such as potassium acetate, bicarbonate, or citrate should be used. (Liquid Potassium Triplex, Lilly, contains these three salts.)

The average daily intake of potassium ions ranges from 50 to 75 mEq. This is equivalent to 3.73 to 5.6 g of potassium chloride. When hypokalemia is present, 100 to 300 mEq of potassium (7.46 to 21.38 g of potassium chloride) can be given daily.

The amount of potassium that is required to correct a potassium deficit cannot be determined by any fixed formula. Average deficits of 200 to 400 mEq are common. However, the deficit may amount to as much as 800 to 1000 mEq of potassium. The deficit should be corrected slowly over a period of days. It may take weeks or months to correct severe potassium loss. However, the patient responds even when a small part of the potassium loss is corrected. Often as little as 30 to 50 mEq potassium daily is adequate to ameliorate symptoms of hypokalemia.

Numerous stock preparations of potassium chloride are now available, including Kay Ciel (10%) Elixir, or Kaochlor (10%) Liquid (each 15 mL supplies 1.5 g potassium chloride, equivalent to 20 mEq potassium and 20 mEq chloride ions), K-Lyte-Cl powder (a unit dose supplies 25 mEq potassium and 25 mEq chloride ions), and many others.

If a patient needs potassium chloride and cannot tolerate it because of gastrointestinal symptoms (which commonly occurs), an extended-release tablet of potassium chloride in a wax matrix can be tried. The following tablets are available: Kaon-Cl (6.67 mEq potassium and chloride ions per tablet), Micro-K Extencaps (8 or 10 mEq potassium and chloride ions per capsule). Slow-K (8 mEq potassium and chloride ions per tablet) and many others. However, complications may occur from the use of these extended-release potassium chloride tablets: they should not be used if a patient has an enlarged left atrium (due to mitral valvular disease), or if esophageal displacement or compression is present, or if a patient has definite or suspected stasis or obstruction of any part of the gastrointestinal tract. In addition, they should be used with extreme caution, if at all, if a patient has a history of a peptic ulcer.

Foods high in potassium content should also be ingested (See Table 26–1, page 247 and Table 30–1).

So-called electrolyte replacement solutions, such as lactated Ringer's solution, contain only 4 mEq potassium ions per liter, and are not suitable to treat hypokalemia.

If the patient cannot take potassium chloride by mouth, it can be given intravenously in a solution containing 39 to 80 mEq potassium (3 to 6 g of potassium chloride) per liter. The rate of infusion should not exceed 20 mEq (rarely 35 mEq) potassium per hour. If 2 liters of solution containing 60 mEq/L are given daily for 2 days, the patient will have received 240 mEq.

The potassium chloride can be added to an infusion of dextrose in water or dextrose in saline solution. When severe hypokalemia is present, it is preferable, if possible, to give the potassium without sodium, because sodium tends to aggravate the potassium deficiency.

Large doses of potassium chloride from 80 to 120 mEq of potassium chloride in 250 mL of 5% dextrose in water or normal saline solution can also be given through a central venous catheter and an infusion pump at a rate up to 20 mEq per hour. Usually 8 to 15 mEq per hour is infused (Cullen).

The intravenous administration of potassium in dextrose solutions may be associated with a transient *lowering* of serum potassium concentration. Kunin and his associates have suggested that this is due to a cellular uptake of potassium with dextrose that is more rapid than the potassium being given.

The rapid intravenous infusion of potassium chloride in a digitalis-toxic patient may precipitate ventricular arrhythmias, such as ventricular premature beats or ventricular tachycardia, or, if AV block is present, it may

TABLE 30–1
POTASSIUM CONTENT (IN mEq) OF SOME POTASSIUM-RICH FOODS

Apricots, 3	11 mEq
Banana	15
Cantaloupe, 1/2	23
Dates, 1 cup	36
Fig, dried, 1 large (1" × 2")	20
Orange	9
Orange juice, 8 oz.	11
Raisins, 1 cup	29
Watermelon, 1/2 slice	10

become more marked. The reason for this is that digitalis toxicity may interfere with the uptake of potassium ions by skeletal muscles. Therefore, the potassium chloride which is infused remains in the bloodstream and may cause an abnormal elevation of serum potassium concentration.

Potassium can also be given rectally. Twenty milliliters of a 25% solution of potassium chloride (5 g) can be instilled into the rectum with a rubber bulb syringe, or a continuous rectal drip of a 10% potassium chloride solution can be given.

Familial periodic paralysis can be prevented by avoiding unusual stresses as much as possible and by avoiding high carbohydrate meals. An attack can be precipitated by rest, especially following vigorous exertion. Severe attacks often occur at night, or in the early hours of the morning. Some patients are able to "walk off" a mild attack. Acetazolamide (Diamox) is the most effective treatment available. Drugs such as epinephrine, thyroid extract, DOCA, and ACTH should be avoided.

Bibliography

Aldinger, KA, et al: Hypokalemia with hypercalcemia. Prevalence and significance in treatment. Ann Intern Med 87:571, 1977.

Babior, BM: Villous adenoma of the colon. Study of a patient with severe fluid and electrolyte disturbances. Am J Med 41:615, 1966.

Bia, MJ, and DeFronzo, RA: Potassium chloride therapy. Questions and Answers. JAMA 248:2501, 1981.

Brown, MJ, et al: Hypokalemia from beta$_2$-receptor stimulation by circulating epinephrine. N Engl J Med 309:1414, 1983.

Carlisle EJF, Donnelly SM, Ethier JH et al: Modulation of the secretion of potassium by accompanying anions in humans. Kidney Int 39:1206, 1991.

Cullen, DJ: Potassium chloride therapy, letter. JAMA 247:2780, 1982.

DeFronzo, RA, and Bia, M: Intravenous potassium chloride therapy. Questions and Answers. JAMA 245:2246, 1981.

DeGraeff, J, Struyvenberg, A, and Lameijer, LDF: The role of chloride in hypokalemic alkalosis. Am J Med 37:778, 1964.

Dyckner, T, and Wester, PO: Potassium deficiency contributing to ventricular tachycardia. Acta Med Scandinav 212:89, 1982.

Feld, M, and Chang, EB: Pancreatic cholera. Is the diarrhea due to VIP? Editorial. N Engl J Med 309:1513, 1983.

Fisher, JR: Hypokalemia in leukemia, comments. Ann Intern Med 86:363, 1977.

Fleming, BJ, et al: Laxative-induced hypokalemia, sodium depletion and hyperreninemia. Ann Intern Med 83:60, 1975.

Fletcher, GF, Hurst, JW, and Schlant, RC: Electrocardiographic changes in severe hypokalemia. A reappraisal. Am J Cardiol 20:628, 1967.

Garella, S, Chazan, JA, and Cohen, JJ: Saline-resistant metabolic alkalosis, or "chloride-wasting nephropathy." Report of four patients with severe potassium depletion. Ann Intern Med 73:31, 1970.

Glazier, WB, and Silen, W: Acute potassium defect. Arch Surg 112:1165, 1977.

Gossain, VV, and Werk, EE: Surreptitious laxation and hypokalemia. Ann Intern Med 76:671, 1972.

Griggs, RC, Engel, WK, and Resnik, JS: Acetazolamide treatment of hypokalemic periodic paralysis. Ann Intern Med 73:39, 1970.

Hoffbrand, BI, and Stewart, JD: Carbenicillin and hypokalemia. BMJ 4:476, 1970.

Jackson, H, and Glassburg, S: Pancreatic cholera. NY State J Med 84:31, 1984.

Jensen, RT, et al: Zollinger-Ellison syndrome. Ann Intern Med 98:59, 1983.

Katz, FH, Eckert, EC, and Gebott, MD: Hypokalemia caused by surreptitious self-administration of diuretics. Ann Intern Med 76:85, 1972.

Knutsen, OH: New method for administering hydrochloric acid in metabolic alkalosis. Lancet 1:953, 1983.

Kraft, AR, Tompkins, RK, and Zollinger, RM: Recognition and management of the diarrheal syndrome caused by nonbeta islet cell tumors of the pancreas. Am J Surg 119:163, 1970.

Kruse, JA, and Carlson, RW: Rapid correction of hypokalemia using concentrated intravenous potassium chloride infusions. Arch Intern Med 150:613, 1990.

Lai, F, et al: Licorice, snuff, and hypokalemia, letter. N Engl J Med 303:463, 1980.

Lawson, DH, et al: Hypokalaemia in megaloblastic anemias. Lancet 2:588, 1970.

Lawson, DH, et al: Potassium supplements in patients receiving long-term diuretics for edema. Q J Med 45:469, 1976.

Maronda, RF, et al: Response of thiazide-induced hypokalemia to amiloride. JAMA 249:237, 1983.

Maronder, RF, Milgrom, M, and Dickey, JM: Potassium loss with thiazide therapy. Am Heart J 78:16, 1969.

McMahon, F, et al: Upper gastrointestinal lesions after potassium chloride supplements, Lancet 2:1059,1982.

Mir, MA, et al: Hypokalaemia in acute myeloid leukaemia. Ann Intern Med 82:54, 1975.

Nagy, M: Dietary means of avoiding potassium deficiency. JAMA 226:87, 1973.

Parker, MS, et al: Chronic hypokalemia and alkalosis. Arch Intern Med 140:1336, 1980.

Perez, GO, et al: Acid-base disturbances in gastrointestinal disease. Dig Dis Sci 32:1033, 1987.

Re, R: Hypokalemia in hypertension. Practical Cardiol 9:103, 1983.

Resnick, JS, et al: Acetazolamide prophylaxis in hypokalemic periodic paralysis. N Engl J Med 278:582, 1968.

Rosen, RA, et al: On the mechanism by which chloride corrects metabolic alkalosis in man. Am J Med 84:449, 1988.

Rovner, DR: Use of pharmacologic agents in the treatment of hypokalemia and hyperkalemia. Rational Drug Ther 6:2, 1972.

Roy, AD, and Ellis, H: Potassium-secreting tumours of the large intestine. Lancet 1:759, 1959.

Salerno, DM: Post-resuscitation hypokalemia in a patient with a normal pre-arrest serum potassium level. Ann Intern Med 108:836, 1988.

Satoyoshi, E, et al: Periodic paralysis in hyperthyroidism. Neurology 13:746, 1963.

Schwartz, AB, and Swartz, CD: Dosage of potassium chloride elixir to correct thiazide-induced hypokalemia. JAMA 230:702, 1974.

Sirota, DK, Gendelman, S, and Huschmand, F: Thyrotoxic periodic paralysis. Mt Sinai J Med 39:165, 1972.

Soffer, A: Potassium therapy for digitalis toxicity. JAMA 183:228, 1963. Also JAMA 180:775, 1962.

Streeten, DHP: Periodic paralysis. In Stanbury, JB, Wyngaarden, JB, and Frederickson, DS, (eds). *The Metabolic Basis of Inherited Disease.* New York: McGraw-Hill, 1966.

Veldhuis, JD: The many faces of hypokalemia. Editorial. Arch Intern Med 143:1521, 1983.

Williams, ME, Gervino, EV, Rosa, RM, et al: Catecholamine modulation of rapid potassium shifts during exercise. N Engl J Med 312:823, 1985.

31

METABOLIC ALKALOSIS
SYNDROMES (Continued)

PRIMARY ALDOSTERONISM

In 1941, Ferrebee found that large doses of desoxycorticosterone acetate (Doca) produced sodium retention, potassium loss, polydipsia, polyuria, and intermittent muscular paralysis in dogs. Other investigators described similar but milder signs in humans who had been given excessive amounts of Doca. In 1955, Conn was able to show that a patient with similar signs had an excessive amount of a sodium-retaining hormone, which he identified as aldosterone. He described the patient as having "primary aldosteronism." The patient was cured by removing an adrenal cortical adenoma. Since then, numerous other reports of primary aldosteronism have been published.

PATHOPHYSIOLOGY

In Chapters 2 and 8 the mechanisms associated with the secretion of aldosterone were described. Aldosterone is the most potent mineralocorticoid secreted by the zona glomerulosa of the adrenal cortex. Its major effect is to increase resorption of sodium ions and to promote the secretion of potassium ions in the distal tubules of the kidneys. (A similar effect occurs in thermal sweat, saliva, and in the stool, causing a decreased sodium-potassium ratio in these fluids.)

The usual stimulus for the secretion of aldosterone is a decrease in the circulating blood volume. However, in primary aldosteronism, aldosterone is secreted by adrenal cortical cells autonomously. This causes a chronic retention of sodium ions and water, and an increased circulating blood volume and extracellular volume. However, edema is typically absent in patients with primary hyperaldosteronism. The reason for this apparently paradoxical absence of edema despite an excessive secretion of a salt-retaining hormone is not clear. Somehow, there is a homeostatic "escape" from the increased sodium resorption. The possibility that atrial natriuretic factor is responsible for this escape phenomenon was mentioned in Chapter 2.

Renin activity is characteristically suppressed in primary aldosteronism, partly because of the increased circulating blood volume.

The diastolic hypertension that occurs in primary aldosteronism may be due partly to an increased concentration of sodium ions and water in the arteriolar walls. This causes the arterioles to swell and the lumina to become smaller. As a result, the peripheral resistance rises and hypertension develops.

The renal loss of potassium ions produced by aldosterone causes a loss of total exchangeable body potassium. This in turn causes a metabolic alkalosis and other disturbances that have been described in Chapter 30. Aldosterone also causes an increased urinary excretion of magnesium ions.

Primary aldosteronism produces a hypokalemic metabolic alkalosis. A similar metabolic alkalosis can occur with Cushing's syndrome, ACTH-secreting tumors (such as adrenal adenocarcinoma or oat-cell carcinoma of the lung), Bartter's syndrome (hyperplasia of the juxtaglomerular apparatus), with the administration of mineralocorticoid steroids such as DOCA, cortisone, hydrocortisone, prednisone, and particularly fludrocortisone (Florinef), or with the excessive ingestion of licorice (20 to 40 g daily). (Glycyrrhizic acid, the active principle of licorice extract, is structurally and chemically similar to aldosterone.) Estrogens can also cause a similar metabolic alkalosis.

The metabolic alkalosis that develops is characterized by the fact that it is *saline resistant;* it cannot be corrected by sodium chloride alone, and requires potassium chloride (see Chapter 29).

PATHOLOGY

Primary aldosteronism is usually produced by a unilateral, benign, adrenal cortical adenoma. Rarely, multiple or bilateral adenomas may be present. In about 15% of patients, the syndrome is associated with diffuse, bilateral, micronodular adrenal cortical hyperplasia. (This has been called idiopathic, nonadenomatous, pseudoprimary, or tertiary aldosteronism.)

The syndrome can also be caused by an adrenal carcinoma that may also produce significant amounts of corticosterone. If the urinary excretion of 17-hydroxycorticosterone is greatly increased, this suggests Cushing's syndrome associated with an anaplastic ACTH-secreting adrenal carcinoma.

Glucocorticoid-remediable hyperaldosteronism is a rare cause of primary aldosteronism. It may be familial and is associated with adrenal hyperplasia. It is characterized by the fact that the hypertension and metabolic abnormalities can often be reversed by a glucocorticoid drug, such as dexamethasone.

SYMPTOMS AND SIGNS

Primary aldosteronism is found most commonly in the fourth and fifth decades, more often in women than in men, although it can occur at any age and in either sex.

Common symptoms include severe "bursting" central headache, fatigue or muscle weakness, which may be episodic with flaccid paralysis, paresthesias, muscle cramps, or frank tetany, increased thirst, and polyuria or nocturia.

Hypertension is present. The blood pressure may be slightly elevated. Occasionally, the diastolic blood pressure may rise to 120 or 130 mm Hg, but, even when this occurs, other signs of malignant hypertension, such as advanced retinopathy, do not usually appear. Peripheral edema, as mentioned above, is not usually noted.

Signs of potassium loss (*potassium wasting*) such as muscle weakness, fatigue, hyposthenia, polydipsia, or polyuria are other common findings.

The electrocardiogram shows signs of hypokalemia.

LABORATORY FINDINGS

The characteristic laboratory findings in patients with primary aldosteronism are: increased plasma aldosterone level (however, urinary aldosterone excretion may be normal or increased), subnormal plasma renin activity, metabolic alkalosis with hypokalemia and hypochloremia, and a slightly elevated serum sodium concentration (usually 145 mEq/L or higher). (In the early stages, the serum electrolyte concentrations may be normal.) The 24-hour urinary excretion of 17-hydroxycorticosteroids is normal, unless the aldosteronism is due to Cushing's syndrome.

Other laboratory findings may include abnormal glucose tolerance (probably due to the hypokalemia) or a maturity-onset type of diabetes mellitus. The sodium-potassium ratio of saliva is characteristically less than 0.25. Serum calcium and magnesium concentrations are almost always normal although hypomagnesemia has been reported.

Urine

The specific gravity is typically below 1.010 because urine concentration ability is reduced. The urine pH is typically alkaline, because of the increased urinary excretion of bicarbonate ions. However, some patients can acidify the urine to a pH of 5.0. (The presence of an alkaline urine associated with hypokalemia does not necessarily indicate aldosteronism, because an alkaline urine can develop as a result of a urinary tract infection.)

The urinary potassium excretion has diagnostic importance. In the usual patient with hypokalemia (for example, secondary to diarrhea, decreased intake, cathartic abuse), urinary potassium excretion is low. However, if hypokalemia is due to primary aldosteronism, the daily urinary potassium excretion is 40 mEq or more.

When the patient has been taking diuretics, the daily urinary potassium excretion may also be abnormally high, and may continue this way for several days to weeks after the diuretic is stopped. Therefore, if primary aldosteronism is suspected, the patient must not receive diuretics for at least 3 or 4 weeks.

Example: Patient with primary aldosteronism
    pH 7.54
    PCO_2 45 mm Hg
    Standard bicarbonate 36.3 mEq/L
    Actual bicarbonate 37 mEq/L
    Base excess +14 mEq/L
    CO_2 content 38.4 mEq/L

The pH is elevated. This indicates an alkalosis. The positive base excess and standard bicarbonate indicate that a metabolic alkalosis is present. The PCO_2 is normal, indicating a respiratory balance. However, the actual bicarbonate level is slightly higher than the standard bicarbonate. This indicates a slight respiratory acidosis. Therefore, a primary metabolic alkalosis is present with a partially compensatory respiratory acidosis (Chapter 15).

Cation-Anion Balance:
Na 146   K 2 HCO_3 37   Cl 96 mEq/L.
Anion gap = $(Na + K) - (HCO_3 + Cl)$.
        = $(146 + 2) - (37 + 96)$.
        = $148 - 133$
        = 15 mEq/L. This is normal.

DIAGNOSIS

Primary aldosteronism must be suspected in any patient, particularly a relatively young person, who shows mild or moderate diastolic hypertension, metabolic alkalosis with a serum potassium concentration of less than 3.5 mEq/L, a urinary potassium loss of 40 mEq/L or more, and who has no obvious reasons (diuretic therapy, vomiting, etc.) for the metabolic findings. Other symptoms and signs include muscular weakness and fatigue, hyposthenuria, polyuria, or nocturia due to potassium loss. (Primary aldosteronism must also be differentiated from the metabolic alkalosis due to potassium loss from other causes [Chapter 30].)

The diagnosis of primary aldosteronism must be confirmed by showing that an increased aldosterone excretion in the urine or an elevated plasma aldosterone level cannot be suppressed by volume loading, together with a low and suppressed plasma renin activity, for example:

1. Testing the effect of volume loading on aldosterone excretion or secretion.

   All diuretic drugs must be stopped for 3 to 4 weeks, because the volume-depleting effect of the diuretics may cause increased aldosterone secretion due to *secondary aldosteronism.*

   An initial screening test for aldosterone production can be done as an out-patient procedure (Bravo et al.). The patient adds 10 to 12 g of salt to the daily intake. After 5 to 7 days of increased salt intake the patient's serum potassium concentration is measured, along with a 24-hour urinary excretion of sodium, potassium, and aldosterone.

   Patients who demonstrate nonsuppressible aldosterone production following the salt loading, namely, an excretion rate of 14.0 μg or more per 24 hours, when the urinary sodium excretion is more than 250 mEq per 24 hours, require further diagnostic tests to determine if primary aldosteronism is present.

   A more specific test to determine whether aldosterone production cannot be suppressed with volume loading is to give the patient a high-sodium diet for 3 to 5 days. Then, 0.9% sodium chloride solution is infused over a 4-hour period in a dose of 25 mg/kg. Patients with primary aldosteronism show a high aldosterone excretion rate, greater than 14.0 μg per 24 hours.

   A patient with primary aldosteronism will show an increased aldosterone excretion or an elevated plasma aldosterone level in spite of the volume loading. Other patients will show decreased aldosterone excretion or plasma levels.

2. Testing for low and suppressed plasma renin activity. It is important that the patient is not receiving any medications that can affect the plasma renin activity for at least 2 weeks.

   (Conditions and drugs that can cause decreased renin release include supine posture; sodium loading [volume expansion]; drugs, such as potassium salts, propranolol, methyldopa, reserpine, ganglionic blockers (except guanethidine), clonidine, and nonsteroidal anti-inflammatory agents; and blockade of the autonomic nervous system. Conditions and drugs that can cause increased renin release include upright posture; sodium restriction [volume depletion]; drugs such as diuretics, including spironolactone, diazoxide, nitroprusside, hydralazine, chlorpromazine, thyroxine, oral contraceptives; and depletion of potassium [McGuffin and Gunnells]).

One should remember that finding a low or suppressed renin activity in a hypertensive patient is not necessarily a sign of primary aldosteronism, because it can occur in patients with low-renin essential hypertension. In order to establish a diagnosis of primary aldosteronism, it is also necessary to show that aldosterone excretion or secretion is nonsuppressible (see above).

Differentiation of Primary Aldosteronism Due to Adrenal Tumor from That Due to Bilateral Adrenal Hyperplasia (Idiopathic Aldosteronism)

When nonsuppression of aldosterone excretion and suppressed plasma renin activity are present, this indicates primary aldosteronism. However, it does not differentiate patients who have an aldosterone-producing tumor from those who have bilateral adrenal hyperplasia (idiopathic aldosteronism). The differential diagnosis is important because patients with an adrenal tumor should have the tumor removed surgically, whereas patients with bilateral hyperplasia should be treated medically. However, the differential diagnosis can be difficult. It has been found (Bravo et al.) that when the spontaneous serum potassium concentration is less than 3.0 mEq/L in a patient with primary aldosteronism, this indicates that an adenoma is present. Another sign of an adenoma is a postural decrease in aldosterone production. However a postural increase in aldosterone production does not exclude an adenoma.

Measurement of plasma 18-hydroxycorticosterone concentration can also be used to differentiate an adenoma from adrenal hyperplasia. Biglieri et al. found that overnight recumbent values greater than 100 ng/dL were considered pathognomonic of an adenoma.

It is important to try to localize the adenoma, which is most easily accomplished by computerized tomography.

Diagnosis of Normokalemic Primary Aldosteronism

Rarely, the serum potassium concentration is normal, in association with hypertension, in the early stages of primary aldosteronism. One can suspect that primary aldosteronism is present in such a patient if there are episodes of spontaneous hypokalemia, if hypokalemia develops shortly after thiazides are used, or if hypokalemia develops after a large amount of salt is ingested.

Low renin activity itself does not indicate primary aldosteronism, because low renin may be present in hypertensive patients who do not have aldosteronism. (These patients also have a normal or low urinary aldosterone excretion.)

Diagnosis of Secondary Aldosteronism

The term "secondary aldosteronism" describes patients in whom aldosterone levels are elevated due to extra-adrenal factors (primary increase in renin activity, decreased aldosterone clearance, etc.). Patients with hypertension associated with renal artery stenosis and patients with malignant hypertension may also have secondary aldosteronism and hypokalemia. Plasma renin activity in these patients with hypertension and secondary aldosteronism, however, will be *high*, in contrast to the low plasma renin activity in patients with primary aldosteronism.

(There have been several reports of aldosteronism secondary to a primary benign renin-secreting tumor of the kidney [juxtaglomerular cell tumor, renal hemangiopericytoma]. These patients show diastolic hypertension, increased plasma aldosterone level, increased plasma renin activity, and hypokalemia. Adrenal arteriography can be used to differentiate renal artery stenosis from a juxtaglomerular tumor. A unilateral high adrenal vein renin activity occurs in both conditions. However, a renal arteriogram will indicate if renal artery stenosis is present.)

Secondary aldosteronism (without hypertension) may also occur in the following situations: sodium depletion due to any cause, hypovolemia due to any cause, nephrotic syndrome, administration of large amounts of potassium salts, cirrhosis of the liver with ascites, congestive heart failure (particularly right-sided failure), idiopathic cyclic edema, Bartter's syndrome, and pregnancy. In all such patients, the plasma renin activity is high.

Differential Diagnosis of Patients with Hypertension, Hypokalemia, and Excessive Urinary Loss of Potassium Ions

These patients can be divided into two main types, depending on the plasma renin activity:

1. Patients with suppressed plasma renin activity include those with primary aldosteronism, aldosteronism due to Cushing's syndrome or tumors associated with excessive glucocorticoid production, excessive intake of licorice, tumors associated with the production of DOCA or corticosteroids, or excessive administration of mineralocorticoids or glucocorticoids, renal parenchymal disease, 11- or 17-hydroxylase deficiency.

2. Patients with elevated plasma renin activity include those with essential hypertension who have received diuretic therapy, malignant hypertension, renovascular hypertension, acute hydronephrosis, renin-producing juxtaglomerular tumors, or sodium-losing renal disease.

TREATMENT

Surgical removal of a single adrenal cortical tumor will cure the metabolic alkalosis and the hypokalemia. In addition, the hypertension will disappear in approximately one half of the patients and will become significantly lower in the others. However, if bilateral adrenal hyperplasia is present, subtotal or total adrenalectomy will restore the metabolic balance, but will not relieve the hypertension. In addition, the surgery may produce adrenocortical insufficiency, which may require mineralocorticoid or glu-cocorticoid therapy indefinitely. It is preferable to treat such patients with spironolactone. A low-sodium, high-potassium diet may also be necessary.

Preoperatively, the serum potassium concentration should be raised to normal. This can be done with potassium chloride, or with the aldosterone antagonist spironolactone (Aldactone). Large doses of 300 to 600 mg daily may be needed for even 1 week or more. As the serum potassium concentration rises, the blood pressure will fall and the weight will also fall because of a large urinary excretion of sodium ions (and water). (When the spirono-lactone is stopped, the serum potassium concentration will fall within 7 to 10 days. Also, when such large doses are used for chronic medical therapy, severe side effects—impotence, symptomatic gynecomastia, intermenstrual bleeding, mild azotemia, and so on—may occur.)

Immediately postoperatively, the patient usually shows signs of de-creased aldosterone secretion, so that hyponatremia and hyperkalemia de-velop. In addition, the electrocardiogram may show ST and T changes that simulate myocardial ischemia. The patient should be treated with both min-eralocorticoid and glucocorticoid steroids until aldosterone secretion re-turns to normal.

A renin-secreting kidney tumor is treated by surgical removal of the kidney.

BARTTER'S SYNDROME

Bartter's syndrome is a rare disorder in which patients show a hy-pokalemic metabolic alkalosis, occasionally with hyponatremia, due to al-dosteronism with increased aldosterone levels but usually without hyper-tension. The plasma renin activity is characteristically elevated. The syndrome is associated with hyperplasia of the juxtaglomerular apparatus. The pathogenesis of Bartter's syndrome remains uncertain; primary tubu-lar chloride wasting is the leading hypothesis. This in turn leads to the in-creased release of renin. Other characteristics include resistance to the pressor effects of intravenous angiotensin, a low serum magnesium con-centration, megacolon, and dilated ureters.

The syndrome often begins in childhood. Patients may show retarda-tion of growth, mental retardation, salt craving, tetany, and signs of hy-pokalemia.

The syndrome may be due to a form of salt wastage in the kidneys caused by defective reabsorption of sodium chloride in the loop of Henle. The loss of sodium chloride produces a sodium loss syndrome with a de-creased blood volume. This stimulates the secretion of aldosterone. In ad-dition, the reabsorption of potassium ions in the kidneys seems to be im-paired, so that an excessive amount of potassium ions are lost in the urine. The combination of potassium loss and increased aldosterone secretion produces a metabolic alkalosis.

Bartter's syndrome can be simulated by pseudo-Bartter's syndrome. Patients with this disease are mostly women who have chronic potassium loss due to long-term use of diuretics, cathartics, and sometimes surreptitious vomiting. As a result there is a loss of potassium and sodium ions and extracellular water, and a resulting secondary aldosteronism.

Treatment of Bartter's syndrome includes the use of spironolactone (Aldactone), which blocks the action of aldosterone, or triamterene (Dyrenium), a potassium-sparing diuretic. Drugs that inhibit prostaglandin synthesis, such as indomethacin, may be helpful. Propranolol (Inderal), which inhibits renin activity, may also be helpful.

Bibliography

Bartter, FC: Bartter's syndrome. Juxtaglomerular hyperplasia, normotension, hypokalemic alkalosis. JAMA 216:152, 1971.

Bartter, FC: So-called Bartter's syndrome. N Engl J Med 281:1483, 1969.

Bravo, DL, et al: The changing spectrum of primary aldosteronism. Am J Med 74:641, 1983.

Biglieri, EG, et al: Plasma aldosterone concentration. Further characterization of aldosterone-producing adenomas. Circ Res (suppl 11) 34:1183, 1974.

Carey, RM: Screening for surgically correctable hypertension caused by primary aldosteronism, Editorial. Arch Intern Med 141:1594, 1981.

Conn, JW, et al: Normokalemic primary aldosteronism. JAMA 193:100, 1965.

Conn, JW, et al: The syndrome of hypertension, hyperreninemia and secondary aldosteronism associated with renal juxtaglomerular cell tumor (primary reninism). J Urol 109:349, 1973.

Conn, JW, Rovner, DR, and Cohen, EL: Licorice-induced pseudoaldosteronism. Hypertension, hypokalemia, aldosteronopenia, and suppressed plasma renin activity. JAMA 205:492, 1968.

Farese, RV, Jr, Biglieri, EG, Schackleton, CHL, et al: Licorice-induced hypermineralocorticoidism. N Engl J Med 325:1223, 1991.

Ganguly, A, and Donohue, JP: Primary aldosteronism. J Urol 129:241, 1983.

Hoefnagels, WHL, and Kloppenborg, PWC: Hazards of long-term dexamethasone treatment in primary aldosteronism, Letter. N Engl J Med 306:427, 1982.

Holifield, JW, et al: Renin-secreting clear cell carcinoma of the kidney. Arch Intern Med 135:859, 1975.

Kassirer, JP, et al: On the pathogenesis of metabolic alkalosis in hyperaldosteronism. Am J Med 49:306, 1970.

Mazzacca, G, et al: Metoclopramide and secondary hyperaldosteronism, Letter. Ann Intern Med 98:1024, 1983.

McGuffin, WL, Jr, and Gunnells, JC, Jr: Primary aldosteronism. Urol Clin N Am 4:227, 1977.

Modlinger, RS, et al: Some observations on the pathogenesis of Bartter's syndrome. N Engl J Med 289:1022, 1973.

Ram, CVS: Primary aldosteronism. Comprehensive Therapy 8:60, 1982.

Torres, VE, Young, WF, Jr, Offord, KP, Hattery, RR: Association of hypokalemia, aldosteronism, and renal cysts. N Engl J Med 322:345, 1990.

Vaisrub, S: Simulacra of Bartter's syndrome, Editorial. JAMA 243:1075, 1980.

Weinberger, MH: Primary aldosteronism. Diagnosis and differentiation of subtypes, Editorial. Ann Intern Med 100:300, 1984.

White, MG: Bartter's syndrome. A manifestation of renal tubular defects. Arch Intern Med 129:41, 1972.

Williams, GH: Hyporeninemic hypoaldosteronism. N Eng J Med 314:1041, 1986.

Young, WR, et al: Primary aldosteronism: Diagnosis and treatment. Mayo Clin Proc 65:96, 1990.

32

SIMULTANEOUS RESPIRATORY AND METABOLIC SYNDROMES OF ACID-BASE BALANCE

It has already been pointed out that a primary respiratory acidosis is usually associated with a compensatory metabolic alkalosis. The reverse is also true. Similarly, a primary respiratory alkalosis is usually associated with a compensatory metabolic acidosis. The reverse is also true. However, primary respiratory and metabolic disturbances of acid-base balance can occur simultaneously and independently.

SIMULTANEOUS RESPIRATORY AND METABOLIC DISTURBANCES CAUSING OPPOSITE CHANGES IN pH

Two types of such disturbances can occur: simultaneous respiratory acidosis and metabolic alkalosis, and simultaneous respiratory alkalosis and metabolic acidosis. When this happens, the two disturbances tend to neutralize the changes in pH. However, the PCO_2 and the CO_2 content and the actual bicarbonate and standard bicarbonate concentrations indicate the two disturbances. This is shown below.

Simultaneous Respiratory Acidosis and Metabolic Alkalosis

This can occur, for example, in a patient with cor pulmonale who shows a respiratory acidosis and who also develops a metabolic alkalosis due to excessive diuretic therapy.

The simultaneous presence of the acidosis and the alkalosis tends to keep the pH within normal. However, the PCO_2 tends to be high due to the respiratory acidosis. The standard bicarbonate level is high because of the metabolic alkalosis. The actual bicarbonate level and the CO_2 content are necessarily high because of the standard bicarbonate concentration. However, the actual bicarbonate concentration is higher than the standard bicarbonate concentration because of the respiratory acidosis.

Example: Simultaneous respiratory acidosis and metabolic alkalosis.
   pH 7.4
   PCO_2 56 mm Hg
   CO_2 content 35.1 mEq/L
   Standard bicarbonate 30 mEq/L
   Actual bicarbonate 33.4 mEq/L
   Base excess +7 mEq/L

The pH is normal. However, the PCO_2 is high, indicating that a respiratory acidosis is present. Similarly, the actual bicarbonate concentration is higher than the standard bicarbonate concentration, because of the respiratory acidosis. The high standard bicarbonate concentration and the positive base excess indicate that a metabolic alkalosis is also present. Therefore, a respiratory acidosis and a metabolic alkalosis are present (Chapter 15).

This type of acid-base pattern can occur as a result of a simultaneous respiratory acidosis and a compensatory metabolic alkalosis, or vice versa. However, in a patient such as this, the history and clinical course would enable one to diagnose that two independent acid-base abnormalities are present.

Confidence bands of pH-PCO_2 relationships have been constructed to differentiate acute from chronic respiratory acidosis or alkalosis patients (Fig. 13–1). These relationships describe 95% of patients. However, they are not diagnostic, particularly when simultaneous mixed respiratory and metabolic disturbances are present.

Simultaneous Respiratory Alkalosis and Metabolic Acidosis

This type of disturbance, for example, can occur in a patient with diabetic (or renal) acidosis who shows hyperventilation for any reason. It also occurs in salicylate poisoning.

Here again, the simultaneous respiratory alkalosis and the metabolic acidosis cause the pH to remain within normal. However, the PCO_2 will tend to be low because of the respiratory alkalosis. The CO_2 content and the actual bicarbonate level will necessarily be low because of the low standard bicarbonate level. However, because a respiratory alkalosis is present, the actual bicarbonate level will be lower than the standard bicarbonate level.

Example: Simultaneous respiratory acidosis and metabolic alkalosis.

pH   7.4
PCO_2 20 mm Hg
CO_2 11 mEq/L
Standard bicarbonate 17 mEq/L
Actual bicarbonate 10 mEq/L
Base excess -10 mEq/L

The pH is normal. However, the PCO_2 is quite low, reflecting a respiratory alkalosis. However, the low CO_2 content, acutal bicarbonate level, and negative base excess all suggest concomitant metabolic acidosis. That the standard bicarbonate exceeds the actual confirms the metabolic acidosis. Examples of such clinical states would include hyperventilation (due to hypoxia, central nervous system disease, or metabolic derangement) associated with lactic acidosis, alcoholic ketoacidosis, salicylate poisoning, diarrhea, and so forth.

SIMULTANEOUS RESPIRATORY AND METABOLIC DISTURBANCES CAUSING SIMILAR CHANGES IN pH

These patients may show a simultaneous respiratory acidosis and a metabolic acidosis, or a simultaneous respiratory alkalosis and a metabolic alkalosis.

In these patients, it is obvious that the respiratory and the metabolic disturbances are not related, because when a respiratory or a metabolic disturbance is compensated, the compensation tends to cause the pH to move in the opposite direction. This type of disturbance is serious because an extreme shift in pH occurs and the patient may die.

Two types of such similar respiratory and metabolic changes can occur: acidosis and simultaneous respiratory and metabolic alkalosis.

Simultaneous Respiratory Acidosis and Metabolic Acidosis

This is an unusual combination. It has been produced experimentally by administering carbon dioxide to a curarized mental patient. It can occur in a patient with a respiratory acidosis due to chronic pulmonary disease and a metabolic acidosis due to excessive treatment with ammonium chloride for congestive heart failure. Severe acute pulmonary edema may cause concomitant respiratory acidosis and lactic acidosis.

In such a patient, the pH may be lowered to an extreme value below 7. The standard bicarbonate level will be low because of the metabolic acidosis. The CO_2 content and the actual bicarbonate level will be necessarily low because the standard bicarbonate level is low. However, the actual bicarbonate level will be higher than the standard bicarbonate level because of the respiratory acidosis.

Example: Simultaneous respiratory acidosis and metabolic acidosis.
pH 7.04
P_{CO_2} mm Hg
CO_2 content 21.9 mEq/L
Standard bicarbonate 14.8 mEq/L
Actual bicarbonate 20.5 mEq/L
Base excess − 12.8 mEq/L

The pH is low. This indicates an acidosis. The low standard bicarbonate level and the negative base excess indicate that a metabolic acidosis is present. However, the high P_{CO_2} and the fact that the actual bicarbonate level is higher than the standard bicarbonate level indicate that a respiratory acidosis is also present. Therefore, a metabolic acidosis and a respiratory acidosis are simultaneously present.

Simultaneous Respiratory Alkalosis and Metabolic Alkalosis

This type of disturbance also occurs rarely. Singer and Hastings produced it experimentally by having a subject ingest sodium bicarbonate (causing a metabolic alkalosis) and simultaneously having the subject hyperventilate (causing a respiratory alkalosis).

It can also be produced therapeutically if metabolic acidosis is treated with an excessive amount of an alkalinizing solution. The patient shows a compensatory respiratory alkalosis, which often persists even when the pH returns to normal. The excessive alkalinizing solution causes the metabolic alkalosis.

Example: Simultaneous respiratory alkalosis and metabolic alkalosis.
pH 7.64
P_{CO_2} 28 mm Hg
CO_2 content 30 mEq/L
Standard bicarbonate 32.5 mEq/L
Actual bicarbonate 29 mEq/L
Base excess + 9.3 mEq/L

The pH is high. This indicates an alkalosis. The high standard bicarbonate concentration and the positive base excess indicate that a metabolic alkalosis is present. However, the low P_{CO_2} and the fact that the actual bicarbonate level is lower than the standard bicarbonate level indicate that a respiratory alkalosis is also present. Therefore, a metabolic alkalosis and a respiratory alkalosis are simultaneously present.

SIMULTANEOUS MIXED METABOLIC DISTURBANCES

A primary metabolic acidosis can be complicated by a primary metabolic alkalosis, or vice versa. This can occur, for example, in a patient with diabetic (or renal) acidosis who develops severe vomiting or receives gastric lavage, which causes a metabolic alkalosis.

Example: Simultaneous metabolic alkalosis and metabolic acidosis.
pH 7.40
PCO_2 40 mm Hg
CO_2 content 26 mEq/L
Standard bicarbonate 24 mEq/L
Actual bicarbonate 24 mEq/L
Base excess — zero

All parameters are apparently normal. However, a high anion (see below) suggests a more complicated process.

Cation-Anion Balance:
Na 139   K 5 HCO_3 24   Cl 85
Anion gap = $(Na + K) - (HCO_3 + Cl)$
     = $(139 + 5) - (24 + 85)$
     = $144 - 109$
     = 35 mEq/L. This is abnormally high, indicating
       accumulation of metabolic acid.

The patient described above suffered from underlying renal failure, complicated by gastric outlet obstruction.

Bibliography

Fulop, M: Metabolic acidosis with alkalemia. New York State J Med 80:1365, 1980.
Gamble, JL: *Chemical Anatomy, Physiology and Pathology of Extracellular Fluid*, 6th ed. Cambridge, Mass: Harvard University Press, 1954.
McCurdy, DK: Mixed metabolic and respiratory acid-base disturbances. Diagnosis and treatment. Chest 62:355, 1972.
Singer, RB, and Hastings, AB: Improved clinical method for estimation of disturbances of acid-base balance of human blood. Medicine 27:233, 1948.

33

SYNDROMES ASSOCIATED WITH CALCIUM AND PHOSPHATE DISTURBANCES

A detailed discussion of syndromes associated with calcium and phosphorus metabolism is outside the scope of this book. However, a few important aspects of the problem can be considered.

CALCIUM

Bone consists of an organic matrix in which a complex calcium phosphate salt, hydroxyapatite $(Ca_{10}[PO_4]_6[OH]_2)$, is deposited. Bone has bone-resorbing and bone-forming surfaces. The kidneys normally regulate the composition of the extracellular fluid in contact with bone in such a way that bone is constantly being resorbed. The rate at which this occurs depends on minor fluctuations in the composition of the extracellular fluid. Bone deposition, on the other hand, occurs in response to stresses and strains whenever bone is needed; this is usually in areas where the bone has been resorbed. As a result of these two processes, about 0.5 g of calcium is renewed each day. This mechanism keeps the structure of the skeleton strong but not bulky. The average adult requires about 0.65 g of elemental calcium a day. A child needs 1 g, and a pregnant or lactating woman needs more.

The major factors that regulate bone resorption and formation are the presence or absence of vitamin D, the availability of parathyroid hormone, the serum concentrations of calcium and phosphate ions, and the ability of the kidneys to excrete or hold calcium or phosphate ions.

Level of Organic Phosphate Ions in the Serum

Normally, calcium and phosphate ions exist in a supersaturated state in the serum. The solubility constant of these ions is relatively fixed, so that an increase or decrease in serum phosphate concentration will tend to be associated with a reciprocal decrease or increase in serum calcium concentration, and vice versa.

Vitamin D

Necessary for the intestinal absorption of calcium, vitamin D also has the capacity to increase phosphate excretion by the kidneys to a lesser degree. Its presence may also be necessary for parathyroid hormone function.

Inactive vitamin D precursor in the skin is transformed into vitamin D_3 (cholecalciferol) as a result of ultraviolet radiation. It is also derived from foods such as milk, eggs, and fish. The vitamin D_3 is transported to the liver where it is hydroxylated to 25-OH-D_3 (25-hydroxycholecalciferol), which is more potent than vitamin D_3. (Anticonvulsive therapy with phenobarbital or phenytoin [Dilantin] interferes with the hydroxylation of vitamin D_3 and can lower the circulating level of 25-OH-D_3 and in this way can produce osteomalacia.) The 25-OH-D_3 is then carried through the blood to the kidneys where it is transformed into 1,25-$(OH)_2D_3$ (1,25 dihydroxy-vitamin D_3), which promotes the absorption of calcium ions in the intestines and mobilizes calcium ions from the bones. 1,25-$(OH)_2D_3$ is the most potent vitamin D metabolite.

When chronic renal disease is present, 1,25-$(OH)_2D_3$ is not formed in adequate amounts. Impaired vitamin D_3 metabolism is probably a significant factor in the pathogenesis of the hypocalcemia, osteomalacia, and secondary hyperparathyroidism that occur in chronic renal disease.

Other causes of a deficiency of vitamin D or its metabolites include dietary deficiency, hyperphosphatemia, intestinal malabsorption, nephrotic syndrome, and chronic renal failure.

It is now possible to measure the blood level of 25-OH-D_3. In patients with overt rickets or osteomalacia, the serum 25-OH-D_3 levels are essentially not detectable. Subnormal blood levels of 25-OH-D_3 can occur when there is a dietary deficiency of vitamin D, or decreased intestinal absorption due, for example, to gastrectomy or intestinal malabsorption, or long-term anticonvulsant therapy.

Parathyroid Hormone

Parathyroid hormone responds to the serum calcium concentration. A low serum calcium concentration stimulates parathyroid secretion, and a high concentration stops its secretion. 1,25 dihydroxy-vitamin D_3 also has an independent suppressive effect on parathyroid hormone release. Parathyroid hormone also is indirectly under the influence of the serum phosphate concentration. A high serum phosphate concentration will cause a secondary lowering of serum calcium concentration, which in turn stimulates the parathyroid hormone. This occurs in patients with severe renal disease and phosphate retention who develop secondary hyperparathyroidism (renal rickets).

The primary action of the parathyroid hormone is to increase the renal excretion of phosphate ions. Normally, most of the phosphate that is lost from the body appears in the urine. The amount excreted depends on the degree of glomerular filtration and the degree of tubular reabsorption. Parathyroid hormone reduces the amount of phosphate ions that are reabsorbed by the kidney tubules. As a result, an increased amount of phosphate is excreted in the urine, and the serum phosphate concentration falls. When parathyroid hormone is absent, the kidney tubules reabsorb an increased amount of phosphate, and the serum phosphate concentration rises. These changes in serum phosphate concentration caused reciprocal changes in serum calcium concentration and thus stimulate or depress the parathyroid gland. Parathyroid hormone also stimulates bone resorption directly and can raise the serum calcium concentration in this way.

Calcitonin

In 1961, Copp described a new calcium-lowering hormone that he called *calcitonin*. More recently, investigators have shown that calcitonin is secreted by specialized parafollicular cells that are embryonically related to the ultimobranchial bodies of birds.

The main action of calcitonin is to control calcium balance by counteracting some of the hypercalcemic effects of parathyroid hormone. For example, parathyroid hormone affects calcium metabolism by increasing resorption of bone, by increasing absorption of calcium ions from the gastrointestinal tract, and by increasing the reabsorption of calcium ions by the renal tubules. Calcitonin prevents the action of parathyroid hormone on bone by inhibiting the *osteoclastic* resorption of bone. Therefore, the serum calcium concentration decreases. Calcitonin secretion is directly stimulated by a high serum calcium concentration.

Calcitonin is a polypeptide and is inactivated by gastric juices. It is now available for clinical use and can be given parenterally. It may be useful in the treatment of hypercalcemic patients with hyperparathyroidism, hypervitaminosis D, osteoporosis, and a tendency to calcium stone formation, although it is recommended only for the treatment of patients with symptomatic Paget's disease. Conversely, the excessive production of calcitonin may be associated with hypocalcemia and increased density of bone.

Renal Excretion of Calcium

Most of the ingested calcium is excreted in the intestines. Less than 1% is excreted in the urine. In an adult, this amounts to about 100 to 150 mg a day. The amount of calcium excreted in the urine depends approximately on the serum calcium concentration. Parathyroid hormone is also able to increase directly calcium reabsorption by the renal tubules.

SIGNIFICANCE AND DETERMINATION OF SERUM CALCIUM CONCENTRATION

Disturbances in calcium metabolism are usually described in terms of hypocalcemia or hypercalcemia. However, determinations of serum calcium concentration may be misleading. The reason for this is that calcium is present in the blood primarily in two forms: (1) ionized calcium, which is physiologically active, and (2) calcium bound to protein. The concentration of bound calcium depends on the concentration of the plasma proteins. Normally, about 50% to 75% of the serum calcium is ionized; the remainder is bound to protein, mostly to the serum albumin. As the total protein in the blood rises, more of the calcium becomes bound.

Clinically it is important to correlate serum calcium concentration with the serum albumin level, because a larger percentage of the serum calcium becomes ionized as the total protein in the blood decreases. Therefore, a low serum calcium concentration in the presence of a low serum albumin level (this can occur with starvation, cirrhosis of the liver, or in the nephrotic syndrome) is associated with an increased concentration of ionized calcium ions, and symptoms of hypocalcemia do not appear. However, a low serum calcium concentration in the presence of a normal serum albumin level is associated with a decreased ionized calcium concentration, so that symptoms and signs of hypocalcemia may develop.

The following simple rule can be used to determine if the measured serum calcium concentration is significant:

Each fall (or rise) of serum albumin level by 1.0 g/dL (beyond the normal range of 4 to 5 g/dL) is associated with a fall (or rise) of serum calcium concentration of approximately 0.8 mg/dL.

It is now possible to measure the ionized calcium ion concentration directly, using a special calcium ion electrode.

HYPOCALCEMIA

Hypocalcemia exists when the serum calcium concentration falls below the lower normal value of 9 mg/dL (4.5 mEq/L). It may be associated with a loss of calcium in both the extracellular fluid and bone (for example in osteomalacia). In other patients, the hypocalcemia may be associated with a retention of phosphate (as in chronic renal disease), or with other factors localized in the extracellular fluid, such as hypomagnesemia or hypermagnesemia, or acute pancreatitis which results in the binding of calcium in the inflammatory exudate in the peritoneal cavity.

Serum calcium determinations should always be made simultaneously with a serum albumin determination, for reasons discussed above.

Etiology

Hypocalcemia can occur in the following situations:

1. Deficiency of vitamin D. This is the cause of childhood rickets, or osteomalacia (adult rickets). It also appears in malabsorption states, such as steatorrhea due to pancreatic insufficiency, sprue, celiac disease, biliary obstruction, or small bowel disease. These patients have decreased fat absorption and an increased amount of fat in the stool. This causes a loss of calcium due to the excretion of calcium salts of fatty acids. Vitamin D is also lost in this way. An excess of phytic acids, a constituent of cereals, can cause a loss of calcium in a similar way.

   In vitamin D deficiency, as in patients with steatorrhea, the poor absorption of calcium from the intestinal tract causes hypocalcemia, and a resultant secondary hyperparathyroidism. This in turn counteracts the decrease in serum calcium concentration. However, it produces a low serum phosphorus concentration.

2. Deficiency of parathyroid hormone (*hypoparathyroidism*). This may be idiopathic (where it may also be associated with adrenocortical insufficiency or with pernicious anemia), or it may develop after thyroid or parathyroid surgery.

3. Inadequate response of the renal tubules to parathyroid hormone (*pseudohypoparathyroidism* and *pseudopseudohypoparathyroidism,* see below).

4. Acute pancreatitis. Hypocalcemia is a common finding in acute pancreatitis. In the past, it was attributed entirely to the precipitation of calcium esters in areas of fat necrosis. It has also been suggested that the hypocalcemia might be due to the excessive secretion of glucagon from the inflamed pancreas, which in turn stimulates the secretion of calcitonin. Studies by Weir and associates indicate that the hypocalcemia of acute pancreatitis is secondary to sequestration of calcium ions outside the skeleton and/or is due to a yet undefined defect of bone metabolism.

   Clinically, a fall in serum calcium concentration below 7 mg/dL is a sign of poor prognosis in acute pancreatitis. A normal or high serum calcium concentration suggests that hyperparathyroidism may be present.

5. Hyperphosphatemia. This occurs in renal insufficiency where phosphate ions are retained in the body. (The hyperphosphatemia is one of the causes of hypocalcemia in these patients.)

   Recently, hyperphosphatemia and hypocalcemia have been reported in patients with acute lymphoblastic leukemia 24 to 48 hours after chemotherapy has been started.

6. Magnesium deficiency. The magnesium deficiency may prevent the action of parathyroid hormone on bone, so that hypocalcemia develops.
7. Excessive secretion of adrenocortical hormones, as in Cushing's syndrome, or when corticosteroids are given therapeutically.
8. Neoplasms of the breast, lung, prostate, associated with *osteoblastic* (bone-forming) metastases. Also, medullary thyroid carcinoma, if calcitonin is secreted by the carcinoma.
9. Renal tubular acidosis.
10. Acute intermittent porphyria with inappropriate secretion of ADH. The usual electrolyte disturbance is hyponatremia due to water excess. However, hypocalcemia and hypomagnesemia may also occur.
11. Drugs, such as the chelating agent disodium ethylenadiaminetetraacetate (disodium EDTA), corticosteroids, mithramycin, glucagon, heparin, loop diuretics, sodium fluoride, sodium nitroprusside, theophylline.

    Hypocalcemia may also develop after an infusion of phosphate or sulfate salts (used to treat hypercalcemia).
12. Nephrotic syndrome or cirrhosis of the liver. The low serum calcium concentration is due to the low protein concentration. The ionized calcium concentration is usually normal, and there are no symptoms or clinical signs of hypocalcemia. However, a small percentage of patients with nephrotic syndrome may develop true hypocalcemia due to vitamin D deficiency resulting from urinary loss of vitamin D–binding proteins.
13. Infusion of ACD (acid-citrate-dextrose) blood. This can occur as a result of the transfusion of a large volume of citrated blood-bank blood.

    When sodium citrate is infused, it is usually oxidized to sodium bicarbonate. (This can produce a transfusion alkalosis.) However, if a large amount of sodium citrate is infused rapidly, or in the presence of shock or liver damage, the excess citrate ions may bind calcium ions, producing hypocalcemia. This may cause tetany and even shock.
14. Parathyroid hormone deficiency. Causes include:
    a. Genetic disturbances, such as congenital absence of parathyroid glands, multiple endocrine deficiency with autoimmune candidiasis (MEDAC syndrome) where patients show chronic mucocutaneous candidiasis, Addison's disease, and other disturbances in association with hypoparathyroidism;
    b. Acquired disturbances, such as surgical removal of the parathyroid glands, irradiation to the glands, iron overload, neoplastic infiltration, suppression by hypercalcemia, hypomagnesemia, transient maternal hyperparathyroidism.

Pathophysiology

Calcium is needed by all tissues. It is needed for normal cardiac function, for the normal functioning of the nervous system, for the normal development of bone, and for normal blood clotting. The characteristic sign of hypocalcemia is an increased neuromuscular irritability that may cause tetany or even epileptiform seizures (see discussion of tetany below). In addition, the intracranial pressure may become elevated, with choked discs. When hypocalcemia persists for any length of time, calcium deposits may occur in abnormal locations, such as the eye lens or the basal ganglia. In addition, the bones may be more dense if the hypocalcemia is due to a lack of parathyroid hormone.

Symptoms and Signs

Tetany is the most characteristic sign of hypocalcemia. This can be caused either by a decreased serum calcium concentration, as in the above patients, or by an increased pH, as in patients with metabolic or respiratory alkalosis. A low pH decreases the tendency to tetany. This is the reason that tetany does not appear in metabolic acidosis due to chronic renal disease, even when the serum calcium concentration is very low. When the pH is increased, as in alkalosis, tetany occurs even if the serum calcium concentration is normal. When both the serum calcium and potassium concentrations are low, tetany is also inhibited. However tetany will appear if the serum potassium concentration is raised in such a patient, but the serum calcium concentration is allowed to remain low. Tetany can also be associated with hypokalemia, hypomagnesemia, or primary aldosteronism.

The patient may show carpopedal spasm, Trousseau's sign, Chvostek's sign, facial muscle spasm, paresthesias, or even convulsions that are often misdiagnosed as idiopathic epilepsy. (However, there is no aura and the patient does not get relief with anticonvulsive drugs.) Spasm of the bronchial muscles can produce an asthmatic attack. Spasm of the muscles of the abdominal viscera can simulate the symptoms and signs of an acute surgical abdominal condition.

Trousseau's sign to detect latent tetany is elicited by applying a blood pressure cuff to an upper extremity and inflating the cuff above the systolic level for 3 minutes. A positive reaction is the development of carpal spasm. However, Trousseau's sign is often absent in patients with latent tetany, and may be present in normal persons.

Chvostek's sign to detect latent tetany is elicited by percussing the facial nerve anterior to the ear. A positive reaction is unilateral contraction of the facial muscles and the muscles of the eyelids. (Contraction of the facial muscles alone may occur normally.)

Mental changes include changes in mood, emotional depression, impairment of memory, confusion, delirium, or even hallucinations.

Hypoparathyroid patients may show *defects in ectodermal structures,* including the skin, nails, hair, and teeth. Coarse, dry skin with patchy or absent axillary or pubic hair may be noted. Various degrees of hypoplasia of the teeth may be present, depending on when the hypoparathyroidism started. Fingernails may be deformed and brittle. Monilial infections of the nails, pharynx, or vagina are common. *Cataracts* may develop within one year. *Papilledema,* with or without an increased cerebrospinal fluid pressure, may also develop and may be associated with symptoms and signs, including convulsions, suggestive of a brain tumor. *Congestive heart failure* that responds to treatment with calcium salts may occur. *Diarrhea* due to intestinal malabsorption of vitamin B_{12} or fats may also manifest itself.

Laboratory Tests

When parathyroid hormone is totally absent, the serum calcium concentration may fall to 4.5 mg/dL, and the serum phosphate concentration may rise even to 12 mg/dL, especially in children.

Parathyroid Hormone (iPTH) Immunoassay in Blood

It is now possible to measure the parathyroid hormone level in serum, using a radioimmunoassay technique. Serum levels obtained in this way should be correlated with the serum calcium level to differentiate different conditions that may be associated with either hypocalcemia or hypercalcemia.

One should be aware that several assays are available (carboxy or nitrogen terminal or intact) and that the sensitivity of iPTH analyses from different laboratories can vary widely.

A metabolic alkalosis may develop. (Barzel and others have pointed out that the parathyroid hormone increases the urinary excretion of bicarbonate ions in association with changes in serum calcium and phosphate concentrations. When hypoparathyroidism is present, the lack of the parathyroid hormone causes a retention of bicarbonate ions and a rise in pH.)

Hypokalemia, hyperphosphatemia, and hypomagnesemia may also occur.

In the urine, there is a threshold for calcium excretion. As a result, calcium will be absent from the urine when the serum calcium concentration falls below 7 to 8 mg/dL. In some diseases, such as sarcoidosis, a high urinary calcium excretion can occur in spite of a normal serum calcium concentration.

The electrocardiogram shows a characteristic prolongation of the QT interval, with normal ST segments and normal T waves.

X-ray examination of the bones may not show abnormal findings. Occasionally, thickening of the lamina dura or calcification in various regions of the brain may occur. (Subcutaneous calcification rarely occurs in idiopathic hypoparathyroidism, but is common in pseudohypoparathyroidism.)

The electroencephalogram may show nonspecific changes.

Diagnosis

Common causes of symptomatic hypocalcemia include azotemia, hypoparathyroidism, osteomalacia (or rickets), and malabsorption syndromes. (Hypocalcemia associated with hypoalbuminemia is asymptomatic, as has been pointed out above.)

The serum phosphate concentration may be helpful in the differential diagnosis of hypocalcemia. For example, it is normal or low in most patients with vitamin D deficiency or with intestinal malabsorption and is elevated in most patients with hypoparathyroidism or azotemic patients (who are hypocalcemic).

Hypoparathyroidism can be simulated by *pseudohypoparathyroidism.* Such patients show a low serum calcium and a high serum phosphate concentration due to a genetic lack of response of the renal tubules to parathyroid hormone rather than to a lack of the hormone. In addition, patients may show short metacarpals, characteristic thickset figure and round face, demonstrable presence of parathyroid gland on biopsy, subcutaneous calcification (this is rare in idiopathic hypoparathyroidism), calcification of the basal ganglia, cataracts, tetany, dental defects, and often mental retardation. Treatment is the same as for hypoparathyroidism.

These patients can be differentiated from those with hypoparathyroidism by means of the Ellsworth-Howard test. The test is based on the fact that parathyroid hormone normally causes a markedly increased urinary excretion of phosphate ions in hypoparathyroid patients and in normal persons, but only a small increased excretion in pseudohypoparathyroid patients.

The term *pseudopseudohypoparathyroidism* has been used to describe patients who show physical signs similar to the pseudohypoparathyroid patients. However, there is no tetany, and the serum calcium and phosphate concentrations are normal. The Ellsworth-Howard test shows a normal phosphate diuresis. This condition is now considered to be merely a variant of pseudohypoparathyroidism.

Treatment

Tetany can be treated by either lowering the pH, if alkalosis is present, or raising the serum calcium concentration, if it is low. Calcium gluconate in a dose of 10 to 20 mL of a 10% solution can be given intravenously. It should be given slowly at a rate not exceeding 2 mL/min.

If symptoms are severe, calcium gluconate can be given by continuous intravenous solution. An average adult will require approximately 100 mL of 10% calcium gluconate dissolved in 1 liter of 5% dextrose in water, given slowly over a period of 4 hours.

Calcium salts should be given orally. Calcium lactate (which contains

13% calcium ions) can be given in a daily oral dose of 12 g. Calcium gluconate (which contains 9% calcium ions) can be given in a daily oral dose of 16 g. (A level teaspoonful of calcium lactate or calcium gluconate contains approximately 3 g.) Calcium carbonate (40% calcium) is also effective, but may cause gastric upset due to carbon dioxide formation in the stomach.

If tetany does not respond to the injection of a calcium salt, this may be a sign that the tetany is due to hypomagnesemia, particularly if the patient shows chronic alcoholism or malabsorption, or is poorly nourished. In such a case, 2 mL of a 50% solution of magnesium sulfate can be given intramuscularly.

Hypoparathyroidism is treated with large doses of calcium salts orally (16 to 32 g calcium lactate daily) plus vitamin D. Usually, large doses of vitamin D (25,000 to 100,000 IU daily) are needed. Various vitamin D preparations can be used. Ergocalciferol (Vitamin D_2: Drisdol, Winthrop) is satisfactory. One can start with a dose of 50,000 IU daily. However, ergocalciferol may not cause the serum calcium concentration to rise for two or more weeks.

If the hypocalcemia appears to be resistant to the action of ergocalciferol, dihydrotachysterol (Hytakerol, Winthrop) or calcitriol ($1,25$-$(OH)_2 D_3$; Rocaltrol, Roche) can be substituted. Conversely, patients who are resistant to dihydrotachysterol may respond to ergocalciferol. One should also remember that apparent resistance to the action of vitamin D may be due to hypomagnesemia. In such a case, the serum calcium concentration will rise only when the magnesium deficit is corrected. Vitamin D requirements will also be higher if the patient is taking estrogens.

If hypercalcemia develops as a result of conventional vitamin D therapy, it may last 2 months or more after the vitamin D is stopped. Hypercalcemia induced by calcitriol usually dissipates within a few days.

The hypocalcemia of hypoparathyroidism can also be treated with a thiazide or similar diuretic, such as chlorthalidone (Hygroton), in conjunction with a salt restricted diet, because the thiazides cause the serum calcium concentration to rise (Porter and associates). (Conversely, a diuretic such as furosemide, which can lower the serum calcium concentration, may worsen hypoparathyroidism.)

Rarely, a patient will respond to calcium salts, without vitamin D. However, it may take 1 or 2 weeks for the oral calcium salts to cause a rise in serum calcium concentration.

Patients may respond clinically even when they remain slightly hypocalcemic (serum calcium concentration 8.5 to 9.0 mg/dL). The effectiveness of calcium supplements and vitamin D should be checked with periodic serum calcium determinations every 3 to 4 months indefinitely. (In this way, the development of drug-induced *hypercalcemia* can be prevented.) The use of the Sulkowitch test to measure urinary calcium excretion is therefore not necessary.

When a patient is given large doses of oral calcium salts, it is not necessary to use a high-calcium diet. It is also not necessary to place the patient on a low-phosphorus diet, or to use aluminum hydroxide gels to prevent absorption of phosphate ions from the gastrointestinal tract.

Hypocalcemia due to hypomagnesemia must be treated by raising the serum magnesium concentration.

Calcium salts should be given cautiously to patients taking digitalis because there is evidence that the calcium can precipitate digitalis toxicity.

Hypocalcemia due to citrate toxicity can be prevented when no more than 1000 to 1500 mL of blood bank blood is given per hour to an adult, and when 10 mL calcium gluconate is given intravenously with each 1500 mL blood. (Howland and his associates found that the administration of calcium salts with blood-bank transfusions of 2500 mL or more can be associated with ventricular fibrillation. They therefore suggest that calcium salts should not be used even with blood-bank blood. Studies by Olinger and associates and others indicate the value of calcium salts during transfusion of blood-bank blood.)

OSTEOPOROSIS

Osteoporosis is due to excessive bone resorption. It is often seen in postmenopausal women, in hypogonadic males, or in elderly persons. However, it may occur at any age (idiopathic osteoporosis). Other causes include long-term corticosteroid therapy, Cushing's syndrome, hyperthyroidism, long-term heparin therapy, steatorrhea and other intestinal malabsorption syndromes, rheumatoid arthritis, vitamin C deficiency, and gastrectomy. It can also be precipitated by long-term immobilization. The mechanism by which it occurs is not clearly understood. A deficiency of calcium absorption from the gastrointestinal tract may be a factor, because there is an abnormally high fecal excretion of calcium ions in osteoporosis, regardless of the cause.

In spite of this, serum calcium, phosphate, and alkaline phosphatase levels are normal in most patients with postmenopausal, senile, or idiopathic osteoporosis. In hyperthyroidism, the serum calcium concentration may become elevated; the serum phosphate concentration may be normal or low. In Cushing's syndrome, the patient may show slight hypocalcemia and hypophosphatemia, with a slight increase in alkaline phosphatase level.

Clinical signs are related to compression of one or more vertebral bodies (however, compression of the spinal cord does not occur) or fracture, particularly of the lower end of a radius, rib, or neck of a femur.

Treatment includes a high calcium intake, approximately 1 to 1.5 g of calcium ions daily. (One quart of milk provides 1 g of calcium ions, plus phosphate ions, which are also helpful in alleviating osteoporosis.) Other foods that have a high calcium content include broccoli, turnip greens (raw or cooked), watercress (raw or cooked), almonds, mackerel, molasses, and dried brewer's yeast.

Estrogens in postmenopausal women are also beneficial, despite a slightly increased risk of uterine cancer even with small doses.

Vitamin D is also helpful, particularly when the osteoporosis is due to corticosteroid therapy. As much as 5,000 to 10,000 IU daily may be needed. (One must check the serum calcium concentration every several months when such high doses of vitamin D are given to prevent hypercalcemia.)

Fluoride salts have also been used but can induce changes in bone structure and can cause secondary hyperparathyroidism. Accordingly, they are unlikely to be released for clinical use.

OSTEOMALACIA

Osteomalacia in adults (or rickets in children) is due to a defective mineralization of osteoid bone. The usual explanation for its development is a decrease of the serum Ca × P product below the critical level of approximately 30 to 40, which is necessary for the growth of hydroxyapatite crystals in bone matrix and epiphyseal cartilage. Therefore, osteomalacia can occur when the serum calcium concentration is low, as in vitamin D deficiency (this may occur as a result of a dietary deficiency of vitamin D, or from steatorrhea or other intestinal malabsorption syndromes, or after gastrectomy), or when the serum phosphate concentration is low (as after excessive intake of aluminum hydroxide gels, in the Fanconi syndrome, or in familial hypophosphatemia [*vitamin D–resistant rickets*]). In addition, osteomalacia can occur when the Ca × P product is normal, as in renal osteodystrophy, renal tubular acidosis, or ureteroenterostomy with acidosis, for reasons which are not clear. Osteomalacia and osteoporosis can coexist.

In the beginning of this chapter it was pointed out that phenobarbital or phenytoin (Dilantin) interferes with the metabolism of vitamin D and can cause osteomalacia. When acetazolamide is given to a patient who is taking phenytoin, the tendency to osteomalacia is increased.

Symptoms include muscular weakness, severe bone pains, worsened by weight lifting, and a waddling gait. Tetany may also occur. Characteristic findings on x-ray examination are linear translucencies (pseudofractures, Looser's zones, Milkman's syndrome). These can be seen in the wings of the scapulae, ribs, pubic and ischial rami, neck of the femurs, proximal third of the ulnae, and other bones. Actual fractures may also develop through these pseudofractures. (X-ray findings of secondary hyperparathyroidism [Chapter 34] may also develop.)

Characteristic laboratory findings include an elevated alkaline phosphatase level and a marked decrease or absence of calcium in the urine. (Hypophosphatemia may be more marked than the hypocalcemia. This is probably due to the development of secondary hyperparathyroidism, which raises the low serum calcium concentration.)

When the osteomalacia is due to vitamin D deficiency or to renal osteodystrophy, vitamin D is effective. Patients with the Fanconi syndrome, renal tubular acidosis, or ureteroenterostomy acidosis can be treated with alkaline salts to correct the acidosis, and with oral phosphate supplements (Chapter 18), to correct the hypophosphatemia (page 302). Vitamin D is probably not necessary in these patients. If osteomalacia due to inadequate calcium absorption from the intestines is also present, the patient should be given a high calcium intake.

Postmenopausal osteoporotic hypertensive women with adequate kidney function can be treated with thiazides, which conserve the urinary excretion of calcium ions, rather than with furosemide, which increases calcium excretion through the kidneys (Norenberg).

HYPERPHOSPHATEMIA

An excess of phosphate ions and hyperphosphatemia are usually due to renal insufficiency. However, hyperphosphatemia may occur as a result of hypoparathyroidism. Clinically, it is associated with tetany. The hyperphosphatemia is usually associated with some degree of hypocalcemia and signs of renal impairment, such as acidosis, azotemia, or high serum creatinine level. Hyperphosphatemia also occurs with excessive bone growth activity, as in acromegalic patients.

Hyperphosphatemia is treated by a low phosphorus diet and phosphate binders (i.e., calcium acetate, calcium carbonate).

Bibliography

Ajlouni, K, et al: Hyperphosphatemia and hypocalcemia in myeloproliferative disorders. Ann Intern Med 81:119, 1974.
Albright, F, and Reifenstein, EC, Jr: *Parathyroid Glands and Metabolic Bone Disease.* Baltimore: Williams & Wilkins, 1948.
Austin, LA, and Heath, H, III: Calcitonin. Physiology and pathophysiology. N Engl J Med 304:269, 1981.
Avioli, LV, guest editor: Vitamin D metabolites. Their clinical importance. Arch Intern Med 138:835, 1978.
Avioli, LV, and Haddad, JG: The vitamin D family revisited. N Eng J Med 311:47, 1984.
Barragry, JM, et al: Vitamin D metabolism in nephrotic syndrome. Lancet 2:629, 1977.
Bartter, FC: Pseudohypoparathyroidism and pseudo-pseudohypoparathyroidism. In Stanbury, JB, Wyngaarden, JB, and Fredrickson, DS, (eds): *The Metabolic Basis of Inherited Disease,* 2nd ed. New York: McGraw-Hill, 1966.
Barzel, US: Treatment of hypoparathyroidism. New York State J Med 76:579, 1976.
Bashour, TT, et al: Hypocalcemic cardiomyopathy. Chest 78:663, 1980.
Bashour, TT, et al: Hypocalcemic acute myocardial failure secondary to rapid transfusion of citrated blood. Am Heart J 108:1040, 1984.
Baylink, DJ: Glucocorticoid-induced osteoporosis (editorial). N Engl J Med 309:306, 1983.

Bikle, DD: Fluoride treatment of osteoporosis (editorial). Ann Intern Med 98:1013, 1983.

Bilezikian, JP: Surgery or no surgery for primary hyperparathyroidism. Ann Intern Med 102:402, 1985.

Carpenter, TO, et al: Hypoparathyroidism in Wilson's disease. N Engl J Med 309:874, 1983.

DeLuca, HF: Vitamin D endocrinology. Ann Intern Med 85:377, 1976.

Dent, CE: Osteomalacia due to phosphate depletion from excessive aluminum hydroxide ingestion. BMJ 1:551, 1974.

Fatourechi, V, and Heath, H, III: Salmon calcitonin in the treatment of postmenopausal osteoporosis. Ann Intern Med 107:923, 1987.

Frame, B, and Marel, GM: Clinical disorders of bone and mineral metabolism, Symposium. Ann Intern Med 99:725, 1983.

Frame, B, and Parfitt, AM: Osteomalacia. Current concepts. Ann Intern Med 89:966, 1978.

Frame, B, and Sudhaker, RD: Calcium-regulating hormones. Symposium. Ann Intern Med 93:928, 1980.

Fraser, DR: The physiological economy of vitamin D. Lancet 1:969, 1983.

Freitag, J, et al: Impaired parathyroid hormone metabolism in patients with chronic renal failure. N Engl J Med 298:29, 1978.

Fulop, M: Hypoparathyroidism after ^{131}I therapy. Ann Intern Med 75:808, 1971.

Gabow, PA, et al: Furosemide-induced reduction in ionized calcium in hypoparathyroid patients. Ann Intern Med 86:579, 1977.

Gravelyn, TR, et al: Hypophosphatemia-associated respiratory muscle weakness in a general inpatient population. Am J Med 84:870, 1988.

Horsman, A, et al: The effect of estrogen dose on postmenopausal bone loss. N Engl J Med 309:1405, 1983.

Juan, D: Vitamin D metabolism. Postgrad Med 68:210, 1980.

Kalu, DN, and Foster, CV: Calcitonin. Its physiologic roles. New York State J Med 76:230, 1976.

Lane, JM, et al: Osteoporosis. Current diagnosis and treatment. Geriatrics 39:40, 1984.

Laymon, CW, and Zelickson, A: Pseudohypoparathyroidism: The Seabright Bantam syndrome. Arch Derm 79:194, 1959.

Levine, MM, and Kleeman, CR: Hypercalcemia. Pathophysiology and treatment. Hosp Pract July 15, 1987, p 93.

Ludbrook, J, and Wynn, V: Citrate intoxication. Br Med J 2:523, 1958.

Lufkin, EG, et al: Parathyroid hormone radioimmunoassay in the differential diagnosis of hypercalcemia due to primary hyperparathyroidism or malignancy. Ann Intern Med 106:560, 1987.

Lutwak, L, Singer, FR, and Urist, MR: Current concepts of bone metabolism. Ann Intern Med 80:630, 1974.

McLean, F, and Hastings, AB: Clinical estimation and significance of the calcium ion concentration in the blood. Am J Med Sci 189:601, 1935. Also J Biol Chem 108:285, 1935.

McPherson, ML, et al: Theophylline-induced hypercalcemia. Ann Intern Med 105:52, 1986.

Moore, FD: The citrate lesion. In *Metabolic Care of the Surgical Patient*. Philadelphia: W.B. Saunders, 1959.

Newmark, SR, and Himathongkam, T: Hypercalcemic and hypocalcemic crises. JAMA 230:1438, 1974.

Norenberg, DD: Furosemide, hypertension, and osteoporosis, letter. JAMA 241:237, 1979.

Olinger, GN, et al: Acute clinical hypocalcemic myocardial depression during rapid blood transfusion and postoperative hemodialysis. J Thoracic Cardiovascular Surg 72:503, 1976.

Parfitt, AM: Adult hypoparathyroidism. Treatment with calcifediol. Arch Intern Med 138:874, 1978.

Parfitt, AM, and Kleenkoper, M: Clinical disorders of calcium, phosphorus, and magnesium metabolism. In Maxwell, MH, and Kleeman, CR, (eds): *Clinical Disorders of Fluid and Electrolyte Metabolism,* 3rd ed. New York: McGraw-Hill, 1980.

Payne, RB, et al: Interpretation of serum calcium in patients with abnormal serum proteins. BMJ 4:643, 1973.

Pepper, GM, et al: Hypocalcemia in metastatic bone disease. NY State J Med 84:41, 1984.

Porter, RH, et al: Treatment of hypoparathyroid patients with chlorthalidone. N Engl J Med 298:577, 1978.

Raisz, LG: The pharmacology of bone. Rational Drug Ther 5:6, 1971.

Raisz, LG, and Kream, BE: Regulation of bone formation. N Engl J Med 309:29:83, 1983.

Raisz, LG, and Smith, J: Prevention and therapy of osteoporosis. Rational Drug Ther 19:1985.

Raskin, P, McClain, CJ, and Medsger, TA, Jr: Hypocalcemia associated with metastatic bone disease. Arch Intern Med 132:539, 1973.

Riggs, LB, and Melton, LJ: The prevention and treatment of osteoporosis. N Engl J Med 327:620, 1992.

Robertson, GM, et al: Inadequate parathyroid response in acute pancreatitis. N Engl J Med 294:512, 1976.

Rushton, AR: Pseudohypoparathyroidism, cimetidine, and neurologic toxicity, letter. Ann Intern Med 98:677, 1983.

Rude, RK, et al: Functional hypoparathyroidism and parathyroid hormone end-organ resistance in human magnesium deficiency. Clin Endocrinol 5:209, 1976.

Silva, OL, et al: Ectopic secretion of calcitonin by oat-cell carcinoma. N Engl J Med 290:1122, 1974.

Spencer, H, and Kramer, L: Antacid-induced calcium loss. Editorial. Arch Intern Med 143:657, 1983.

Spiegel, AM, et al: Pseudohypoparathyroidism. Editorial. N Engl J Med 307:679, 1982.

Tapia, J, Stearns, G, and Ponseti, IV: Vitamin D-resistant rickets. J Bone Joint Surg 46A:935, 1964.

Uhr, N, and Bezahler, HB: Pseudo-pseudohypoparathyroidism. Ann Intern Med 54:443, 1961.

Walter, RM: A strategy for the management of osteoporosis. Modern Med 55:84, 1987.

Weir, GC, et al: The hypocalcemia of acute pancreatitis. Ann Intern Med 83:185, 1975.

Zimmerman, J, et al: Normocalcemia in a hypoparathyroid patient with sarcoidosis. Evidence for parathyroid-hormone-independent synthesis of 1,25 dihydroxyvitamin D. Ann Intern Med 98:338, 1983.

Zsigmond, EK: Hypocalcemic hypotension. JAMA 226:355, 1973.

Zusman, J, Brown, DM, and Nesbit, ME: Hyperphosphatemia, hyperphosphaturia and hypocalcemia in acute lymphoblastic leukemia. N Engl J Med 289:1335, 1973.

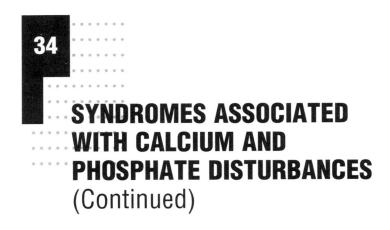

SYNDROMES ASSOCIATED WITH CALCIUM AND PHOSPHATE DISTURBANCES
(Continued)

HYPERCALCEMIA

Hypercalcemia exists when the serum calcium concentration rises above the upper normal value of 10.5 mg/dL (5.25 mEq/L). It may be associated with an excess of calcium in both extracellular fluid and in bone (for example, due to excessive intake of vitamin D or calcium). In other patients, the hypercalcemia is associated with a localized or generalized deficit of calcium in bone (as in hyperparathyroidism).

Etiology

The most common causes of hypercalcemia are neoplasms (with or without bone metastases), hyperparathyroidism, multiple myeloma, sarcoidosis, excessive vitamin D therapy, the milk-alkali syndrome, and prolonged immobilization.

Hypercalcemia can also be classified in the following ways:

1. More calcium is absorbed from the gastrointestinal tract than can be stored in the bones, or excreted by the kidneys. This occurs in:
    a. Excessive administration of vitamin D (usually 50,000 IU or more daily) for several months or more. The hypercalcemia may occur as early as 2 weeks or as late as years after the vitamin D therapy has started.
    b. Sarcoidosis. Hypercalcemia can occur in the absence of bone involvement. It is probably due to excessive absorption of calcium

from the bowel, related to increased sensitivity to exogenous or endogenous vitamin D. (Hypercalciuria is also common and may occur in sarcoid patients who do not have hypercalcemia.)

  c. Milk-alkali syndrome. This can occur in patients with peptic ulcer treated with an excessive amount of milk and alkaline antacids, particularly calcium carbonate, for a long time. (Excessive calcium carbonate intake, without milk, can also cause the syndrome.) These patients show a metabolic alkalosis in association with the hypercalcemia. If the syndrome persists, the hypercalcemia may cause severe renal failure. Vomiting is common and aggravates the metabolic alkalosis.

    (The hypercalcemia, due to the increased intake of calcium salts, suppresses the secretion of parathyroid hormone. As a result, the urinary excretion of phosphate salts decreases, so that hyperphosphatemia may develop. The combination of hypercalcemia and hyperphosphatemia can produce nephrocalcinosis, metastatic calcification, and progressive renal failure.)

  d. Lymphoma. Some variants may be associated with excessive calcium absorption due to hydroxylation of vitamin D by the lymphoma cells, but most lymphoma-induced hypercalcemia is due to bone destruction (see 2b below).

2. Bone destruction may exceed bone production so much that the kidneys are unable to excrete the excessive calcium ions. This occurs in:

  a. Primary hyperparathyroidism. This is usually due to a single parathyroid adenoma. In about 10% of patients, it is due to hyperplasia of the four parathyroid glands. Carcinoma of the parathyroid is a rare cause of hyperparathyroidism.

    Occasionally, hyperparathyroidism occurs in association with other endocrine disorders (multiple endocrine adenomatosis). For example, Sipple's syndrome refers to the triad of hyperparathyroidism, pheochromocytoma, and medullary carcinoma of the thyroid. Hyperparathyroidism also may occur in association with a pituitary adenoma. Severe peptic ulcer may be present, because parathyroid hormone induces hyperplasia of pepsin-secreting cells in the stomach. Other hyperparathyroid patients may show signs of a Zollinger-Ellison syndrome or WDHA syndrome.

  b. Malignant neoplasms. Hypercalcemia may occur in patients with many types of neoplasms, especially carcinoma of the breast and lung, hypernephroma, multiple myeloma, and lymphomas and leukemias. The hypercalcemia of these patients may be due to diverse causes. In some, the hypercalcemia occurs with osteolytic metastases. Immobilization of a cancer patient may also contribute to the hypercalcemia. Some neoplasms may produce a parathormone-like hormone. Other patients can produce a hormonal substance (or substances), such as prostaglandins and growth factors, not related to parathormone, that causes calcium resorption from bone. In many patients with neoplasms, hypercalcemia is present without obvious signs of bony metastases.

   c. Disseminated tuberculosis of the bones.

3. Decreased bone formation may be present. This can occur if a patient is immobilized for a long time, particularly if Paget's disease is present. It can occur, however, in any patient who is immobilized.

4. A persistent, excessive secretion of parathyroid hormone may be present. This occurs in:

   a. Primary hyperparathyroidism.

   b. Secondary hyperparathyroidism. This can occur when the serum calcium concentration is lowered by such conditions as renal glomerular insufficiency with phosphate retention, renal tubular insufficiency with urinary loss of calcium, rickets or osteomalacia, or pregnancy. However, even when secondary hyperparathyroidism develops and the serum calcium concentration rises, it does not become abnormally high.

   c. Irreversible secondary hyperparathyroidism (previously called "tertiary" hyperparathyroidism). This may develop in patients with secondary hyperparathyroidism when the parathyroid glands become autonomous. These patients show both hypercalcemia and hyperphosphatemia.

5. Hypercalcemia due to inadequate renal excretion of calcium salts.

6. Familial hypocalciuric hypercalcemia. This is a genetic disturbance showing an autosomal dominant syndrome of hypercalcemia, hypophosphatemia, and signs of parathyroid overactivity. In contrast to hyperparathyroidism, there is a markedly reduced urinary excretion of calcium. Chondrocalcinosis and pancreatitis are common. Ordinarily, no treatment is needed. However, if acute pancreatitis develops, total parathyroidectomy is recommended (Marx et al.).

7. Hypercalcemia may also occur as a result of the following miscellaneous causes:

   a. Endocrine disturbances such as hyperthyroidism, hypothyroidism, adrenocortical insufficiency, acromegaly, pheochromocytoma.

   b. Diuretics. Thiazides and chlorthalidone potentiate the action of parathyroid hormone on the kidneys, resulting in a retention of calcium ions. They are therefore helpful in treating idiopathic hypercalciuria. They rarely cause hypercalcemia. (When this occurs, hyperparathyroidism should be suspected.)

   c. Hypervitaminosis A. Hypercalcemia may occur as a result of increased bone resorption.

   d. After the use of calcium exchange resins in hemodialysis, the diuretic phase of acute renal failure, after renal transplantation, and in hypophosphatasia.

e. Lithium salt intake.
f. After the use of oral isotretinoin for acne.
g. Tuberculosis, beryllosis.
h. Artifactual hypercalcemia. This can occur, for example, in multiple myeloma, where one of the abnormal globulin molecules binds calcium ions. In such cases, the value of ionized calcium is normal.

Pathophysiology

Hypercalcemia causes decreased neuromuscular excitability, in contrast to hypocalcemia. In addition, marked hypotonicity of the muscles occurs.

Hypercalcemia may be associated with an increased calcium excretion in the urine (hypercalciuria). As a result, calcium stones can form in the kidney pelves, and calcium deposits can develop in the collecting tubules of the kidneys. These tubular injuries are probably the cause of the decreased ability of the kidneys to form a concentrated urine. Hypercalcemia can cause severe anatomical injury to the kidneys, especially in the ascending limb of Henle, the distal convoluted tubules, and the collecting tubule. Epithelial degeneration, necrosis, and calcification have also been found.

In addition, metastatic calcification in various organs of the body (the lung, gastric mucosa, and kidneys) may develop, particularly where the local pH of the body is elevated. Calcification can also occur in arterial walls, around joints, in the cornea (producing a "band" keratitis), and in the conjunctiva.

If the hypercalcemia is due to hyperparathyroidism and if the patient is in negative calcium balance due to a low-calcium diet, osteolytic bone lesions may develop.

Hypercalcemia (or parenteral calcium salts) can precipitate digitalis toxicity.

Symptoms and Signs

Some of the symptoms, such as muscular weakness or incoordination, loss of appetite, and constipation, may be due to decreased tone in smooth and striated muscle. Generalized muscle weakness is common, with or without muscle incoordination. The patient may drop things with the hands or trip with the feet. Ataxia may be present, and the patient may develop a loss of pain or vibration sense. Hypotonia may be present, and the patient may show hyperextensible limbs. Muscle aches and pains may be severe. Deep tendon reflexes may be increased or abnormal, and a positive Babinski reflex may be present. The electroencephalogram may show diffuse slow activity.

The cerebrospinal fluid protein level may be elevated. Therefore, when a patient with cancer develops disturbed consciousness, headache, and increased cerebrospinal fluid protein, this may be due to hypercalcemia alone rather than to cerebral metastases.

Gastrointestinal symptoms are also common—anorexia, nausea, vomiting, and constipation. Occasionally, increased salivation and dysphagia may be noted. Severe abdominal pain, abdominal distention, and ileus may simulate an abdominal emergency. (However, acute pancreatitis may develop as a complication of hyperparathyroidism.) Thirst may be severe. The increased incidence of peptic ulcers in hyperparathyroid patients has already been mentioned.

Itching may develop with chronic hypercalcemia. This may be due to calcium deposits in the skin.

Characteristic ocular signs of hypercalcemia may be found, including gray or white opaque granular bands in the cornea (band keratopathy). These have a crescent shape and follow the arc of the limbus. They resemble arcus senilis, but are more marked in the lateral and medial margins of the cornea. (Arcus senilis is more prominent at the superior and inferior borders of the cornea.) Small, clear, glasslike deposits may also develop in the conjunctivae, near the palpebral fissures.

Incomplete or complete AV block may occur. Cardiac standstill occurs when the serum calcium concentration is approximately 18 mg/dL.

Psychoneurotic and neurological signs are often prominent. The patient may show mental confusion, impairment of memory, slurred speech, acute psychotic behavior, lethargy, or coma. Convulsions are rare. The more severe signs occur when the serum calcium concentration is approximately 16 mg/dL or higher. If hypercalcemia persists for a long time, mental retardation may occur.

Polyuria and polydipsia, with clinical signs of water loss, may occur, due to disturbed renal tubular function produced by the hypercalcemia. When kidney damage is marked, azotemia may develop. This may then cause a secondary hyperparathyroidism.

Renal colic due to kidney stones is very common. (X-ray signs of calcification in the kidneys may also be present.) The stones are usually composed of calcium oxalate or calcium phosphate, or both. However, if a chronic urinary tract infection has been present, the stones may be covered with a layer of triple phosphates.

If hyperparathyroidism is present, a palpable mass, often tender, may be found in the region of the thyroid gland in about one third of patients.

Hyperparathyroid patients may also show other endocrine abnormalities (see Etiology, above).

Hypercalcemic Crisis

Hyperparathyroid and other hypercalcemic patients may develop a hypercalcemic crisis associated with an acute rise in serum calcium concentration. The critical level of serum calcium is approximately 17 mg/dL. At this concentration, calcium salts precipitate in the kidneys and in other organs.

Symptoms include muscular weakness, intractable nausea, abdominal cramps, obstipation or diarrhea, peptic ulcer symptoms, or bone pain. Severe thirst and polyuria are characteristic. These findings may quickly lead to signs of severe water loss, including fever, lethargy, mental confusion, delirium, or coma. Azotemia is present. The serum phosphate concentration may be normal or high. Hypokalemia or hypomagnesemia may be present due to increased urinary excretion of these ions. Hypernatremia may be present due to a loss of water from vomiting or from the excessive volume of urine.

Laboratory Tests

Blood

The serum calcium concentration is usually elevated above 11 mg/dL. However, Yendt has pointed out that the serum calcium concentration is *below* 11 mg/dL in approximately one third of hyperparathyroid patients. He believes that the normal upper range of serum calcium concentration is 10.3 to 10.5 mg/dL for males, and slightly lower for females.

(Occasionally, primary hyperparathyroidism may occur with periods of normal calcium concentration. However, these patients will show an increased urinary excretion of calcium ions—see idiopathic hypercalciuria, below.)

The serum phosphate concentration is often low when hyperparathyroidism is present. However, hyperphosphatemia may be present if the hypercalcemia is due to vitamin D intoxication, the milk-alkali syndrome, sarcoidosis, multiple myeloma, or hyperthyroidism. The serum alkaline phosphatase level varies. It is high when bony changes are present. However, it may be high when bone disease is not evident. It is normal or low when vitamin D intoxication is present. It is normal in multiple myeloma. It often is elevated if the hypercalcemia is due to sarcoidosis or osteolytic metastases.

For serum parathyroid hormone assay, see page 304.

A hyperchloremic metabolic acidosis with a low serum bicarbonate concentration is often present in patients with hypercalcemia due to hyperparathyroidism. This is due to increased urinary excretion of bicarbonate ions produced by parathyroid hormone. Patients with hypercalcemia due to other causes tend to show instead a metabolic alkalosis with a low serum chloride concentration and a high serum bicarbonate concentration. Therefore, the presence of a metabolic alkalosis in a patient with hypercalcemia who has no other cause for the alkalosis suggests that hyperparathyroidism is not the cause of the hypercalcemia.

Similarly, the serum chloride phosphate ratio can also be used to differentiate hypercalcemia due to hyperparathyroidism from hypercalcemia due to other causes. In hyperparathyroidism, the chloride-phosphate ratio ranged from 31.8 to 80 and was almost always more than 33, whereas in hypercalcemia due to other causes it ranged from 17.1 to 32.3 and was almost always less than 30 (Palmer and associates). (These investigators also found a high chloride-phosphate ratio in some neoplastic patients, due to the ectopic secretion of parathormone by the neoplasm.)

Urine

The urine may show an increased calcium content. (Normally, the daily urinary calcium excretion is less than 300 mg in males, and 250 mg in females, when the diet is unrestricted.) However, an increased calcium excretion in the urine can occur in idiopathic hypercalciuria (page 324), after excessive calcium intake, excessive vitamin D ingestion, as a result of furosemide or ethacrynic acid. It may also occur in the Fanconi syndrome, renal tubular acidosis, and in some cases of osteoporosis. (Urinary calcium excretion is usually less than 400 mg a day in primary hyperparathyroidism, but is usually more than 500 mg a day in cancer, sarcoidosis, or with excessive vitamin D intake.)

The urine osmolality and specific gravity are low, secondary to the decreased ability of the kidneys to concentrate water produced by the hypercalcemia.

The urinary excretion of cyclic AMP (cAMP) is usually high in primary hyperparathyroidism. However, it may also be abnormally high in other causes of hypercalcemia.

The electrocardiogram shows a characteristic shortened QT interval, with rounding of the T waves and normal ST segments.

X-Ray Findings

Hyperparathyroid patients usually show characteristic x-ray findings, including areas of subperiosteal demineralization, especially on the lateral aspects of the middle phalanges. Similar periosteal demineralization may also occur in other bones, including the lateral ends of the clavicles, symphysis pubis, and sacroiliac joints. Generalized osteitis fibrosa cystica may also develop. The lamina dura of the teeth may disappear. (However, this is not pathognomonic of hyperparathyroidism and may occur in osteomalacia or even in pyorrhea.)

Diagnosis

Hyperparathyroidism should be suspected when the serum calcium concentration is elevated in a patient with peptic ulcer, pancreatitis, kidney stones (consisting of calcium salts), renal insufficiency where the cause is not obvious, or when generalized weakness or vague psychoneurotic symptoms are present.

X-ray findings of generalized osteitis fibrosa, such as subperiosteal resorption of bone in the phalanges, are further diagnostic signs.

The serum chloride concentration and the serum chloride-phosphate ratio (just discussed) are also helpful in differential diagnosis.

Sarcoidosis can simulate hyperparathyroidism because hypercalcemia and bony changes may be present. (However the pulmonary hilar adenopathy of sarcoidosis does not appear in hyperparathyroidism.)

The preoperative use of new diagnostic techniques (parathormone radioimmunoassay, thyroid arteriography, computed tomography, and selective venous catheterization of the thyroid veins) has been very helpful. Discussion of these techniques, however, is outside the scope of this book.

The *milk-alkali syndrome* can be differentiated from primary or secondary hyperparathyroidism because the urinary calcium excretion remains normal in spite of hypercalcemia. In addition, there is the history of prolonged milk and alkali ingestion.

Course and Prognosis

The course and prognosis depend on the etiology of the hypercalcemia. However, an acute hypercalcemic crisis may occur, especially in hyperparathyroid patients, with intractable nausea, vomiting, decreasing urine volume, progressive azotemia with rising serum calcium and phosphate concentrations, progressive drowsiness, and coma. Such patients may die in a few days.

Treatment

The serum calcium concentration can be used as a general guide to determine the urgency of treatment. A serum calcium concentration less than 12 mg/dL indicates that treatment of the hypercalcemia can be postponed while one searches for the cause of the hypercalcemia, unless azotemia or hypercalcemic symptoms or signs are present. A serum calcium concentration more than 12 mg/dL should be treated. A serum calcium concentration of 15 mg/dL or higher requires emergency treatment.

Hyperparathyroidism, acute adrenocortical insufficiency, or hyperthyroidism, if present, should be promptly treated. If a patient with neoplasm has been receiving estrogens or androgens, these should be promptly stopped. If the patient has been immobilized, he or she should be made ambulatory as quickly as possible.

Symptomatic primary hyperparathyroidism requires surgical removal of the parathyroid tumor. One must remember that removal of a parathyroid tumor does not always cure the patient—a hyperfunctioning gland may still be present, or an aberrant parathyroid gland (or glands) may be present in the mediastinum, within or near the thymus. Such a patient may require re-operation.

After a successful parathyroidectomy, the serum calcium concentration usually falls to normal within 24 hours. Transient hypocalcemia may also develop approximately 4 to 10 days after surgery. This hypocalcemia usually does not require treatment. However, if hypocalcemic symptoms develop, calcium salts and vitamin D should be started. (Postoperative hypoparathyroidism and hypocalcemia may last as long as 4 years.)

Hypomagnesemia may also develop postoperatively, particularly if bone disease is present. Acute pancreatitis, acute hyperchloremic acidosis, or pseudogout may also occur postoperatively.

If surgical exploration of the neck has been done and no parathyroid tumor has been found but symptoms continue, long-term medical treatment with phosphate salts may be helpful.

If the patient is taking digitalis, the dosage should be temporarily reduced until the serum calcium concentration falls.

If the patient has been taking too much vitamin D, calcium salts, or milk, these should be stopped immediately. In addition, the daily dietary calcium intake should be reduced to approximately 150 to 200 mg. Table 34–1 is an example of a low-calcium diet.

Emergency Treatment of Hypercalcemia

Drugs can also be used to treat hypercalcemia. Dosage and route will depend on the urgency of the clinical situation. A serum calcium concentration of 15 mg/dL or higher is an indication for emergency treatment.

Isotonic sodium chloride infusion is particularly helpful in a hypercalcemic crisis, particularly if the BUN concentration is less than 50 mg/dL. The sodium chloride increases urinary calcium excretion and lowers the serum calcium concentration, and the water alleviates the marked water loss that is present. (Dextrose in water infusions may also be necessary.) Two to three liters daily can be used for 1 to 2 days. However, the sodium chloride solution may precipitate acute congestive heart failure. Therefore, it may be advisable to use CVP (central venous pressure) monitoring. If the CVP rises above 15 cm water, half-strength sodium chloride solution can be used instead. In addition, the patient can be given a diuretic such as furosemide or ethacrynic acid concomitantly.

Suki and associates have also used large doses of intravenous furosemide alone (80 to 100 mg at intervals of 1 to 2 hours) to increase urinary calcium excretion and to lower the serum calcium concentration. However, such large doses produce severe losses of water, sodium, potassium, magnesium, and chloride ions, and require continued measurement

TABLE 34–1
A LOW-CALCIUM DIET (APPROXIMATELY 150 mg)

BREAKFAST

Orange juice—1 small glass
Cooked farina or rice—1/3 cup after cooking
Uneeda biscuits—4 (or 1 to 2 slices of Italian or French bread that is made without milk)
Margarine
Coffee or tea
Sugar
Coarse salt (ordinary table salt often contains calcium to prevent lumping)

LUNCH

Lean meat or chicken—medium-size serving
Potato—1 medium size
Uneeda biscuits—2 (or 1 or 2 slices of Italian or French bread)
Margarine
Apple—1
Coffee or tea
Sugar
Coarse salt

SUPPER

Lean meat or chicken—medium-size serving
Macaroni—1/3 cup (cooked)
Uneeda biscuits—4 (or 1 or 2 slices of Italian or French bread)
Banana—1 medium size
Coffee or tea
Sugar
Coarse salt

Use margarine and sugar generously to maintain weight. No butter, milk, cheese, cream or egg yolk allowed. Avoid cereals, margarine, or other foods to which calcium has been added.

of urinary and serum electrolytes so that the excreted electrolytes (with the exception of calcium) can be replenished intravenously.

Inorganic phosphate salts can be given orally or intravenously. They are contraindicated when hypocalcemia is due to vitamin D intoxication, because of the dangers of metastatic calcification. They are also contraindicated if renal failure and hyperphosphatemia (serum phosphorus concentration more than 5 mg/dL before treatment) are present. The phosphate salts lower the serum calcium concentration by inhibiting bone resorption and by forming a calcium-phosphate complex that is deposited in soft tissue and/or bone.

Fleet Phospho-Soda is a palatable phosphate preparation. Each teaspoonful (5 mL) contains approximately 645 mg elemental phosphorus. One-half teaspoonful (2.5 mL), 2 times a day, can be prescribed as a starting dose. Not more than 5 mL 3 times a day (approximately 2 g of elemental phosphorus) should be prescribed. (Vomiting or diarrhea will occur when a large dose is used, and may even occur with very small doses.) The serum calcium concentration begins to decrease in approximately 1 to 3 days. However, a normal calcium concentration may not appear for approximately 10 days. Long-term oral phosphate therapy has been given to hyperparathyroid patients who cannot be treated surgically. However, extraskeletal calcification and pancreatitis may develop.

Other phosphate preparations are listed in Table 34–2.

Inorganic phosphate salts can also be given intravenously if an acute hypercalcemic crisis is present, or if the patient is comatose or is vomiting. A 0.1 molar solution of sodium phosphate and potassium bi-phosphate can be prepared in the hospital pharmacy. This contains 0.081 mole of dibasic sodium phosphate and 0.019 mole of monobasic potassium phosphate, dissolved in 1 liter of distilled water. The solution has a pH adjusted to 7.4, an osmolality of 240 mOsm/kg, and each liter contains 100 millimoles (3.1 g) of elemental phosphorus, 162 mEq sodium, and 19 mEq potassium ions.

The solution is given slowly intravenously over a period of approximately 12 hours. Not more than one infusion of phosphate salts should be given in a 24-hour period, and treatment should not be continued for more than two days. If renal disease is present, 15 to 30 millimoles of phosphorus, rather than 100 millimoles, should be infused, and the serum calcium and phosphorus concentrations should be checked frequently during the infusion.

The serum calcium concentration may begin to decrease in a few minutes. A normal calcium concentration usually appears within 24 hours. However, in some patients, the serum calcium concentration may not decrease to normal for almost a week. The serum phosphorus concentration rises because of the infusion of the phosphate salts. The effects of the phosphate infusions may last as long as two weeks.

Intravenous phosphate therapy can cause calcification in the vein used for the infusion, and metastatic calcification in various tissues. In addition, hypocalcemia with tetany or hypotension or shock may occur. Acute renal

TABLE 34–2
SOME PHOSPHATE SALTS FOR ORAL USE

Name	Content of Elemental Phosphorus (P)	Content of Other Electrolytes
K-Phos Neutral	250 mg P per tablet	approx. 45 mg potassium and 298 mg sodium per tablet
Neutra-Phos-K	250 mg P per capsule	approx. 15 mEq potassium per tablet. No sodium.
Phospho-Soda	645 mg P per 5 mL (a teaspoonful)	approx. 40 mEq sodium ions per 5 mL

failure may also occur if the serum calcium concentration decreases acutely.

Diphosphonates have recently become available for the treatment of hypercalcemia. Etidronate and pamidronate are effective in virtually all types of hypercalcemia. Severe reductions in glomerular flow rate are a contraindication.

Corticosteroids have been found helpful in treating the hypercalcemia of patients with sarcoidosis, myelomas, lymphomas and leukemias. Patients with solid carcinomas are less responsive, and hyperparathyroid patients usually do not respond. The corticosteroids probably act by decreasing resorption of bone and reducing the intestinal absorption of vitamin D. The serum calcium concentration may not decrease for 1 to 2 weeks after the corticosteroids are given. In addition, prolonged use of corticosteroids will produce osteoporosis. Therefore, they should be used only for a limited time.

Prednisone can be given orally in a daily dose of 40 to 80 mg until a satisfactory decrease in serum calcium concentration occurs. Then the dosage is gradually reduced. Parenteral corticosteroid therapy is used mostly in patients with renal insufficiency and hypercalcemia who have not responded to other medical therapy. Hydrocortisone sodium succinate, 100 to 500 mg daily, or prednisolone sodium phosphate, 20 to 100 mg daily, can be given intramuscularly, intravenously, or preferably by intravenous infusion.

Mithramycin (Mithracin), now also called plicamycin, a cytotoxic drug, is also able to lower the serum calcium concentration, probably by acting directly on the bones. One fifth to one tenth of the antineoplastic dose is used to minimize toxic reactions. The serum calcium concentration may not decrease for 24 to 48 hours after an intravenous injection, but it may remain normal for one to three weeks. Mithramycin is useful to treat hypercalcemia associated with neoplastic diseases.

Mithramycin can cause severe thrombocytopenia and bleeding as well as liver and renal toxicity. It should not be used if the patient has pancytopenia, decreased liver function, or severe renal insufficiency.

Disodium EDTA (disodium edetate, endrate, sodium versenate), a chelating agent, can lower the serum calcium concentration rapidly. However, its effects are transient and it is nephrotoxic. This seriously limits its usefulness. A dose of 40 to 50 mg per kg body weight is infused in a liter of 5% dextrose in water or isotonic saline solution over a period of 4 to 6 hours. The total dose must not exceed 3 g.

Calcitonin can transiently lower the serum calcium concentration within several hours. However, its use for this purpose is still investigational. It also has been used in conjunction with prednisone, to treat the hypercalcemia of parathyroid carcinoma.

Propranolol has also been used to treat hypercalcemia due to hyperthyroidism (Rude and associates).

Treatment of Hyperparathyroidism

If a patient with primary hyperparathyroidism has significant hypercalcemia (greater than 1 mg/dL above the upper limits of normal) and shows symptoms or signs of hypercalcemia, surgical removal of the parathyroid adenoma should be done.

Surgery for hyperparathyroidism is not always successful because an aberrant parathyroid adenoma may be missed at operation. In addition, a patient may refuse surgery. Also, a patient may have a coexisting medical problem that makes a neck operation a serious risk.

If medical therapy for hyperparathyroidism is necessary, the patient must be adequately hydrated and encouraged to walk. Diuretic therapy may be dangerous if dehydration develops. Thiazide diuretics particularly should be avoided because they reduce urinary calcium excretion and may cause the serum calcium concentration to rise. Also the patient should be on a low-calcium diet (see Table 34–1).

Oral phosphates may be helpful (see Table 34–2). Estrogens may be helpful in postmenopausal women with primary hyperparathyroidism. Diphosphonates have been used experimentally.

IDIOPATHIC HYPERCALCIURIA

Idiopathic hypercalciuria is a metabolic abnormality characterized by excessive 24-hour urinary calcium excretion (greater than 300 mg in males, 250 mg in females, on a normal diet). Hypercalcemia is *not* present, alkaline phosphatase level is normal, and the serum phosphate concentration is usually normal. Occasionally it is low.

Idiopathic hypercalciuria is the most common cause of calcium-containing kidney stones. An effective treatment is the long-term use of the thiazide diuretics, for example, hydrochlorothiazide (Hydro-DIURIL, Esidrix) 50 mg orally, twice a day. (Some patients may develop hypercalcemia on this regimen. If this occurs, it suggests that the hypercalciuria is not idiopathic but is due to latent hyperparathyroidism.)

PHOSPHORUS

Just as potassium ions are the major intracellular cations, phosphorus ions are the major intracellular anions. Phosphorus is found in the body in the form of inorganic and organic phosphate salts. However, only inorganic phosphate salts are present in the extracellular water and blood.

Phosphorus is needed in many stages of intermediary metabolism, in bone formation. It is a constituent of nucleic acids. It has an important role in the delivery of oxygen to the tissues by regulating the levels of 2,3-DPG (2,3-diphosphoglycerate), and ATP (adenosine triphosphate) in red blood cells. Therefore, when hypophosphatemia is present, these levels fall. This interferes with the oxygen exchange in the red blood cells. Greater binding of oxygen to hemoglobin occurs and there is a decreased release of oxygen from the red blood cells. This leads to cellular anoxia. Lowering the ATP content of the red blood cells may also cause hemolysis and a hemolytic anemia.

Phosphate ions are also an important buffer mechanism in the kidneys for the elimination of fixed acids. Hypophosphatemia also depresses the bactericidal, phagocytic, and chemostatic activity of the white blood cells and is one of the factors that decrease resistance to infections.

Phosphate homeostasis is affected by several hormonal mechanisms: Growth hormone and probably vitamin D increase phosphate reabsorption from the gastrointestinal tract and kidneys. Parathyroid hormone increases the excretion of phosphate ions by the kidneys. Parathyroid hormone and vitamin D shift phosphate ions from bone to the extracellular water.

Phosphate balance is maintained by an intake of approximately 1 g of elemental phosphorus a day. Pregnant and lactating women have a greater need for phosphorus than other adults.

HYPOPHOSPHATEMIA

Hypophosphatemia or depletion of phosphate stores (phosphorus depletion syndrome) can occur from a loss of phosphate ions in the urine or intestines, from decreased absorption from the intestines, or from intracellular shifts of phosphate ions, and can be found in the following conditions:

1. Low intake of phosphorus-containing foods, such as milk, meat, vegetables, due to anorexia, starvation, vomiting, prolonged diarrhea.
2. Poor absorption from the gastrointestinal tract, due to a lack of vitamin D, or to steatorrhea.
3. Increased renal excretion of phosphate ions, as in primary or secondary hyperparathyroidism, hypokalemia, hypomagnesemia.
4. Excessive ingestion of phosphate-binding antacids, such as magnesium-aluminum hydroxides (Amphogel, Gelusil, Maalox, and many other preparations).
5. Diabetic acidosis. The osmotic diuresis that occurs with the diabetic acidosis is associated with an increased excretion of phosphate ions in the urine.
6. Hyperventilation and acute respiratory alkalosis. When respiratory alkalosis occurs, carbon dioxide moves out of the cells to compensate for the loss of carbon dioxide in the extracellular water. As a result, the pH of the cells becomes higher. This is associated with an increased formation of phosphorylated carbohydrate compounds in the cells. As a result, the serum phosphate concentration falls.

Hyperventilation is one of the causes of hypophosphatemia seen in patients with bacteremia due to gram-negative sepsis.

7. Renal tubular acidosis (Chapter 18).
8. Administration of insulin, glucose, glucagon, lactate salts, fructose, intravenous sodium chloride, sodium bicarbonate, or sodium lacate solutions, diuretics, anabolic steroids, corticosteroids, androgens, epinephrine.
9. Intravenous hyperalimentation. As the patient receives the intravenous nourishment, extensive tissue repair occurs, and phosphate ions are withdrawn from the blood and extracellular water into the cells.
10. Nutritional recovery syndrome. This occurs when persons who have been starved or severely malnourished, such as military prisoners or concentration camp victims, are suddenly given food with a high carbohydrate content. Edema, ascites, pleural effusions, and even death may occur, unless foods with a high phosphate content are included in the diet.
11. Alcoholic withdrawal. Chronic alcoholics who eat well do not show hypophosphatemia. However, severe hypophosphatemia can occur when alcohol is withdrawn suddenly. The mechanism by which this occurs is not clearly understood. Chronic alcoholics often have hypomagnesemia, which may be a factor in the loss of an excessive amount of phosphate ions in the urine.
12. Salicylate poisoning.
13. Acute gout.
14. The diuretic-recovery phase after a severe burn (see Chapter 9).
15. Primary hypophosphatemia.

Symptoms and Signs

Since phosphate ions are found in all cells, the symptoms and signs of phosphate loss and hypophosphatemia can involve numerous organ systems:

Central nervous system symptoms include mental irritability, apprehension, malaise, numbness, paresthesias around the mouth, dysarthria, confusion, obtundation, convulsive seizures, or coma. The clinical findings may resemble delirium tremens, but characteristic hallucinations of delirium tremens do not appear. (Both conditions may coexist.) Cranial nerve palsies may also develop.

Muscle weakness, myopathy, or rhabdomyolysis may occur. EMG abnormalities may be present. Gastrointestinal symptoms include anorexia and dysphagia. Skeletal symptoms include joint stiffness and aching bone pains. Osteomalacia and pseudofractures may also occur. Severe congestive heart failure may develop. Respiratory muscle weakness with resultant respiratory failure has also been reported.

Laboratory Tests

The normal serum phosphate concentration ranges from 2.7 to 4.5 mg/dL. (The blood should be drawn before breakfast, to prevent a high phosphate concentration due to food.) When moderate hypophosphatemia is present, the serum phosphate concentration ranges from 1.0 to 2.5 mg/dL. When severe hypophosphatemia is present, the serum phosphate concentration is less than 1.0 mg/dL and may fall to even less than 0.2 mg/dL.

A hemolytic anemia may develop.

Treatment

An attempt should be made to eliminate the factors that can contribute to the hypophosphatemia. Phosphate salts should be included in an intravenous hyperalimentation regimen. Antacids containing aluminum or magnesium that bind phosphates should be eliminated.

Numerous preparations containing phosphate ions are available (Table 34–2). One should remember that one 8-ounce glass (250 mL) of skim or low fat milk contains approximately 250 mg elemental phosphorus and is useful if a patient can tolerate oral feedings and if calcium salts are not contraindicated.

An attempt should be made to raise the serum phosphate concentration to between 3 and 4 mg/dL. This may require 1000 mg or more elemental phosphorus a day.

Contraindications to the use of phosphate salts include hypercalcemia from any cause, hyperphosphatemia (usually due to renal failure or hypoparathyroidism), oliguria, or obvious tissue necrosis.

In extreme clinical circumstances, intravenous phosphorus can be administered as potassium phosphate or sodium phosphate. (The latter is relatively unavailable in many hospital pharmacies.) A dose of 0.1 mmol/kg given over 1 hour is generally recommended to avoid transient hyperphosphatemia and resultant hypocalcemia. Multiple doses (after repeat serum values) are often necessary.

Bibliography

Calcium

Agna, JW, and Goldsmith, RE: Primary hyperparathyroidism associated with hypomagnesemia. N Engl J Med 258:222, 1958.
Akgün, S, and Ertel, NH: Chloride : phosphate ratio in hypercalcemia. Comments. Ann Intern Med 81:129, 1974.
AMA Drug Evaluations: Acton, Mass: Publishing Sciences Group, April, 1995.
Annesley, TM, et al: Artifactual hypercalcemia in multiple myeloma. Mayo Clin Proc 57:572, 1982.

Arnaud, CD: Familial benign hypercalcemia. Nature's solution to neonatal hyperparathyroidism (editorial). Mayo Clin Proc. 59:864, 1984.

Aro, A, et al: Hypercalcemia. Serum chloride and phosphate (letter). Ann Intern Med 86:664, 1977.

Aurbach, GD, et al: Hyperparathyroidism. Recent studies. NIH Conference. Ann Intern Med 79:566, 1973.

Barzel, US: The differential diagnosis of hypercalcemia. Ann Intern Med 76:825, 1972.

Barzel, US: Calcitonin therapy for bone disease and hypercalcemia. Editorial. Arch Intern Med 142:2076, 1982.

Bayat-Mokhtari, F, et al: Parathyroid storm. Arch Intern Med 140:1092, 1980.

Bechtel, JT, White, JE, and Estes, EH, Jr: The electrocardiographic effects of hypocalcemia induced in normal subjects with ethamil disodium. Circulation 13:837, 1956.

Bilezikian, JP: The medical management of primary hyperparathyroidism. Ann Intern Med 96:198, 1982.

Bilezikian, JP: Drug therapy: Management of acute hypercalcemia. N Engl J Med 326:1196, 1992.

Bilezikian, JP et al: Pseudogout after parathyroidectomy. Lancet 1:445, 1973.

Brown, JE, and Palmisano, DJ: Rapid identification of parathyroid adenoma by angiography. JAMA 231:177, 1975.

Burman, KD, et al: Ionized and total serum calcium and parathyroid hormone in hyperthyroidism. Ann Intern Med 84:666, 1976.

Caulfield, JB, et al: Blood calcium levels in the presence of arteriographic contrast material. Circulation 52:119, 1975.

Chakmakjian, ZH, and Bethune, JE: Sodium sulfate treatment of hypercalcemia. N Engl J Med 275:862, 1966.

Chaplin, H, Clark, LD, and Ropes, MW: Vitamin D intoxication. Am J Med Sci 221:369, 1951.

Christensson, T, et al: Hypercalcemia and primary hyperparathyroidism. Prevalance in patients receiving thiazides as detected in a health screen. Arch Intern Med 137:1138, 1977.

Coe, FD: Magnitude of metabolic acidosis in primary hyperparathyroidism. Arch Intern Med 134:262, 1974.

Cushard, WG, Jr, et al: Parathyroid function in sarcoidosis. N Engl J Med 286:395, 1972.

Davies, P: Vitamin D poisoning. Ann Intern Med 53:1250, 1960.

deMorgan, NP, and Waterhouse, C: A case of tertiary hyperparathyroid crisis. Am J Med Sci 256:322, 1968.

Dent, DE: Emergency treatment of hypercalcemia. Lancet 2:613, 1967.

DeTorrente, A, et al: Hypercalcemia of acute renal failure. Am J Med 61:119, 1976.

Duarte, CG, et al: Thiazide-induced hypercalcemia. N Engl J Med 284:828, 1971.

Dudley, FJ: Extraskeletal calcification complicating oral neutral phosphate therapy. Lancet 2:628, 1970.

Editorial: Tertiary hyperparathyroidism after renal transplantation. JAMA 209:2048, 1969.

Edmonson, JW: Relationship of serum ionized and total calcium in primary hyperparathyroidism. J Lab Clin Med 87:624, 1976.

Elias, EG, and Evans, JT: Hypercalcemic crisis in neoplastic diseases. Management with mithramycin. Surgery 71:631, 1972.

Esselstyn, C, Jr., et al: Hyperparathyroidism after radioactive therapy for Graves' disease. Surgery 92:811, 1982.

Fialkow, PJ, et al. Multicellular origin of parathyroid adenomas. N Engl J Med 297:696, 1977.

Gabow, PA, et al: Furosemide-induced reduction in ionized calcium in hypoparathyroid patients. Ann Inter Med 86:579, 1977.

Gallagher, JC, and Nordin, BEC: Treatment with oestrogens of primary hyperparathyroidism in postmenopausal women. Lancet 1:503, 1972.

Gardner, RJ, and Koppel, DM: Hyperparathyroid crisis. Arch Surg 98:674, 1969.

Ginsberg, H, and Schwartz, KV: Hypercalcemia and complete heart block. Ann Intern Med 79:903, 1973.

Goldsmith, RS, and Ingbar, SH: Inorganic phosphate treatment of hypercalcemia of diverse etiologies. N Engl J Med 274:1, 1966.

Halver, B: Phosphates and hypercalcemia, letter. JAMA 233:551, 1975.

Heath, H, III: What is "normal" serum calcium? Ann Intern Med 77:329, 1972.

Heinemann, HO: Metabolic alkalosis in patients with hypercalcemia. Metabolism 14:1137, 1965.

Hodgkinson, A, Peacock, M, and Nordin, BEC: Asymptomatic hyperparathyroidism. Lancet 2:49, 1971.

Hossain, M: Vitamin D intoxication during treatment of hypoparathyroidism. Lancet 1:1119, 1970.

Kaplan, EL, et al: Acid-base balance and parathyroid function. Metabolic alkalosis and hyperparathyroidism. Surgery 70:198, 1970.

Keynes, WM, and Caird, FI: Hypocalcemic primary hyperparathyroidism. BMJ 1:208, 1970.

Kutner, FR: Parathyroid crisis. Arch Surg 91:71, 1965.

Lentz, RD, et al: Treatment of severe hypophosphatemia. Ann Intern Med 89:941, 1978.

Leonard, A, and Helms, RJ, Jr: Hypercalcemia in diuretic phase of acute renal failure. Ann Intern Med 73:137, 1970.

Lerner, R: Tenderness above parathyroid adenoma. JAMA 221:716, 1972.

Livesay, JJ, and Mulder, DC: Recurrent hyperparathyroidism. Arch Surg 111:688, 1976.

Low, JC, et al: Ionic calcium determination in primary hyperparathyroidism. JAMA 223:152, 1973.

Mahadevia, PS, et al: Hypercalcemia in prostatic carcinoma. Arch Intern Med 143:1339, 1983.

Mallette, LE, et al: Neuromuscular disease in secondary hyperparathyroidism. Ann Intern Med 82:474, 1975.

Marx, SJ, et al: Familial hypocalciuric hypercalcemia. The relation to primary hyperparathyroidism. N Engl J Med 307:416, 1982.

Massry, SG, et al: Inorganic phosphate treatment of hypercalcemia. Arch Intern Med 121:307, 1968.

Massry, SG, et al: Metabolic acidosis of hyperparathyroidism. Arch Intern Med 134:385, 1974.

McMillan, DE, and Freeman, RB: The milk-alkali syndrome. Medicine 44:485, 1965.

Moreau, J-F, et al: Localization of parathyroid tumors by ultrasonography (letter). N Engl J Med 302:582, 1980.

Moses, AM, and Notman, DD: Secondary hyperparathyroidism caused by oral contraceptives. Arch Intern Med 142:128, 1982.

Muggia, FM, and Heinemann, HO: Hypercalcemia associated with neoplastic disease. Ann Intern Med 73:281, 1970.

Muggia, FM, Chia, GA, and Mickley, DW: Hyperphosphatemia and hypocalcemia in neoplastic disorders. N Engl J Med 290:857, 1974.

Mundy, CR, et al: The hypercalcemia of cancer. N Engl J Med 310:1718, 1984.

Mundy, GR, and Yates, AJP: Recent advances in pathophysiology and treatment of hypercalcemia of malignancy. Am J Kidney Dis 14:2, 1989.

Orwoll, ES: The milk-alkali syndrome. Current concepts. Ann Intern Med 97:242, 1982.

Nathaniels, EK, Nathaniels, AM, and Wang, CA: Mediastinal parathyroid tumors. Ann Surg 171:165, 1970.

Newmark, SR, and Himathongkam, T: Hypercalcemic and hypocalcemic crises. JAMA 230:1438, 1974.

Paloyan, E, and Lawrence, AM: Primary hyperparathyroidism. Pathology and therapy. Editorial. JAMA 246:1344, 1981.

Pak, CY, et al: A simple and reliable test for the diagnosis of hyperparathyroidism. Arch Intern Med 129:48, 1972.

Palmer, FJ, et al: The chloride-phosphate ratio in hypercalcemia. Ann Intern Med 80:200, 1974.

Petersen, P: Psychiatric disorders in primary hyperparathyroidism. J Clin Endocrinol 28:1491, 1968.

Purnell, DC, et al: Primary hyperparathyroidism. A prospective clinical study. Am J Med 50:670, 1971.

Rubens, RD, et al: Dissimilar adenomas in four parathyroids presenting as primary hyperparathyroidism. Lancet 1:596, 1969.

Rude, RK, et al: Treatment of thyrotoxic hypercalcemia with propranolol. N Engl J Med 294:431, 1976.

Samaan, NA, et al: Hyperparathyroidism and carcinoid tumor. Ann Intern Med 82:205, 1975.

Sataline, LR, Powell, C, and Hamwi, GJ: Suppression of the hypercalcemia of thyrotoxicosis by corticosteroids. N Engl J Med 267:646, 1962.

Segal, AJ, Miller, M, and Moses, AM: Hypercalcemia during the diuretic phase of acute renal failure. Ann Intern Med 68:1066, 1968.

Shen, F-H, and Sherrard, DJ: Lithium-induced hyperparathyroidism. Ann Intern Med 96:63, 1982.

Sherwood, LM: Hypernatremia during sodium sulfate therapy. N Engl J Med 277:314, 1967.

Siddiqui, AA, and Wilson, DR: Primary hyperparathyroidism and proximal renal tubular acidosis. Can Med Assoc J 100:654, 1972.

Silva, OL, and Becker, KL: Salmon calcitonin in the treatment of hypercalcemia. Arch Intern Med 132:337, 1973.

Singer, FR, et al: Mithramycin treatment of intractable hypercalcemia due to parathyroid carcinoma. N Engl J Med 283:634, 1970.

Spiegel, AM, et al: Intrathyroidal parathyroid adenoma or hyperplasia. An occasionally overlooked cause of surgical failure in primary hyperparathyroidism. JAMA, 234:1029, 1975.

Spiegel, AM, et al: Persistent hyperparathyroidism caused by incomplete parathyroid resection and a hyperfunctioning parathyroid autograft. JAMA 250:1896, 1983.

Stamp, TCB: The hypocalcemic effect of intravenous phosphate administration. Clin Sci 40:55, 1971.

Suki, WN, et al: Acute treatment of hypercalcemia with furosemide. N Engl J Med 283:836, 1970.

Torring, O, et al: Urinary cyclic AMP corrected for glomerular filtration rate in the differential diagnosis of hypercalcemia. Acta Med Scand 211:401, 1982.

Twycross, RG, and Marks, V: Symptomatic hypercalcemia in thyrotoxicosis. BMJ 2:701, 1970.

Walsh, FB, and Howard, JE: Conjunctival and corneal lesions in hypercalcemia. J Clin Endocrinol 7:644, 1947.

Weinberger, A, et al: Chlorthalidone-induced hypercalcemia. JAMA 231:134, 1975.

Wells, SA, Jr, et al: Repeated neck exploration in primary hyperparathyroidism. Localization of abnormal glands by selective thyroid arteriography, selective venous sampling, and radioimmunoassay. Surgery 74:678, 1973.

Wills, MR, and McGowan, GK: Plasma chloride levels in hyperparathyroidism and other hypercalcemic states. BMJ 1:1153, 1964.

Yendt, ER: Disorders of calcium, phosphorus, and magnesium metabolism. In Maxwell, MH, and Kleeman, CR (eds): *Clinical Disorders of Fluid and Electrolyte Metabolism,* 2nd ed. New York: McGraw-Hill, 1972.

Zweig, JI: Treatment of hypercalcemia with etidronate disodium, letter. JAMA 244:437, 1980.

Phosphorus

Betro, MG, and Pain, RW: Hypophosphatemia and hyperphosphatemia in hospital population. BMJ 1:273, 1972.

Darsee, JR, and Nutter, DO: Reversible severe congestive cardiomyopathy in three cases of hypophosphatemia. Ann Intern Med 89:867, 1978.

Fisher, J, et al: Respiratory illness and hypophosphatemia. Chest 83:504, 1983.

Jacobs, HD, and Amsden, T: Acute hemolytic anemia with rigid red cells in hypophosphatemia. N Eng J Med 285:1446, 1971.

Knochel, JP: The pathophysiology and clinical characteristics of severe hypophosphatemia. Arch Intern Med 137:203, 1977.

Knochel, JP: The clinical status of hypophosphatemia. N Engl J Med 313:447, 1985.

Lichtman, MA, Miller, DR, and Freeman, RB: "Mountain sickness" at low altitude due to hypophosphatemia. N Engl J Med 281:567, 1969.

Lotz, M, Zisman, E, and Bartter, FC: Evidence for a phosphorus-depletion syndrome in man. N Engl J Med 278:409, 1968.

Schonfeld, Y, et al: Hypophosphatemia as diagnostic aid in sepsis. NY State J Med 82:163, 1982.

Territo, MC, and Tanaka, KR: Hypophosphatemia in chronic alcoholism. Arch Intern Med 134:445, 1974.

Young, DS: "Phosphorus" or "phosphate" (editorial). Ann Intern Med 93:631, 1980.

Yu, GC, and Lee, DB: Clinical disorders of phosphorus metabolism. Western J Med 147:569, 1987.

Zamkoff, KW, and Kirshner, JJ: Marked hypophosphatemia associated with myelomonocytic leukemia. Arch Intern Med 140:1523, 1980.

35

SYNDROMES ASSOCIATED WITH HYPOMAGNESEMIA AND HYPERMAGNESEMIA

The human body contains a large store of magnesium ions. Like potassium, magnesium is found primarily intracellularly. Magnesium has many functions. It acts as an activator for all the enzymes that require thiamine pyrophosphate as a cofactor, and plays a role in both carbohydrate and protein metabolism.

The intravenous injection of magnesium sulfate in the dog causes peripheral muscular paralysis. This is due to the curare-like effect of magnesium. This effect is due to a decreased liberation of acetylcholine at the neuromuscular junction and at sympathetic ganglia. It can be antagonized by an excess of calcium and by anticholinesterases such as physostigmine or neostigmine, or by the simultaneous administration of potassium.

In addition, the central nervous depression caused by magnesium ions is so great that magnesium can be used as a general anesthetic.

Magnesium produces a fall in blood pressure and can cause cardiac arrest in diastole. Toxic electrocardiographic signs include a prolongation of the PR interval, widening of the QRS interval, and premature ventricular contractions.

Although there are similarities between the actions of magnesium and calcium, there are also curious differences between these two ions. Both a low serum magnesium and a low serum calcium concentration increase neuromuscular irritability, and a high concentration of these ions has a reverse effect. Magnesium narcosis, produced by injecting a magnesium preparation, can be promptly antagonized by the parenteral administration of calcium. However, the toxic effects of hypomagnesemia can be aggravated by calcium or phosphorus in the diet.

Most of the factors that control magnesium metabolism are not known.

In humans, hypomagnesemia may reduce parathyroid gland secretion and may prevent the action of parathyroid hormone on bones, so that hypocalcemia may develop as a result of the hypomagnesemia. The renal excretion of magnesium ions is probably under the control of aldosterone. The normal serum magnesium concentration varies from approximately 1.5 to 2.5 mEq/L (1.8 to 3.0 mg/dL). A portion of the magnesium, approximately 35%, is bound to protein.

The normal diet supplies approximately 25 mEq (3.1 g) of magnesium ions daily. This is slightly more than the normal daily requirement. A large source of dietary magnesium is the chlorophyll in green vegetables. It is plentiful in nuts and legumes, fruits such as bananas, grapefruits, and oranges, and also in peanut butter and chocolate.

The kidneys are able to conserve magnesium ions, so that renal excretion may be less than 1 mEq a day, even when the patient is on a magnesium-free diet.

HYPOMAGNESEMIA

Hypomagnesemia is present when the magnesium serum concentration is less than 1.5 mEq/L (1.8 mg/dL). However, when symptomatic hypomagnesemia is present, the serum magnesium concentration is usually less than 1 mEq/L. (One should remember that there is no direct correlation between serum magnesium concentration and the body stores of magnesium ions.)

Etiology

Hypomagnesemia can occur in the following situations:

1. Impaired intake of magnesium salts, or impaired intestinal absorption of magnesium salts. It is difficult to produce magnesium deficiency or hypomagnesemia by means of dietary restriction. However, it can occur with prolonged malnutrition or starvation, or when a patient is given magnesium-free fluids intravenously, in association with no oral intake of food, and/or with nasogastric suction, for more than a week.

   Impaired intestinal absorption of magnesium ions occurs in steatorrhea and other intestinal absorption syndromes. In these conditions, the magnesium ions are excreted in the stool in the form of magnesium soaps. A high calcium intake or a low protein intake exacerbates the loss of magnesium ions this way. Magnesium ions are also lost with diarrhea, gastrointestinal fistulas, and so on.

2. Excessive urinary excretion of magnesium ions. The usual cause of this is diuretic therapy with the loop or thiazide diuretics, or ammonium chloride. Hypomagnesemia produced this way may be clinically significant because many of these patients are also taking digitalis, and there is evidence that digitalis toxicity can be precipitated or aggravated by hypomagnesemia.

Hypomagnesemia due to excessive urinary losses also occurs for 24 hours after major surgery. It also occurs in primary aldosteronism, diabetic acidosis, primary hyperparathyroidism and other hypercalcemic states, acute intermittent porphyria with the syndrome of inappropriate secretion of ADH, acute pancreatitis, acute renal failure during the diuretic phase, renal tubular acidosis, chronic renal disease.

3. Other causes. Hypomagnesemia may occur in hypoparathyroidism in association with hypocalcemia, or postoperatively when all four parathyroid glands are removed, possibly due to some internal shift of magnesium ions from the extracellular water into bones ("hungry bones"). Excessive lactation may produce hypomagnesemia. Finally, hypomagnesemia due to renal magnesium wasting may occur from drugs such as gentamicin, amphotericin B, carbenicillin, cisplatin, and cyclosporine.

4. Chronic alcoholism with or without cirrhosis or delirium tremens. This is a common cause of hypomagnesemia. It is due to reduced caloric intake, including reduced intake of magnesium-containing foods, intestinal malabsorption, and even a direct effect of alcohol in enhancing urinary magnesium excretion. (Hypomagnesemia may exacerbate the increased neuroirritability of patients with delirium tremens.)

The cause of the decreased serum concentration of magnesium is not always clear. During the treatment of a patient with diabetic acidosis, for example, part of the magnesium passes from the extracellular water into the cells, but part is also excreted in the urine and lost. In patients with chronic lesions, malnutrition may be associated with a decreased intake of magnesium in the food. Patients with steatorrhea excrete a large amount of magnesium soaps in the stool. Another factor that may contribute to the loss of magnesium ions is a high intake of calcium salts when the diet is lacking in magnesium salts, because absorption of magnesium ions from the intestines varies inversely with the uptake of calcium salts. In hyperthyroidism, there is an increased protein-bound fraction of magnesium. Aldosteronism may cause increased fecal as well as urinary loss of magnesium ions. Alcoholic patients may develop hypomagnesemia because of chronic inadequate food intake.

Hypokalemia and a negative potassium balance may also occur because a diet that is lacking in magnesium salts is usually lacking in potassium salts also. Hypomagnesemia may also be associated with hypocalcemia or hypophosphatemia.

Pathology

In animals, experimental magnesium deficiency has resulted in pathological changes in the heart, vascular system, kidneys, liver and brain. Necrotic lesions without calcification have been found in the kidney glomeruli and tubules. In addition, tubular degeneration and fibrosis with calcium casts in the medullary loops and collecting tubules have been observed.

Symptoms and Signs

Investigators do not agree on the clinical picture that magnesium deficiency produces in humans. The following psychiatric and neurological symptoms and signs have been described: personality changes with agitation, mental depression or confusion, hallucinations (usually auditory or visual), convulsions (grand mal or multifocal), increased reflexes, clonus, a positive Babinski sign, coarse tremor, athetoid and/or choreiform movements, ataxia, nystagmus, tetany with a positive Chvostek sign (usually with a negative Trousseau sign), muscle fasciculations, muscle cramps, paresthesias of the feet and legs, abnormal electroencephalographic signs such as diffuse slow waves.

Cardiovascular signs include tachycardia with atrial or ventricular premature contractions, hypotension, vasomotor changes such as painful cold hands and feet or increased perspiration, and nonspecific T-wave changes in the electrocardiogram.

Gastrointestinal symptoms such as dysphagia may develop.

Hypomagnesemia and hypocalcemia may coexist, especially in patients with an excessive loss of gastrointestinal fluids. The tetany of some of these patients responds to calcium rather than magnesium salts.

Hypomagnesemia and hypercalcemia may also coexist, not only in hyperparathyroid patients but also in neoplastic patients with osteolytic metastases.

Hypomagnesemia, rather than hypokalemia, may be a factor in some patients with digitalis toxicity.

Treatment

In the present state of our knowledge, it is questionable whether a patient, such as one with diabetic acidosis during the course of treatment, requires treatment for the hypomagnesemia. A parenteral solution such as Butler's solution contains about 2mEq/L of magnesium.

Hypomagnesemia can be treated with magnesium salts intramuscularly, intravenously, or orally. Magnesium sulfate (hydrated), the most commonly used magnesium salt, contains 8.13 mEq magnesium ions per gram.

Magnesium sulfate can be given intramuscularly in a dose of 2 g (16.3 mEq) (4 mL of a 50% solution) every 8 hours, for 3 or more days, when significant hypomagnesemia is present. Serial serum magnesium concentrations can be used to regulate the dosage.

Magnesium balance can be maintained by giving as little as 25 mEq magnesium ions (6 mL of 50% magnesium sulfate) daily, if there are no abnormal losses.

Repeated intramuscular injections should be given at different sites because the injections may be painful. Procaine hydrochloride (1%) can be added to the injection if a large dose is used.

Magnesium sulfate can also be given intravenously when severe hypomagnesemia, associated with convulsions, for example, is present. A dose of 4 mL of 50% magnesium sulfate solution (16.3 mEq), diluted to 100 mL should be given in 10 minutes (Parfitt and Kleerekoper).

Magnesium sulfate can also be given IV as a 1% solution (by adding 10 mL of a 50% magnesium sulfate solution (40.7 mEq) to 490 mL of 5% dextrose in water), in a period of 4 to 6 hours.

In patients with normal renal function, up to 50 mEq elemental magnesium can be given IV over 4 to 6 hours, not to exceed 100 mEq every 12 hours.

When renal insufficiency is present, the dose should be reduced by 25% or 50%, depending on the severity of the renal impairment.

Magnesium salts can also be given orally to counteract continuous excessive losses, as in steatorrhea. For example, magnesium sulfate 2 g (16.3 mEq) can be given three times a day without producing a diarrhea. Magnesium citrate solution, N.F., can also be used in a dose of 15 mL three times a day, for example. (Each 100 mL contains 1.5 to 1.9 g of magnesium oxide with citric acid and sodium bicarbonate for effervescence.) Magnesium lactate is also available.

The principal dietary sources of magnesium ions are green vegetables, nuts and legumes, and fruits, as mentioned above.

One should remember that even if magnesium is given to a patient with magnesium deficiency, symptoms and signs may not be relieved for 60 to 80 hours.

HYPERMAGNESEMIA

An excess of magnesium can cause cardiac effects, such as a prolonged PR interval, prolonged QRS interval, tall T waves, various degrees of AV block, or ventricular premature contractions.

Hypermagnesemia is present when the serum magnesium concentration rises above 2.5 mEq/L (3.0 mg/dL).

Etiology

The most common cause of hypermagnesemia is renal failure. This can be aggravated when such a patient is given either magnesium sulfate to control convulsions or one of the many commercial antacids that contain magnesium salts—Aludrox, Camalox, Delcid, Gaviscon, Gelusil, Kolantyl, Maalox, Mylanta, and others.

It is possible that some of the clinical signs of uremia are due to hypermagnesemia.

Hypermagnesemia may also occur in diabetic acidosis when water loss is severe. It has also been reported as a result of frequent magnesium sulfate enemas, used in congenital megacolon, and after excessive intake of Epsom salts in the home treatment of constipation.

Hypocalcemia may occur in association with hypermagnesemia. This may be due to the suppressive effects of hypermagnesemia on parathyroid hormone secretion, or the hypermagnesemia may be associated with a shift of calcium ions into either the intracellular space or bone.

Clinical Signs

When the serum magnesium concentration is between 3 and 5 mEq/L, there is a tendency to hypotension due to peripheral dilatation. In addition, the patient may experience a sense of heat and thirst. Nausea and vomiting may also occur.

When the concentration is 5 to 7 mEq/L, drowsiness appears. Deep tendon reflexes are lost at a serum magnesium concentration of 7 mEq/L. The respiratory center is depressed at a concentration of 10 mEq/L. Coma occurs at a concentration of 12 to 15 mEq/L, and cardiac arrest at a concentration of 15 to 20 mEq/L.

Prophylaxis

Magnesium salts should not be given to patients with acute or chronic renal disease.

Treatment

Magnesium toxicity can be treated by correcting water loss, if it is present, improving renal function, if possible, and the parenteral use of calcium gluconate (page 305). Artificial respiration may be necessary if respiratory failure occurs. Hypermagnesemia can also be corrected by dialysis.

Bibliography

Aikawa, JK: *The Relationship of Magnesium to Disease in Domestic Animals and Humans.* Springfield, Ill: Charles C Thomas, 1971.

Baldwin, TE, and Chernow, B: When to suspect hypomagnesemia in critically ill patients. J Crit Ill June 1987, p. 60.

Bar, RS, et al: Hypomagnesemic hypocalcemia secondary to renal magnesium wasting. A possible consequence of high-dose gentamycin therapy. Ann Intern Med 82:646, 1975.

Barton, C, et al: Renal magnesium wasting associated with amphotericin B therapy. Am J Med 77:471, 1984.

Beller, GA, et al: Correlation of serum magnesium levels and cardiac digitalis intoxication. Am J Cardiol 33:225, 1974.

Burch, GE, and Giles, TD: The importance of magnesium deficiency in cardiovascular disease. Am Heart J 94:649, 1977.

Cholst, IN, et al: The influence of hypermagnesemia on serum calcium and parathyroid hormone levels in human subjects. N Engl J Med 310:1221, 1984.

Dyckner, T, and Wester, PO: Clinical significance of diuretic-induced magnesium loss. Pract Cardiol 10:124, 1984.

Ferdinandus, J, et al: Hypermagnesemia as a cause of refractory hypertension, respiratory depression, and coma. Arch Intern Med 141:669, 1981.

Flink, EB: Role of magnesium depletion in Wernicke-Korsakoff syndrome, letter. N Engl J Med 298:743, 1978.

Flink, EB, and Jones, JE, Editors: The pathogenesis and clinical significance of magnesium deficiency. Ann New York Acad Sci 162:705, 1969.

Gerlach, K, et al: Symptomatic hypomagnesemia complicating regional enteritis. Gastroenterology 59:567, 1970.

Hall, RCW: Hypomagnesemia. Physical and psychiatric symptoms. JAMA 224:1749, 1973.

Hamed, IA, and Lindeman, RD: Dysphagia and vertical nystagmus in magnesium deficiency. Ann Intern Med 89:222, 1978.

Iseri, LT, and French, JH: Magnesium. Nature's physiologic calcium blocker. Editorial. Am Heart J 108:188, 1984.

Juna, D: Clinical review. The clinical importance of hypomagnesemia. Surgery 91:510, 1982.

Laban, E, and Charbon, GA: Magnesium and cardiac arrhythmias, nutrient or drug. Am Coll Nutrit 5:521, 1986.

Lim, P: Magnesium deficiency in patients on long term diuretic therapy for heart failure. BMJ 3:626, 1972.

Lyman, NW, et al: Cisplatin-induced hypocalcemia and hypomagnesemia. Arch Intern Med 140:1513, 1980.

Massry, SG, Coburn, JW, and Kleeman, CR: Evidence for suppression of parathyroid gland activity by hypermagnesemia. J Clin Invest 49:1619, 1970.

Monif, GRG, and Savory, J: Iatrogenic maternal hypocalcemia following magnesium sulfate therapy. JAMA 219:1469, 1972.

Mordes, JP, et al: Extreme hypermagnesemia as a cause of refractory hypotension. Ann Intern Med 83:657, 1975.

Parfitt, AM, and Kleerekoper, M: Clinical disorders of calcium, phosphorus, and magnesium metabolism. In Maxwell, MH, and Kleeman, CR, (eds): *Clinical Disorders of Fluid and Electrolyte Metabolism,* 3rd ed. New York: McGraw-Hill 1980.

Randall, RE, Jr, et al: Hypermagnesemia in renal failure. Ann Intern Med 61:73, 1967.

Rosler, A, and Rabinowitz, D: Magnesium-induced reversal of vitamin D resistance in hypoparathyroidism. Lancet 1:803:1973.

Sawyer, RB, et al: Postoperative magnesium metabolism. Arch Surg 100:343, 1970.

Seelig, MS, and Berger, AR: Range of normal serum magnesium values. N Engl J Med 290:974, 1974.

Shils, ME: Experimental human magnesium depletion. Medicine 48:61, 1969.

Specter, MJ, et al: Studies on magnesium's mechanism of action in digitalis-induced arrhythmias. Circulation 52:1001, 1975.

Triger, DR, and Jockes, AM: Severe muscle cramps due to acute hypomagnesemia in hemodialysis. BMJ 2:804, 1969.

Vallee, BL, Wacker, WEC, and Ulmer, DD: The magnesium-deficiency tetany syndrome in man. N Engl J Med 262:155, 1960.

Wacker, WEC, Moore, FD, Ulmer, DD, and Vallee, BL: Normocalcemic magnesium deficiency tetany. JAMA 180:161, 1962.

Wacker, WEC, and Parisi, AF: Magnesium metabolism. N Engl J Med 278:658, 712, 772, 1968.

Wan-chun, C, et al: ECG changes in early stage of magnesium deficiency, letter. Am Heart J 104:1115, 1982.

Wong, ET, et al: A high prevalence of hypomagnesemia and hypermagnesemia in hospitalized patients. Am J Clin Path 79:348, 1983.

Wiegmann, T, and Kaye, M: Hypomagnesemic hypocalcemia. Arch Intern Med 137:953, 1977.

Wilson, TA, et al: Hypermagnesemia, serum calcium, and parathyroid hormone levels, letter. N Engl J Med 311:601, 1984.

Zimmet, P: Role of magnesium in tetany. N Engl J Med 279:109, 1968.

THE PRINCIPLES
OF FLUID
THERAPY

36

GENERAL PRINCIPLES OF WATER AND ELECTROLYTE THERAPY

In the preceding pages of this book, it has been emphasized that the *patient* must be treated, not an electrolyte or chemical disturbance. In this way, the physician will avoid many errors in therapy, which would otherwise result.

The aims of water and electrolyte therapy are:

1. To treat shock.
2. To replace electrolyte and water deficits.
3. To provide water, electrolytes, and nutriments for maintaining the daily needs of the patient.
4. To avoid creating new disturbances as a result of the therapy.

In the previous chapters, the daily requirements of water and the various electrolytes have been described. This information can now be summarized.

ROUTE OF ADMINISTRATION

Food and fluids should be given by the oral route (either by mouth or by nasogastric tube). If this is not possible, intravenous therapy, rather than subcutaneous therapy (hypodermoclysis), should be used.

Hypodermoclysis

Hypodermoclysis is the administration of a solution subcutaneously. The most commonly used solution for this purpose is isotonic sodium chloride solution, with or without 5% dextrose. Stronger strengths of dextrose should not be used. Half-isotonic (0.45%) sodium chloride solution, with or without 5% dextrose, can also be used. Other solutions that can be given subcutaneously are Darrow's solution, Ringer's solution, lactated Ringer's solution, and 1/6 molar sodium lactate. However, dextrose in water, or any solution without sodium chloride or other extracellular electrolyte in at least half-isotonic concentration, should never be given subcutaneously. If this is done, extracellular water and electrolytes will diffuse into the hypodermoclysis area. When this happens, the circulating blood volume will decrease and shock may occur or become aggravated.

The lateral chest, lateral abdomen, or lateral thigh areas can be used for the hypodermoclysis.

When one needle is used for the hypodermoclysis, 250 to 500 mL of the solution can be administered in 1 hour. This volume can be doubled by injecting the solution in two separate areas.

The rate of absorption of the solution can be greatly increased by injecting the enzyme hyaluronidase into the injection area. One hundred fifty turbidity reducing units (1 mL) can be used for each liter of solution injected. Hypodermoclysis is valuable when it is impossible to find a patient's vein. However, the procedure may allow a staphylococcus skin infection to develop.

RATE OF ADMINISTRATION

The rate of administration depends on the need for fluids and the nature of the fluid. It is important for the physician to prescribe exactly how fast the fluid should be given intravenously. Infusion sets from various manufacturers deliver different-sized drops. Therefore, it is necessary to know how many drops are required to deliver 1 mL of fluid.

The rate of administration of fluids intravenously can be determined from the follow rule:

Drops per minute × drop factor = mL per hour

The *drop factor* is obtained by dividing 60 by the number of drops that are needed to deliver 1 mL. For example, if 15 drops from an infusion set deliver 1 mL, the drop factor is 60/15 = 4. Therefore, if the infusion drips at a rate of 25 drops per minute, 25 × 4 = 100 mL of fluid will be infused in 1 hour. If a different infusion set is used with a smaller aperture, so that 20 drops are required to deliver 1 mL (drop factor 60/20 = 3) and the infusion drips at a rate of 25 drops per minute, only 75 mL (25 × 3) will be infused in 1 hour.

If the number of drops that deliver 1 mL is not known, one can assume that the drop factor is 4. However, the volume of fluid infused in 1 hour should be checked with the number of drops flowing per minute.

Microdrip bulbs are also available. They deliver 60 drops per minute.

Such microdrip bulbs are helpful when a "KVO" ("Keep vein open") order is written and one does not want an excessive amount of fluid infused. (When a microdrip bulb is used, the 24-hour intravenous fluid volume can be maintained at approximately 350 mL. If a regular drip bulb had been used, the patient would receive a liter or more in this time.)

DAILY WATER AND ELECTROLYTE REQUIREMENTS
Daily Water Requirements

Approximately 30 mL per kg body weight (15 mL per pound). Thus, a 70-kg adult would require 2000 mL of water daily.

Fever will increase the water needs by approximately 15% for each 1°C rise in the patient's temperature.

Daily Electrolyte Requirements

Sodium, 100 mEq (5.9 g NaCl) (also see below). If fever and sweating are present, sodium chloride will be needed in addition to water. It is difficult to determine volume losses of sweat (which may vary from 0 to 1000 mL/hr). A significant volume of sweat will be lost if the patient's temperature is above 38.3°C (101°F), or if the room temperature is 32°C (90°F) or higher.

One can replace the lost sweat by infusing 1 part isotonic saline solution and 2 parts dextrose in water (or a solution of one-third strength saline) that has the approximate composition of sweat. The daily volume needed may vary from 500 to 2000 mL.

Potassium, 60 mEq daily (4.5 g KCl). If fever or sweating is present, 4 mEq more potassium ions will be needed.

Magnesium, 8 to 20 mEq daily (1 to 3 g $MgSO_4$).

The use of multiple electrolyte solutions is described below.

Calorie Requirements

During fasting, an average 70-kg male loses approximately 80 g of body protein daily. If 100 g or more of dextrose is given, the protein loss decreases by one half. Therefore, 100 to 150 g of dextrose should be infused daily when the patient is not able to eat. This supplies 340 to 510 kilocalories (kcal). (One gram of *hydrous* dextrose supplies 3.4 kcal.) This is equivalent to 1000 to 1500 mL of a 10% solution of dextrose in water, or 2000 to 3000 mL of a 5% solution.

(One gram of carbohydrates provides 4 kcal, 1 g of ethyl alcohol provides 7 kcal; 1 g of fat provides 9 kcal; and 1 g of protein provides 4 kcal.)

When a patient is unable to eat or drink for a period of 4 to 8 days, a high-calorie solution can be infused, with or without electrolytes, as needed. For example, a solution of 20% dextrose in water provides 200 g of dextrose—680 kcal/L. Two liters will therefore provide 1360 kcal. This is adequate to prevent ketosis and the breakdown of protein temporarily. However, such a concentrated dextrose solution is irritating and will frequently cause a local thombophlebitis or thrombosis when it is used for more than several days. Therefore, it should be infused, if possible, into a large vein, such as the subclavian vein or superior vena cava.

Regular crystalline insulin can be added to such a concentrated dextrose solution to increase the metabolism of the infused dextrose and to decrease hyperglycemia and/or glycosuria. Usually, 1 unit of regular insulin to every 4 g of dextrose is used. When a concentrated dextrose solution infusion is stopped, it should be followed by an infusion of 5% to 10% dextrose solution, to prevent a reactive hypoglycemia.

(Insulin is stable in a solution of 5% or 10% dextrose in water, with or without electrolytes. However, up to 30% of the added insulin can adhere to the glass infusion flask or to the intravenous tubing. The insulin, of course, can be given intramuscularly or subcutaneously.)

A liter of 5% amino acids in 5% dextrose in water can also be infused daily when the patient has not been able to eat for several days.

Commercial solutions containing ethyl alcohol can be used for short-term intravenous infusion, because each 1 g ethyl alcohol provides 7 kcal.

When a patient is unable to eat for 8 or more days, nasogastric tube feeding with ordinary liquefied food and added vitamin supplements, or with an elemental diet, can be used. An alternative is peripheral parenteral nutrition (see below), or total parenteral nutrition (intravenous hyperalimentation). Tube feedings or total parenteral nutrition can be continued for months.

Protein Requirements

40 g a day. This can be supplied by 1000 mL of 5% amino acids in 5% dextrose.

Vitamins

A daily dose of 2 mL parenteral vitamin B complex and 500 mg vitamin C can be added to the infusion.

Summary

Therefore, the following solutions can be given daily for the first 2 or 3 days:

1. 1500 mL 10% dextrose in water.
2. 500 mL isotonic sodium chloride (or lactated Ringer's) solution in 5% dextrose.
3. 3 g potassium chloride (added to a liter of the dextrose solution, or to the sodium chloride solution).
4. Vitamin B complex, 2 mL; vitamin C, 500 mg, added to one of the infusion bottles.
5. If there is fever add 500 mL 10% dextrose in water, plus 500 mL isotonic sodium chloride solution.

If the patient is receiving parenteral therapy for 3 or more days and is not taking food orally, 1000 mL 5% amino acids in 5% dextrose in water can be added.

One should remember that errors may occur in calculating fluid intake and output: a liter bottle of an intravenous fluid may actually contain 1100 mL, a pint bottle of blood or plasma may contain 600 mL and a sip of water or mouth rinsing, if repeated often, may add up to 1000 mL per day.

CHARTING WATER AND ELECTROLYTE BALANCES

It is important to keep accurate and adequate records of the patient's water and electrolyte intake and output. If this is done, the physician will frequently be able to prevent many of the water and electrolyte syndromes from developing.

In the research laboratory, complicated measurements can be done. In the hospital, simple methods must be used. The following simple procedures are of great value:

1. Daily weight, if possible.
2. Daily intake of both water and electrolytes.
3. Daily urine volume, including the specific gravity (or osmolality) of the urine.
4. Serum sodium, potassium, bicarbonate, chloride, and osmolality determinations, on admission and as often as necessary.

Bibliography

Abbott, WE, Levey, S, Foreman, RC, Krieger, H, and Holden, WD: Danger of administering parenteral fluids by hypodermoclysis. Surgery 32:305, 1952.
Bridenbaugh, PO, et al: Limitations of lactated Ringer's solution in massive fluid replacement. JAMA 206:2313, 1968.
Brooke, CE, and Anast, CS: Oral fluid and electrolytes. JAMA 179:792, 1962.
Gamble, JL: *Chemical Anatomy, Physiology and Pathology of Extracellular Fluid,* 6th ed. Cambridge, Mass: Harvard University Press, 1954.
Glick, SM: Insulin. Not recommended in infusions. JAMA 230:468, 1974.

Rigor, B, Bosomworth, P, and Rush, BF, Jr: Replacement of operative blood loss of more than 1 liter with Hartmann's solution. JAMA 203:399, 1968.

Tarail, R: Practice of fluid therapy. JAMA 171:131, 1959.

Trudnowski, RJ: Hydration with Ringer's lactate solution. JAMA 195:545, 1966.

Weisberg, HF: *Electrolyte and Acid-Base Balance,* 2nd ed. Baltimore: Williams & Wilkins, 1962.

37

PARENTERAL THERAPY IN SURGICAL PATIENTS

PATHOPHYSIOLOGY

A major surgical operation, trauma, or other acute stress can produce numerous physiological changes, including the following:

Even before an operation, there is increased sympathetic stimulation and increased secretion of catecholamines (epinephrine and norepinephrine), which last at least 2 to 3 days and are associated with tachycardia, vasoconstriction, and an increased blood sugar, even to diabetic levels.

Stimulation of the anterior pituitary gland causes numerous effects. Increased secretion of anterior pituitary growth hormone also raises the blood sugar level. More importantly, an increased secretion of ACTH (corticotropin) occurs. This stimulates the adrenal glands to secrete large amounts of hydrocortisone and other corticosteroids to combat the stress. This hypersecretion lasts for approximately 1 to 2 days or more.

In addition, the stress stimulates the posterior pituitary gland to secrete ADH. As a result, water retention occurs and the urinary output the first day postoperatively may become as low as 500 mL or less. The serum sodium concentration also becomes low due to the dilution of the plasma with water. The hypersecretion of ADH usually lasts approximately 2 to 4 days.

Increased secretion of aldosterone by the adrenal glands also occurs. This is partly due to stimulation of the adrenals by ACTH. Aldosterone secretion also occurs as a result of the decreased circulating blood volume and/or loss of extracellular fluids that are often present after a major operation. The aldosterone secretion causes an increased diuresis of potassium ions and a retention of sodium ions. However, the serum sodium concentration remains low. The increased aldosterone secretion usually also lasts 2 to 4 days.

There may also be a marked increase in oxygen consumption and a rise in body temperature so that the caloric needs after a major surgical operation may rise to more than 3000 kcal a day, for the first 4 to 5 days. These calories are usually supplied by the metabolism of body fat. For example, 250 to 500 g of fat can be oxidized daily after major surgery. Since each gram of fat produces 9 kcal, 250 g of fat would produce 2250 kcal. The oxidation of lean muscle also occurs. (Each gram of protein provides 4 kcal.) As a result, a patient usually loses 0.5 kg daily in the first 5 days after surgery.

Disturbances in water and electrolyte balance also occur postoperatively. The antidiuresis due to ADH has already been mentioned. The metabolism of body fat and protein produces approximately 460 mL water of oxidation daily (Chapter 3). In addition, there is a moderate retention of sodium and chloride ions and a loss of potassium ions (due to aldosterone). These electrolyte changes usually disappear within 3 to 6 days.

WATER AND ELECTROLYTE SYNDROMES IN SURGICAL PATIENTS
Preoperative Water and Electrolyte Management

It is not unusual for preoperative patients to have severe water and/or electrolyte losses due to inadequate intake of water or food, vomiting, nasogastric suction, diarrhea, diuretics, and so on. These losses should be replaced prior to surgery to prevent hypotension or acute renal failure during or immediately after the operation.

Intraoperative Fluid Therapy

Many different routines are used for giving IV fluids intraoperatively. These range from no fluids at all in minor operations to various combinations of saline, other electrolytes, blood, and colloid expanders. The apparent success of these various regimens indicates that patients can adapt to various fluid and electrolyte treatment.

The following regimen (adapted from Giesecke) applies to adult patients with no pre-existing fluid or electrolyte imbalance. It may require changes depending on the clinical situation.

Stage 1. At the start of a general anesthesia, a 70-kg patient can receive 500 mL of 5% dextrose in water in the first 30 to 45 minutes of anesthesia.

A patient who has been without oral intake for 6 or more hours ("NPO after midnight" order) will show an insensible water loss of 2 mL/kg/hr. This can be replaced with the above hypotonic maintenance solution.

Stage 2. The IV replacement treatment depends on the type of surgery.

1. *Hypotonic maintenance* fluid therapy, using 5% dextrose in water, or 0.45% sodium chloride solution in 5% dextrose in water, given at a rate of 2 mL/kg/hr, is continued in patients when there is minimal loss of

blood or fluids. Such operations include most ophthalmic surgery, cystoscopy, and so on.

2. Minimal *replacement* fluid therapy using lactated Ringer's solution with or without 5% dextrose, 0.9% sodium chloride (full strength saline), or similar solutions, given at a rate of 6 mL/kg/hr. Such operations include those with minimal surgical traumas, such as tonsillectomy and plastic operations.

3. Moderate *replacement* fluid therapy, using lactated Ringer's solution with or without 5% dextrose, 0.9% sodium chloride, or similar solutions given at a rate of 8 mL/kg/hr. Such operations include herniorrhaphy, appendectomy (without peritonitis), and thoracotomy.

4. Severe *replacement* fluid therapy using lactated Ringer's solution with or without 5% dextrose, 0.9% sodium chloride, or similar solutions, given at a rate of 10 mL/kg/hr. Such operations include bowel resection for intestinal obstruction, total hip replacement, radical mastectomy, and so on.

Regardless of the type of surgery, the patient's vital signs and circulation should be continuously monitored. A urine output of 1 mL/kg/hr should be maintained.

Special operations require changes in this regimen. For example 5% dextrose in water should be omitted in a transurethral prostatectomy because such patients will absorb a large amount of hypotonic irrigating solution during the resection. Such patients should receive initially lactated Ringer's solution with or without 5% dextrose, 0.9% sodium chloride, or similar solutions.

Similarly, additional fluids must be given IV for third-space fluid losses.

Third-Space Fluid Losses

In addition, so-called third-space fluid losses, due to sequestration of fluids in the body, may be present. This can occur in the following conditions: acute intestinal obstruction (as much as 5 liters or more can accumulate within the lumen of the obstructed intestines); acute gastric dilatation; acute peritonitis or acute pancreatitis; burns, crush injuries, acute spreading cellulitis; following abdominal surgery, particularly pelvic surgery (the fluid accumulates in the peritoneum, bowel wall and other traumatized tissues); and following surgery on the abdominal aorta after the aortic clamp has been released (*declamping phenomenon*) (the fluid accumulates in the ischemic lower extremities).

The sequestration of fluids in these patients will decrease the circulating blood volume and produce signs of hypotension or shock, since, when plasma exudes out of the bloodstream into a sequestered third space, the red blood cells are now suspended in a smaller volume of plasma. Therefore, the hematocrit rises. This rise in hematocrit can be used to determine the extent of the plasma loss, namely,

$$\text{Plasma deficit (mL)} = \text{normal blood volume} -$$

$$\frac{\text{normal blood vol.} \times \text{normal (or initial) HCT}}{\text{measured HCT}}$$

It is assumed that the normal blood volume equals approximately 7% of body weight, and that the normal hematocrit is 45%.

Example: Patient with acute intestinal obstruction, weight 70 kg. Measured HCT, 55%. The normal blood volume in this patient is $70,000 \times 0.07 = 4900$ mL

$$\text{Plasma deficit} = 4900 - \frac{4900 \times 0.45}{0.55}$$

$$= 4900 - 4000$$

$$= 900 \text{ mL}$$

Theoretically, a third-space fluid loss should be treated with plasma or another colloid solution. However, as was pointed out in the treatment of burns (Chapter 9), this may not be necessary. A multiple electrolyte solution, such as lactated Ringer's solution, can be infused instead. The volume of solution needed can be calculated in a general way by infusing 2½ times the estimated plasma volume deficit.

Thompson and his associates have used the following regimen for their patients undergoing major aortoiliac reconstructive surgery: At the start of the operation, a liter of 5% dextrose in lactated Ringer's solution is infused rapidly as the abdomen is opened and the initial dissection is started. Then the solution is given throughout the operation at a rate of 500 mL for every hour of surgery. Blood loss is replaced volume for volume simultaneously with the infusion. The patient also receives approximately 250 mL of 5% dextrose in water during surgery.

The principal criterion for the rate of infusion of the lactated Ringer's solution during the operation is to maintain a satisfactory blood pressure without using vasoconstrictors, and a urinary output between 30 and 50 mL/hr.

Similar third-space fluid losses occur in medical patients with marked ascites or pleural effusion. However, the decreased circulating blood volume and hypotension occur after the sequestered fluid has been rapidly removed, because the fluid reaccumulates quickly. It is better to treat these patients medically, using water restriction if necessary, digitalis if indicated, increasing the sodium content of the diet, and so on.

Blood Losses

During the operation, blood loss can be calculated in the following ways:

If 500 mL or more of blood is lost, it should be replaced immediately. (If blood cannot be given because of a patient's religious convictions, for example, lactated Ringer's solution can be infused, equal to 2½ times the volume of blood lost. However, if more than 1000 or 1200 mL of blood has been lost, the patient should also receive supplemental plasma or another colloid solution to maintain the circulation. No specific rules can be given for the volume of colloid solution needed. Empirically, one can give 500 mL colloid solution for each 1500 mL lactated Ringer's solution infused.)

A simple way to estimate blood loss during a surgical operation is to weigh the sponges before and after use. The difference in grams is equivalent to the volume in milliliters of blood they have absorbed. Add to this the volume of blood in the operating-room suction bottle. Then increase the total by one half to approximate the actual blood loss.

Postoperative Water and Electrolyte Management

There is also controversy about the volume and type of intravenous fluids needed postoperatively. The immediate goal of postoperative fluid therapy is to maintain a blood pressure of approximately 90/60, a pulse rate of less than 120 per minute, and an hourly urine flow between 30 and 50 mL in association with an adequate level of consciousness, pupillary size, patent airway and breathing pattern, warm skin and skin color, and normal body temperature (Shires).

If an uncomplicated operation has been performed, and if there have been no third-space fluid losses and if acute renal failure is not anticipated, it is necessary only to supply an adequate amount of water. If the patient is able to take 500 mL water by mouth and retain it the first day, there is no need for parenteral water. However, if an abdominal or anastomotic operation has been performed and oral intake is forbidden, from 500 to 1000 mL of water is adequate.

Water needs will be greater if fever, dyspnea, or other causes of water loss are present. Similarly, electrolytes will be needed if abnormal electrolyte losses are present. For example, nasogastric suction drainage can be replaced volume for volume with half-strength saline solution. (Each liter contains 77 mEq sodium and 77 mEq chloride ions.) Potassium chloride should not be added the first postoperative day. From the second postoperative day, 20 mEq potassium ions (1.5 g of potassium chloride) per liter can be added to the half-strength saline solution.

When pyloric obstruction or postoperative malfunction of a gastrointestinal stoma is present, massive volumes of gastric juice can be withdrawn by nasogastric suction. Attempts to replace this loss with a large volume of intravenous fluids, particularly sodium- and potassium-free fluids such as dextrose in water, can cause a self-perpetuating, abnormal, high-output, high-intake cycle that is similar to the situation that may develop during the diuretic phase of acute renal failure when too many fluids are given intravenously. Electrolyte balance does not occur in these patients with a large volume of gastric aspirate. Instead, water excess with hyponatremia, hypochloremia, and hypokalemia may develop, and renal blood flow may decrease, so that the BUN concentration may rise and urine output may decrease.

Berry suggests that when the gastric aspirate reaches 2500 mL or more in a 24-hour period, the nasogastric suction should be stopped temporarily, the volume of intravenous fluids should be decreased by one half, and the patient's clinical condition and electrolyte concentrations should be carefully observed. If severe water excess has developed, hypertonic sodium chloride intravenously may be necessary. If mechanical gastrointestinal obstruction is present, it must be corrected surgically. The use of pharmacological blockers of gastric acid production effectively minimizes these electrolyte problems.

Some surgeons give isotonic sodium chloride solution postoperatively or lactated Ringer's solution, even on the first postoperative day. We prefer to use a quarter-strength sodium chloride solution in dextrose. Each liter supplies water and, in addition, 38.5 mEq sodium and 38.5 mEq chloride ions. Most postoperative patients are able to tolerate this amount of sodium chloride without developing pulmonary edema or edema of the lower extremities. (This volume should be considered as part of the total water intake.)

By the second or third postoperative day, the routine maintenance requirements, described on page 343, can be supplied.

If a complicated operation has been performed with third-space losses or if there is a possibility of acute renal failure, a large amount of fluids and electrolytes may be required to prevent hypotension and renal failure.

Thompson uses the following regimen *postoperatively* for his patients who have undergone abdominal aortic surgery:

1. The intravenous fluids are continued at a rate of approximately 125 mL/hr. The rate of infusion is varied, depending on the blood pressure, urinary output, and any unusual extrarenal losses.

2. In the first 24 hours postoperatively, the patient receives approximately 1 liter of lactated Ringer's solution and 2½ liters of 5% dextrose in water.

3. In the second 24 hours postoperatively, the patient receives approximately 500 mL of 5% dextrose in *isotonic sodium chloride,* and 2000 mL of 5% dextrose in water.

4. On the third postoperative day, the nasogastric tube is removed and fluids are given orally, but 1 to 2 liters of 5% dextrose in water are infused. Thereafter the infusions are stopped.

Many other water, electrolyte, and acid-base syndromes may occur in surgical patients. Acute respiratory acidosis may occur during operation; metabolic acidosis is common after any general surgical operation; operations on the upper gastrointestinal tract may induce an acute hypokalemic alkalosis; respiratory alkalosis is common, particularly if the patient is receiving assisted respiration; the liberal administration of fluids intravenously to postoperative patients frequently produces hyponatremia due to water excess and occasionally water intoxication. These have been discussed in various chapters of this book.

Bibliography

Berry, REL: The "third kidney" phenomenon of the gastrointestinal tract. A complication of parenteral fluid therapy and intestinal trauma. Arch Surg 81:193, 1960.

Duncalf, D, and Underwood, PS: Transfusion during and after surgical operations. In Laufman, H, and Erichson, RB, (eds): *Hematologic Problems in Surgery*. Philadelphia: WB Saunders, 1970.

Giesecke, AH: Perioperative fluid therapy-crystalloids. In RD Miller (Ed.) *Anesthesia,* New York: Churchill Livingstone, vol 2, 1981.

Goggin, MJ, and Joekes, AM: Gas exchange in renal failure. 1. Dangers of hyperkalemia during anaesthesia. BMJ 2:244, 1971.

Gollub, S, et al: Electrolyte solution in surgical patients refusing transfusion. JAMA 215:2077, 1971.

Hogbin, BM, et al: An evaluation of peripheral essential amino acid infusion following major surgery. J Parenteral and Enteral Nutrition 8:511, 1984.

Irvin, TT, et al: Plasma volume deficits and salt and water excretion after surgery. Lancet 2:1159, 1972.

Lauria, JI: Intraoperative management of fluids deficits. New York State J Med 72:691, 1972.

Mason, EE: *Fluid Electrolyte and Nutrient Therapy in Surgery*. Philadelphia: Lea & Febiger, 1974.

Moore, FD: *Metabolic Care of the Surgical Patient*. Philadelphia: WB Saunders, 1959.

Orloff, MJ, and Hutchin, P: Fluid and electrolyte response to trauma and surgery. In Maxwell, MH, and Kleeman, CR (eds). *Clinical Disorders of Fluid and Electrolyte Metabolism*, 2nd ed. New York: McGraw-Hill, 1972.

Rigor, B, Bosomworth, P, and Rush, BF, Jr: Replacement of operative blood loss of more than 1 liter with Hartmann's solution. JAMA 203:111, 1968.

Shires, GT: Fluid and electrolyte therapy. In *American College of Surgeons Committee on Manual of Preoperative and Postoperative Care*, 2nd ed. Philadelphia: WB Saunders, 1971.

Shires, TC, and Canizaro, PC: Fluid, electrolyte and nutritional management of the surgical patient. In Schwartz, SI, (ed): *Principles of Surgery*, 3rd ed. New York: McGraw-Hill, 1979.

Tasker, PRW, et al: Prophylactic use of intravenous saline in patients with chronic renal failure undergoing major surgery. Lancet 2:911, 1974.

Underwood, PS: Fluid management in the recovery room. In Frost, EAM, and Andrews, IC, (eds): *Recovery Room Care*. Int Anesthesiol Clin 21, Spring 1983.

38

SOLUTIONS AVAILABLE FOR FLUID THERAPY

The term *tonicity* is usually used to describe the osmolality of a parenterally given solution in relation to the normal osmolality of the blood and extracellular water. A solution is described as *isotonic* or *isosmotic* when it has the same osmolality of the blood and extracellular water. Therefore, when such a solution is infused, it will not cause the red blood cells to swell or to shrink. A *hypotonic* solution has an osmolality less than that of blood and extracellular water. A *hypertonic* solution has a greater osmolality. Usually, isotonic solutions are infused. However, hypotonic or hypertonic solutions can be used under special conditions.

CARBOHYDRATE IN WATER SOLUTIONS

Physiological Properties

Carbohydrate in water solutions can be used in the following ways:

1. They supply water. Pure water cannot be given parenterally because it is markedly hypotonic and would cause the red blood cells to swell and hemolyze. It therefore must be given with carbohydrates or electrolytes, or other substances, in an isotonic solution.

   A 5% dextrose (glucose) solution in water is approximately isotonic. However, a 10% dextrose, a 10% fructose, or a 10% invert sugar (which is half dextrose, half fructose) solution, or even 20%, 25%, or 50% dextrose solutions can be given intravenously if given slowly. When this is done, adequate mixing and dilution of the sugar solution with blood occur. This prevents local phlebitis.

   Carbohydrates supply water in the following way: The oxidation of each gram of dextrose or fructose supplies 0.6 mL of water of oxidation per gram (Chapter 3). Therefore, the oxidation of 100 g of dextrose, which is present in an infusion of 1 liter of 10% dextrose in water, would supply 60 mL of water in addition to the 1000 mL of water in the solution.

2. In addition, the dextrose or fructose provides calories for part of the daily metabolic needs of the patient. An average adult at rest requires approximately 1500 calories a day. Since each gram of dextrose provides 4.1 calories, a total of approximately 375 g of dextrose would be needed if the dextrose were the only source of calories. This would be equivalent to 3750 mL of a solution of 10% dextrose in water. However, such a large amount of dextrose in water daily is dangerous, and therefore dextrose should not be used primarily for caloric purposes.

3. The ingestion of 100 to 150 g of dextrose decreases the catabolism of endogenous protein. In this way, it decreases the amount of water needed by the kidneys for the excretion of waste products (Chapter 3). The dextrose also prevents depletion of liver glycogen and therefore prevents the production of an excessive amount of ketone acids.

4. Fructose theoretically has the following advantages over dextrose:
   a. Fructose can be metabolized in the absence of insulin. Therefore, it can be utilized more rapidly than dextrose in a patient with diabetic acidosis or with disturbed liver function, as postoperatively, during fevers, and in liver disease.
   b. A 10% fructose solution can be given at the same rate as a 5% dextrose solution, without any of the sugar spilling into the urine.
      However, recent studies in children indicate that fructose may cause a transient increase in the lactic acid content of the blood, and a decrease in the CO_2 content. A fructose infusion can also cause hypophosphatemia.

Dextrose in water solutions may have a pH as low as 4 to 5 to minimize degradation and the resulting caramelization of the dextrose during sterilization. This may be one of the reasons for the development of postinfusion thrombophlebitis. The danger of this can be decreased by using small scalp-vein needles, and by changing the infusion site every 3 days.

Solutions Available

Dextrose in water is available in the following strengths: 2.5%, 5%, 10%, 20%, 25%, and 50%; fructose in water is available in a 10% solution; *invert sugar* (half dextrose–half fructose) is available in a 5% or 10% solution.

Volume of Solution Needed

This is discussed in Chapter 37. In addition, the administration of an excessive amount of dextrose in water may actually cause a loss of water from the body, rather than water excess. This will occur if the circulating blood volume is increased to such an extent that aldosterone secretion stops. As a result, the kidneys may begin to excrete a large amount of sodium ions and water.

Route of Administration

Dextrose or fructose in water should be given intravenously, and should never be given subcutaneously.

Rate of Administration

Dextrose in water can be given intravenously at a rate of 0.5 g per kg body weight, per hour, without causing glycosuria. Therefore, it requires about 3 hours for the infusion of 1000 mL of a solution of 10% dextrose in water. This is equivalent to 333 mL/hr. A 5% dextrose solution, or a 10% fructose or invert sugar solution, can be given at twice this rate, namely, 666 mL/hr (see page 372).

Some patients may be able to tolerate 0.85 g dextrose per kg body weight (1000 mL of a 10% dextrose solution in 2 hours, or 1000 mL of a 5% dextrose solution in 1 hour). It is useful to test the urine for sugar at regular intervals when dextrose is being infused. A moderate glycosuria of 3 plus or less may develop. This will not cause a urinary loss of water or electrolytes because not enough dextrose is being lost in the urine to act as an osmotic diuretic.

If dextrose is infused too rapidly, it may cause a transient reactive hyperinsulinism and the patient may experience weakness, apprehension, sweating, decreased blood pressure, and even disorientation or a convulsive seizure. These symptoms disappear if the infusion is discontinued.

A solution of 20% dextrose in water can be used when carbohydrates are needed, but the intake must be kept low. One liter of 20% dextrose in water can be given in a period of 6 hours. It should be infused into a large vein, such as the superior vena cava, to prevent thrombosis.

ISOTONIC AND HYPOTONIC SODIUM CHLORIDE SOLUTIONS

Physiological Properties

Isotonic sodium chloride solution, or saline, is often called "physiological" or "normal" saline, or salt solution. However, these terms are not correct, because 1 liter of blood contains approximately 142 mEq sodium and approximately 103 mEq chloride, but isotonic saline solution contains approximately 150 mEq sodium and 150 mEq chloride per liter. Therefore, only the sodium concentration of isotonic sodium chloride solution is similar to that of blood. Its chloride concentration is much higher than the chloride concentration of blood. Therefore, if a large amount of isotonic sodium chloride solution is given to a patient who has lost more sodium than chloride (as in diarrhea, for example) and if the kidneys are not able to excrete the excess chloride ions, a severe hyperchloremic metabolic acidosis can occur (Chapter 17). However, it is isosmotic, and will not cause hemolysis of the red blood cells when infused, either alone or with 2.5%, 5%, or 10% glucose, 5% fructose or 5% or 10% invert sugar, or with potassium, alcohol, plasma expanders such as dextran, vitamins, or other electrolytes.

Composition	% Sol.	Grams per liter	Concentration mEq/L Na+	Cl⁻
NaCl	0.9	9.	154	154
NaCl	0.45	4.5	77	77
NaCl	0.33	3.3	56	56
NaCl	0.3	3.	51	51
NaCl	0.2	2.	34	34

Isotonic sodium chloride solution contains sodium and chloride ions, and has been used principally in syndromes associated with sodium loss, such as diabetic acidosis, loss of gastrointestinal fluids, adrenocortical insufficiency, and burns. It should not be used to replace water loss.

Solutions Available

The following types of isotonic and hypotonic sodium chloride solutions are available:

Sodium chloride, 0.9% solution: plain or with 5 or 10% dextrose.

Sodium chloride, 0.45% (half strength): plain or with 2.5, 5, or 10% dextrose.

Sodium chloride, 0.33% (slightly more than third strength): with 5% dextrose.

Sodium chloride, 0.3% (third strength): with 5% dextrose.

Sodium chloride, 0.2% (slightly less than quarter strength): with 5% dextrose.

Volume of Solution Needed

This is discussed in various chapters throughout the book.

Route of Administration

Isotonic 0.9% sodium chloride or hypotonic 0.45% saline solution can be given intravenously or subcutaneously, either alone or with 5% dextrose. A 10% dextrose, fructose, or invert sugar in sodium chloride solution should not be used subcutaneously, because it is hypertonic and will cause water to leave the bloodstream and accumulate in the injection area. This may precipitate or worsen shock. Dextrose in 0.33%, 0.3%, 0.225% or 0.2% sodium chloride solution should only be given intravenously.

Rate of Administration

Isotonic sodium chloride solution is usually given at a rate up to 400 mL/hr. However, if shock due to sodium loss is present, it can be given at a rate of 2000 mL/hr.

HYPERTONIC SODIUM CHLORIDE SOLUTIONS
Physiological Properties

Hypertonic sodium chloride solution is indicated when there is a severe sodium loss in association with a relative water excess, or when there is primary water excess (water intoxication). In these cases, it raises the osmotic pressure of the extracellular water.

Solutions Available

Hypertonic sodium chloride solution is available in 3% and 5% concentrations.

Composition	% Sol.	Grams per liter	Concentration mEq/L Na+	Cl−
NaCl	3	30	513	513
NaCl	5	50	855	855

Route of Administration

Hypertonic sodium chloride solution can only be given intravenously.

Rate of Administration

Hypertonic sodium chloride solution must be given slowly, because it can precipitate pulmonary edema. The rate of infusion is described in Chapters 6 and 7.

ACIDIFYING SOLUTIONS

Ammonium chloride is the solution commonly used.

Physiological Properties

When ammonium chloride is administered, the ammonium ion is converted to urea by the liver. The chloride ion reacts with hydrogen ions in the extracellular water, forming hydrochloric acid that is able to correct a metabolic alkalosis, particularly if the alkalosis is associated with a loss of chloride ions.

Ammonium chloride has been used in the treatment of patients with metabolic alkalosis, due to vomiting and loss of hydrochloric acid. However, in these patients, a solution containing isotonic or hypotonic sodium chloride solution with potassium chloride (see Chapter 29) is usually more effective.

Ammonium chloride is contraindicated in patients with disturbed liver function and a high blood ammonia content, as in right-sided heart failure, cirrhosis of the liver, or azotemia. If an excessive amount of ammonium chloride is given, a metabolic acidosis may develop with drowsiness, mental confusion, disorientation, hyperpnea, and coma. In patients with liver disease, the ammonium chloride can precipitate hepatic coma.

Solutions Available

Ammonium chloride is available as a hypertonic, 2.14% solution in water.

Composition	% Sol.	Grams per liter	Concentration mEq/L Na+	Cl−
NH_4Cl	2.14	21.4	400	400

Ammonium chloride concentrate can also be added to isotonic sodium chloride solution. It is available in 20-mL vials. Each milliliter contains 5 mEq ammonium ions and 5 mEq chloride ions. (To prepare a solution containing approximately 400 mEq/L (2.14%) for example, 80 mL of ammonium chloride concentrate is added to 920 mL isotonic sodium chloride solution.)

Volume of Solution Needed

This is discussed in Chapter 29.

Route of Administration

Ammonium chloride solutions should only be given intravenously. If an excessive amount of ammonium chloride is infused, signs of ammonia intoxication (Chapter 29) can develop.

Rate of Administration

The 2.14% ammonium chloride solution can be given at a rate up to 120 mL/hr (see Chapter 29).

ALKALINIZING SOLUTIONS

These solutions (Table 38–1) contain sodium bicarbonate, or sodium racemic lactate, or acetate, which is oxidized in the body to bicarbonate. THAM (tromethamine) is also an alkalinizing salt.

Physiological Properties

Alkalinizing solutions can be used in the treatment of metabolic acidosis. It is important not to raise the CO_2 content above 18 mEq/L, because of the danger of producing a metabolic alkalosis and tetany. In addition, to prevent tetany calcium salts should also be given when alkalinizing solutions are used.

Sodium bicarbonate is the drug of choice in the treatment of metabolic acidosis. If the acidosis is not severe it can be given orally, or it can be given intravenously as a 1.5% solution in 5% dextrose in water, or in lesser concentrations (see Chapter 17).

When a severe metabolic acidosis is present, hypertonic 7.5% sodium bicarbonate solution can be given intravenously. It is usually diluted with at least a similar volume of dextrose in water. However, in an emergency, as in cardiac arrest, it can be given intravenously undiluted. Hypertonic sodium bicarbonate solution can also be given to a patient with renal failure and metabolic acidosis who develops sodium loss and hyponatremia.

TABLE 38–1
ALKALINIZING SOLUTIONS

Composition	% Sol	Gram per liter	Concentration mEq/L Na+	HCO₃
Sodium bicarbonate, isotonic	1.5*	15.	178	178
Sodium bicarbonate, hypertonic NaHCO₃	7.5	†	†	†
Sodium r-lactate 1/6 molar (isotonic) NaC₃H₅O₃	1.72	17.2	167	167

*A 1.5% solution of sodium bicarbonate can be prepared by adding 4 ampuls of the hypertonic 7.5% solution to 800 mL 5% dextrose in water. Less concentrated solutions, using 1, 2, or 3 ampuls in 1000 mL dextrose in water, can also be prepared. (Two ampuls in a liter will supply approximately 88 mEq sodium and bicarbonate ions; 3 ampuls in a liter will supply approximately 133 mEq sodium and bicarbonate ions.)
†Hypertonic sodium bicarbonate is commercially available in 50-mL ampuls, containing 3.75 g of sodium bicarbonate (45 mEq sodium, and 45 mEq bicarbonate). It should be diluted with at least an equal volume of dextrose in water solution before use.

One-sixth molar (isotonic) sodium racemic lactate, which consists of equal parts of D- and L-lactate, can be used if there is no need for fluid restriction. The lactate ions in sodium lactate are metabolized by the liver into bicarbonate ions, so that the effect of using a lactate salt is the same as using sodium bicarbonate.

One-sixth molar lactate should not be used if liver disease, shock, or right-sided heart failure is present, because the metabolism of lactic acid is impaired. Lactate and bicarbonate solutions are also contraindicated in respiratory alkalosis, where the low CO_2 content may simulate a metabolic acidosis (Chapter 28).

Volume of Solution Needed

To raise the CO_2 content 1 mEq/L, give 1.2 mL of the 1/6 molar sodium lactate per kg body weight.

This rule is derived in the following way: An adult has an extracellular water content of 20% of the body weight. Therefore, there is 0.2 liter extracellular water for every 1 kg body weight. If an ion, such as lactate, has a concentration in the extracellular water of 1 mEq/L, there would be 0.2 mEq of the ion per kg body weight.

If one uses a solution of 1/6 molar sodium lactate, which contains 167 mEq/L of solution, 1 mL of the solution contains 0.167 mEq of the lactate ion. Therefore, 1.2 mL of the 1/6 molar solution will contain 0.2 mEq/L.

If 1.2 mL of the 1/6 molar sodium lactate solution per kg body weight is now given, this would raise the lactate concentration 0.2 mEq per kg of body weight, or 1 mEq/L of extracellular water. The bicarbonate concentration would be raised similarly, because 1 mEq sodium lactate is converted into 1 mEq sodium bicarbonate.

When the patient's water intake must be restricted, as in acute renal failure, hypertonic sodium bicarbonate can be used instead of the 1/6 molar sodium lactate.

Route of Administration

The 1/6 molar sodium lactate or the isotonic (1.5% sodium bicarbonate is given intravenously.

Rate of Administration

Either of these solutions can be given at a rate up to 300 mL/hr.

Molar lactate of hypertonic bicarbonate should be given at the same rate as hypertonic sodium chloride solution (Chapter 1).

SPECIAL SOLUTIONS

Ringer's Solution

Ringer's solution (triple chloride solution) is essentially an isotonic saline with potassium and calcium in concentrations approximately equal to their concentrations in the blood and extracellular water. However, if potassium or calcium loss is present, a much larger amount of these ions will be needed than is present in the Ringer's solution.

Ringer's solution can be given intravenously in the same way as isotonic saline.

	% Sol.	Grams per liter	Na+	Concentration mEq/L K+	Ca+	Cl−
NaCl	0.86	8.6	147.5			147.5
KCl	0.03	0.3		4		4
CaCl₂	0.033	0.33			4.5	4.5
Total			147.5	4 (156)	4.5	156

Saline-Lactate Solutions

Hartmann devised the first practical saline-lactate solution to avoid the excessive chloride content of isotonic saline solution and to supply bicarbonate ions. It consisted of 6 g of sodium chloride (103 mEq sodium and 103 mEq chloride ions) and 5.6 g of sodium lactate (51 mEq sodium and 51 mEq lactate ions) per liter. Bicarbonate ions were formed from the metabolism of the lactate ions. This solution, however, has been superseded by a modified form, which is commercially available. It is called lactated Ringer's solution (Hartmann's modified solution).

	% Sol.	Grams per liter	Na+	Concentration mEq/L K+	Ca++	HCO₃−	Cl−
NaCl	0.6	6.	102				102
KCl	0.03	0.3		4			4
CaCl₂	0.02	0.2			3		3
Sodium lactate	0.3	3.	28			28	
Total			130	4 (137)	3	28	109 (137)

An acetated Ringer's solution is also available. It is similar to Ringer's lactate solution except that the sodium lactate is replaced by sodium acetate.

Theoretically, sodium acetate is preferable to sodium lactate because acetate ions are not metabolized by the liver, but by muscles and other peripheral tissues. In addition, the acetate ions are metabolized in a different way from the lactate ions and require less oxygen for their metabolism to carbon dioxide and bicarbonate ions. This may be important if shock is present.

Several of the pharmaceutical firms are now using sodium acetate instead of sodium lactate in various electrolyte replacement solutions.

Lactated Ringer's solution is superior to isotonic sodium chloride solution because its electrolyte concentration is similar to that of blood. For example, the sodium concentration is higher than the chloride concentration; and the lactate supplies bicarbonate in a concentration that is similar to that present in normal plasma.

Lactated Ringer's solution can be used in place of isotonic sodium chloride solution. It is particularly valuable in metabolic acidosis syndromes.

MULTIPLE ELECTROLYTE SOLUTIONS

Physiological Properties

Talbot and Butler devised multiple electrolyte solutions that are based on the concept that the amount of water and electrolytes that the patient retains is not related to the amount of water and electrolytes received, but instead is dependent on the regulatory mechanisms of the body. In other words, they believe that the apparent success of many different types of fluid therapy has been due not to the types of solutions used, but to the regulatory or homeostatic mechanism of the body, especially of the kidneys. In this way, needed amounts of water and electrolytes are utilized, and what is not needed is excreted. These "multiple electrolyte solutions" are available with modifications under numerous trade names. They are hypotonic and therefore contain free water in addition to electrolytes. They contain sodium, chloride, and lactate ions, which are extracellular electrolytes, as well as potassium and phosphate ions, which are intracellular ions. Some of the solutions also contain magnesium ions.

Originally it had been hoped that a "multiple electrolyte solution" could be used as an "all-purpose" solution, regardless of the water and electrolyte deficit. Multiple electrolyte solutions have been used successfully in the following situations:

1. For water and electrolyte maintenance in patients who are not taking fluids orally.
2. When gastrointestinal fluids are lost, as by vomiting, gastric suction, diarrhea, or fistulas.
3. In moderate sodium loss syndromes.
4. In moderate potassium loss syndromes.
5. In metabolic acidosis syndromes, as in diabetic acidosis, due to excessive administration of chloride ions, and severe infections.
6. In metabolic alkalosis syndromes, due to excessive administration of alkali, or loss of hydrochloric acid and potassium ions from vomiting or gastric suction.

However, multiple electrolyte solutions are contraindicated in the following situations:

1. When severe sodium loss is present, especially if the serum sodium concentration is below 125 mEq/L. These patients may require a hypertonic sodium chloride solution.
2. When a severe burn is present. The serum potassium concentration may be abnormally high due to tissue destruction and acidosis. In addition, these patients require large amounts of a solution such as lactated Ringer's solution rather than a hypotonic solution.
3. In adrenocortical insufficiency. These patients have an abnormally high serum potassium concentration and should not receive fluids with potassium.
4. With severe water loss, or diabetes insipidus. These patients primarily require water without electrolytes.
5. When water excess (water intoxication) is present. These patients require cessation of water therapy, and may require hypertonic sodium chloride solution.
6. When a severe metabolic acidosis or metabolic alkalosis is present.
7. When renal insufficiency is present.
8. When a severe calcium loss is present with tetany. Such patients should receive 10% calcium gluconate intravenously.
9. When hypoparathyroidism is present. These patients have an abnormally high phosphate concentration and should not receive a phosphate salt, which is present in the multiple electrolyte solutions.

Solutions Available

In general, two types of multiple electrolyte solutions are available:

Maintenance Therapy Solutions

This type of *hypotonic* multiple electrolyte solution has been used as a substitute for dextrose and water when the patient cannot take fluids orally, as after surgery. Table 38–2 shows the composition of available maintenance solutions.

A similar maintenance solution can be prepared as follows:

830 mL 5% dextrose in water.

20 mL molar potassium chloride solution. (This supplies 20 mEq potassium ions and 20 mEq chloride ions.)

150 mL 1/6 molar sodium lactate, *or* 150 mL isotonic (1.5%) sodium bicarbonate solution. (This supplies 26 mEq sodium ions and 26 mEq lactate *or* bicarbonate ions.)

VOLUME OF SOLUTION NEEDED. The maintenance therapy solutions contain a large amount of potassium. Therefore, they can be used only when the pa-

TABLE 38–2
MAINTENANCE THERAPY (HYPOTONIC MULTIPLE ELECTROLYTE) SOLUTIONS

Solution	Manufacturer	mEq/L							Carbohydrate
		Na^+	K^+	Ca^{++}	Mg^{++}	Cl^-	HCO_3^-	HPO_4^-	
Isolyte R	American McGraw	40	16	5	3	40	24 (acetate)		5% dextrose plain or 5% dextrose
Normosol M	Abbott	40	13	—	3	40	16 (acetate)	—	
Maintenance solution	Self-prepared	25	20			20	25 (bicarbonate, or lactate)		5% dextrose

tient is passing an adequate amount of urine. If kidney function is not adequate, the patient should receive 1/2 isotonic or 1/4 isotonic saline solution, or dextrose in water, depending on the disturbance present, until the circulation improves and adequate urine output returns.

The required volumes of maintenance therapy solution can be calculated on the basis of the surface area of the body.

A *maintenance* 24-hour volume is approximately 1500 mL/m² of body surface. Table 38–3 shows the approximate relations between body weight and surface area.

When a *moderate* fluid deficit is present (weight loss up to 5%), a 24-hour volume of approximately 2400 mL/m² of body surface will provide the maintenance volume needs and correct the fluid deficit.

When a *severe* fluid deficit is present (weight loss more than 5%), a 24-hour volume of approximately 3000 mL/m² of body surface will provide the maintenance volume needs and correct the fluid deficit.

ROUTE OF ADMINISTRATION. Maintenance therapy solutions should be given only intravenously.

RATE OF ADMINISTRATION. One method of calculating the rate of administration is to divide the total daily volume of the solution by 24 (hours).

In adults, up to 400 mL/hr can be given.

Replacement Therapy Solutions.

This type of *isotonic* multiple electrolyte solution has been used as a substitute for isotonic saline solution, when there is a marked loss of water and electrolytes, as in severe vomiting or diarrhea, or after surgery, burns, trauma. Table 38–4 shows the composition of available replacement solutions.

The "1-2" solution is a similar replacement solution. It can be prepared by mixing 1 part of 1/6 molar sodium lactate with 2 parts of isotonic saline. (This supplies 150 mEq sodium ions, 100 mEq chloride ions, and 50 mEq bicarbonate ions [as lactate].)

VOLUME OF SOLUTION NEEDED. This depends on the clinical condition and the serum electrolyte concentrations. The general rules will have to be modified for each patient.

ROUTE OF ADMINISTRATION. Replacement therapy solutions should be given only intravenously.

RATE OF ADMINISTRATION. Up to 400 mL/hr can be given. One method of calculating the rate of administration is to divide the total daily volume of the solution by 24 (hours).

POTASSIUM-CONTAINING SOLUTIONS

Physiological Properties

Potassium-containing solutions supply potassium ions that are necessary for cellular metabolism. Potassium chloride is generally used. However, potassium acetate or potassium phosphate can also be used.

TABLE 38–3
RELATIONS BETWEEN BODY WEIGHT AND APPROXIMATE SURFACE AREA

| Weight | | Approximate surface area* |
kg	lb	(square meters)
50	110	1.50
60	132	1.65
70	154	1.75
80	176	1.85
90	198	1.95
100	220	2.05

*For adults of average height.

Theoretically, it would seem that potassium phosphate should be more valuable than the potassium chloride because there is usually phosphate loss in association with the potassium loss. However, potassium chloride is satisfactory for most patients. In addition, it is extremely important to use potassium *chloride* and not any of the other potassium salts in patients who have been receiving the thiazide diuretics, furosemide, or ethacrynic acid.

Potassium acetate can be used in patients with potassium loss associated with metabolic acidosis, as in renal tubular acidosis, and potassium-losing nephritis. The acetate is metabolized to bicarbonate that helps restore the pH to normal.

Solutions Available

Potassium chloride ampuls are available, and the required amount of the potassium ion can be added to dextrose in water, or to isotonic saline solution. However, one should remember that if a severe potassium loss is present the administration of sodium ions aggravates the potassium loss.

Numerous solutions are available for IV use containing 10, 20, 30, or 40 mEq K/L with varying concentrations of sodium chloride and 5% dextrose in water.

Volume of Solution to Be Given

The amount of potassium salt to be used is discussed in Chapter 30.

Route of Administration

Potassium-containing solutions should be given intravenously or orally.

TABLE 38–4
REPLACEMENT THERAPY (ISOTONIC MULTIPLE ELECTROLYTE) SOLUTIONS

Solution	Manufacturer	mEq/L						Carbohydrate
		Na^+	K^+	Ca^{++}	Mg^{++}	Cl^-	HCO_3^-	
Hartmann's	Several	130	4	3	—	109	28 (as lactate, or acetate)	None, or 5% dextrose
Normosol-R	Abbott	140	5	—	3	98	50 (acetate 27, gluconate 23)	None, or 5% dextrose
Plasmalyte	Travenol	140	10	5	3	103	47 (acetate 47) dextrose	None, or 5%
Isolyte E	American McGraw	140	10	5	3	103	57 (acetate 49, citrate 8)	None, or 5% dextrose
"1–2"	Self-prepared	150	—	—	—	100	50 (lactate)	None

Rate of Administration

Potassium salts should not be prepared in a concentration greater than 80 mEq/L, and should not be given at a rate greater than 20 mEq/hr (rarely 40 mEq/hr). In addition, no potassium-containing solution should be used until there is an adequate urine output.

COLLOIDAL SOLUTIONS

Physiological Properties

Whole blood, plasma, packed red blood cells, concentrated albumin, or colloidal plasma expanders such as dextran are valuable for increasing the circulating blood volume when shock is present (Table 38–5). Because most of these solutions are retained within the vascular system, they increase the osmotic pressure of the blood above that of the extracellular fluid spaces. As a result, water passes from the extracellular fluid space into the blood, increasing the circulating blood volume.

Solutions Available

Whole Blood

One unit of blood will raise the hemoglobin from 1 to 1.5 g/dL. Common dangers of blood transfusion are serum hepatitis, transient fever due to bacterial contamination, incompatible transfusion reactions, allergic reactions, sensitization to Rh or other blood factors, or acute pulmonary edema due to overtransfusion. The latter can occur either during the transfusion or 1 hour afterward. In addition, a large transfusion of citrated blood can also cause hypocalcemia (page 302). Although whole blood was the solution of choice in shock due to hemorrhage or severe anemia, whole blood is no longer recommended to minimize potential risks of viral transmission.

TABLE 38–5
ELECTROLYTE COMPOSITION OF COLLOIDAL SOLUTIONS

	Volume (mL)	Concentration (mEq per stated volume)		
		Na+	K+	Cl−
Whole blood	1000	142	5	103
Packed red blood cells	250	5	20	13
Plasma	250	38	1	25
Albumin	100	16	0	2
Dextran in isotonic saline	250	36	0	36

Packed Red Blood Cells

Blood can be centrifuged and the plasma drawn off. The packed red cells can then be transfused, either with the small amount of plasma remaining, or they can be resuspended in a small volume of isotonic saline solution or 5% dextrose in saline solution. Packed red blood cells are valuable when patients who show congestive heart failure or sodium excess require blood.

Plasma

A good physiological plasma expander, plasma is better than blood because it is not necessary to type and cross-match the patient. Also, the risk of transmitting viral hepatitis is reduced by the freezing process. Nonetheless, albumin is preferred as a colloid expander to minimize viral risk (see below).

Albumin

When rapid volume expansion is essential, albumin solutions are ideal, particularly in patients with low oncotic pressure due to liver disease, nephrotic syndrome, or malnutrition. Albumin is available as 5% and 25% solutions.

Dextran

Dextran is available in two forms, with a molecular weight of 70,000 (dextran 70) or 75,000 (dextran 75), or with a molecular weight of 40,000 (low-molecular-weight dextran, dextran 40).

DEXTRAN 70 OR 75. This is used to expand the plasma volume as an adjunct treatment of shock or impending shock when the circulating blood volume is low, as in burns, hemorrhage, or surgery, and when blood or blood products are not available. However, dextran is not a substitute for whole blood because it has no oxygen-carrying properties. It is also not a substitute for plasma proteins because its effects are limited.

Adverse effects include hypersensitivity reactions, such as nasal congestion, urticaria, tightness in the chest and wheezing, and hypotension. Severe anaphylactoid reactions with shock and even death have also occurred. Anaphylactoid reactions can be treated with the administration of 1:1000 epinephrine, 0.5 mL subcutaneously, followed, if necessary, by IV injection of 0.25 to 0.5 mL of a 1:10,000 solution.

Because death from an anaphylactic reaction can occur after as little as 10-mL dextran 75 has been given, blood pressure should be monitored and the patient observed closely during at least the first 30 minutes of infusion of any dextran preparation.

Dextran can interfere with platelet function and can increase the bleeding time, especially if the dose exceeds 1 to 1.5 L. This reaction may not appear for 6 to 9 hours after the infusion and bleeding may occur. The hematocrit should be checked after a dextran infusion and care should be taken not to depress the hematocrit below 30%.

Dextran is contraindicated with patients who are hypersensitive to it, and in patients with severe bleeding disorders or severe cardiac or renal failure. It can cause circulatory overload, particularly if dextran in 0.9% sodium chloride solution is used.

Dextran 70 or 75 is given IV as a 6% solution. The total dose should not exceed 1.2 g/kg (20 mL/kg) in the first 24 hours. If dextran is needed after this, the dosage should not exceed 0.6 g/kg (10 mL/kg). In adults, the usual dose is 30 g (500 mL). In an emergency, dextran can be given to adults at a rate of 1.2 to 2.4 g (20 to 40 mL) per minute. If the patient has normal or near normal blood volume, the rate of infusion should not exceed 0.24 g (4 mL) per minute.

Dextran 70 and dextran 75 are available in 5% dextrose in water, or in a 0.9% sodium chloride solution. The containers have no preservatives and any unused solution should be discarded.

(The numerical designation: 70, 75, 40, is simply the weight-average molecular weight divided by 1000.)

DEXTRAN 40. Dextran 40 has a molecular weight of approximately 40,000. Its uses are similar to those of dextran 70 or 75. In addition, it can be used as a priming fluid, alone, or with additives for pump oxygenators during extracorporeal circulation.

It can cause the same kind of anaphylactoid reactions as dextran 70 or 75.

When dextran 40 is given by rapid IV infusion, it may cause the central venous pressure (CVP) to rise precipitously and may provoke congestive heart failure, especially if it is given in a 0.9% sodium chloride solution.

It must be given cautiously to patients with active bleeding because it improves the microcirculation and may increase the bleeding. It is contraindicated in patients with thrombocytopenia or hypofibrinogenemia, and in patients with severe dehydration.

The dosage depends on the patient's needs. A total dose of 10% solution should not exceed 2 g/kg (20 mL/kg) in the first 24 hours. If it is continued beyond this time the dose should not exceed 1 g/kg (10 mL/kg). Therapy should not be continued longer than 5 days.

The first 500 mL of dextran 40 can be infused rapidly while the CVP is monitored. The remaining dose should be infused slowly.

Dextran 40 is available as a 10% solution in 5% dextrose in water, or in 0.9% sodium chloride solution. The containers have no preservative and any unused solution should be discarded.

Mannitol

Mannitol is a low-molecular-weight hexahydric alcohol. It has marked hydroscopic activity, and acts as an osmotic diuretic by raising the osmotic pressure of the glomerular filtrate to such an extent that there is a decrease in the tubular reabsorption of water and ions such as sodium, potassium, chloride, calcium, and magnesium, which are excreted in the urine. Also, if the patient is taking lithium, an increased urinary excretion of this also occurs. When given intravenously, it is associated with a rapid rise in serum osmolality. As a result, water moves from the cells into the extracellular water and the blood, and the serum sodium concentration falls. Mannitol is also able to increase renal blood flow and urine volume even when an antidiuretic state is present, as postoperatively, and after trauma to the kidneys.

Mannitol has been used under the following conditions:

1. In acute renal failure treatment should be started as soon as possible after oliguria is noted. A test dose is necessary, approximately 0.2 g/kg, or 12.5 g—62.5 mL—as a 20% solution, infused in 3 to 5 minutes to produce an adequate urine flow—at least 30 to 50 mL/hr. If the urine flow does not increase within 2 to 3 hours, a second test dose can be given. If there is an inadequate response, no further mannitol should be given until the patient is reevaluated.

   If there is an adequate response to mannitol, a regular dose of 100 g can be given as a 15% or 20% solution in a period of 90 minutes to several hours.

2. To prevent oliguria or acute renal failure, 50 to 100 g of mannitol may be given. Generally, a concentrated solution is given initially, followed by a 5% or 10% solution. When used prophylactically in surgical operations, the mannitol may be started before or immediately after surgery and may be continued postoperatively.

3. A dose of 100 g of mannitol, given in a period of 2 to 6 hours, has been used in nephrotic, cardiac, or cirrhotic patients who show refractory edema and ascites. Either the 10% or 20% solution can be used. However, the physician should observe these patients carefully for signs of increasing edema or the development of pulmonary edema.

4. A 5% to 10% solution of mannitol can be used as an adjuvant treatment of exogenous poisoning, as long as indicated clinically, and as long as the urinary output remains at a high level, or until a maximum of 200 g is given.

5. Mannitol has also been used in ophthalmology and in neurological surgery to reduce elevated intraocular pressure, cerebrospinal pressure, and cerebral edema, as a 20% solution.

Mannitol in water is available in concentrations of 5%, 10%, 15%, 20%, and 25%. It is chemically stable. However, the 20% and 25% solutions have a tendency to crystallize when exposed to a low temperature. If this occurs, the bottle should be warmed to 60°C in a water bath and then cooled to body temperature (38°C) before administering. As the bottle cools enough to be handled, it should be shaken vigorously several times. An alternate method, if a 20% or 25% solution is used, is to administer it with a filter to prevent mannitol crystals from entering the circulation. This problem will not occur if solutions of 15% or less concentration are used.

The usual adult dose of mannitol is 100 g in 24 hours. Doses as high as 200 g per 24 hours and even higher have been given. However, when large doses are used, a water excess syndrome (Chapter 6) may develop. The mannitol can be stopped when the patient is able to maintain a urine flow of 100 mL/hr. If he or she cannot produce more than 100 mL/hr in response to mannitol, he or she should not receive more than 100 g in any 24-hour period. The physicians should also give the patient water and other electrolytes that may be needed.

Side reactions may occur. Thirst is common. Headache, chills, an anaphylactoid reaction, a sensation of constriction or pain in the chest may occur if a large amount of mannitol is given rapidly; convulsions due to water excess may occur, or the patient may develop pulmonary edema due to the sudden increase in circulating blood volume. If repeated doses of mannitol are given, they may produce such an extensive osmotic diuresis that a water loss syndrome (Chapter 4) develops. Although urine that is formed as a result of mannitol infusion shows a low sodium concentration, significant hyponatremia may occasionally develop. Renal changes consisting of swelling of the epithelium of the proximal convoluted tubules may occur in patients who receive more than 100 g of mannitol. Extravasation of the solution may cause local edema or thrombophlebitis.

Mannitol should not be combined with packed red blood cell infusion.
Mannitol intoxication is treated with hemodialysis.
Mannitol infusions are contraindicated if the patient does not respond to a test dose, or if a small dose precipitates or increases pulmonary edema. They should also not be used in metabolic edema associated with abnormal capillary fragility or membrane permeability, where the heart, liver, and kidneys are normal.

Hetastarch

Hetastarch is a synthetic polymer derived from a waxy starch composed mostly of amylopectin. It closely resembles glycogen and has a range of molecular weights ranging from 10,000 to 1,000,000. The smaller molecules are excreted in the urine. The larger molecules require enzymatic degradation before they are excreted.

Hetastarch expands the circulating plasma volume like serum albumin and dextran. It has a calculated osmolality of approximately 310 mOsm/L, and the expansion of plasma volume is slightly in excess of the volume infused. Maximal plasma volume expansion occurs a few minutes after the infusion. The expanded plasma volume may last for 24 hours or longer. However, small amounts of the hetastarch may persist for weeks in the body.

Hetastarch increases the sedimentation rate when added to whole blood. It also raises the blood sugar concentration as it is metabolized and the blood amylase concentration because it binds amylase and prevents its normal excretion in the urine. This increased amylase concentration may persist for 3 to 5 days after the hetastarch is stopped. Therefore blood amylase concentration cannot be used to diagnose acute pancreatitis during this time.

Hetastarch is not antigenic. However, allergic or sensitivity reactions can occur, for example, vomiting, slight rise in temperature with flu-like symptoms, enlargement of submaxillary and parotid glands, urticaria, wheezing. The blood platelet count and hematocrit can decrease as a result of the volume-expanding effects of hetastarch. One should avoid having the hematocrit fall below 30% after an infusion.

Hetastarch is contraindicated in patients with bleeding disorders, congestive heart failure, or impaired renal function.

The dose of hetastarch depends on the patient's needs. The usual adult dose of the hetastarch 6% solution is 30 to 60 g (500 mL to 1 liter). The total daily dose should not exceed 1.2 g/kg (20 mL/kg), or 90 g (1500 mL). In patients in hemorrhagic shock, it can be given at a rate approaching 1.2 g/kg/hr (20 mL/kg/hr). Slower rates are generally used in patients with burns or septic shock.

In patients with severe renal impairment or a creatinine clearance less than 10 mL/min the usual initial dose can be given, but subsequent doses should be reduced to about 1/4 or 1/2 of the usual dose.

Hetastarch is available as Hespan (American Critical Care) as a 6% solution in 0.9% sodium chloride solution. It has no preservatives and any unused solution should be discarded.

Urea

Urea, like mannitol, is an osmotic diuretic. It is not metabolized and it diffuses rapidly through the glomeruli. Therefore, when it is given orally or intravenously, it is associated with the passage of a large amount of water from the extracellular spaces into the bloodstream, and, when it is excreted by the kidneys, it carries along a large amount of water and sodium ions.

Urea can be given IV or orally. IV urea has been used to lower intracranial and intraocular pressure, and also to treat the syndrome of inappropriate secretion of antidiuretic hormone (SIADH).

Oral urea has also been used to treat SIADH and also as a diuretic in refractory heart failure. It can be used in conjunction with furosemide.

In treating SIADH, it can be given IV as a 30% solution, in a dose of 80 g infused over 6 hours. Or it can be given orally as two or three 30-g doses in 24 hours.

When used as an oral diuretic, large doses, 45 to 90 g a day, can be used. It has a bitter taste that can be masked by putting the urea in grape juice. Or, 30 g of urea crystals and 10 mL of an aluminum and magnesium hydroxide antacid, such as Maalox, can be dissolved in 100 mL of water.

For IV use, urea is available in vials of 40 g of lyophilized urea (Ureaphil-Abbott). 105 mL of a 5 or 10% dextrose in water solution, or 10% invert sugar solution is added to the 40 g of lyophilized urea. The resultant solution contains 300 mg urea per mL (30% solution).

The solution is irritating and may result in thrombosis, thrombophlebitis, or sloughing of the tissues. Therefore, it should not be given in the veins of the lower limbs of elderly patients. It should not be given faster than 4 mL of the 30% solution per minute to prevent side effects such as nausea, vomiting, nervousness, tachycardia, hypotension, syncope, mental confusion, or hyperthermia. The infusion should not be stopped abruptly. No more than 1.5 g/kg or 120 g should be given IV in a 24-hour period. Headache may also occur as a result of excessive diuresis, and intraocular hemorrhage may occur in patients with absolute glaucoma, if the urea is infused too rapidly. Abnormal ECG changes may also occur.

Urea is contraindicated in patients showing a severe decrease in renal or hepatic function, or if marked sodium or water loss or active intracranial hemorrhage is present.

PARENTERAL SOLUTIONS THAT PROVIDE NOURISHMENT
Carbohydrate Solutions

These have already been described in the beginning of this chapter.

Alcohol Solutions
Physiological Properties

Intravenous alcohol can be used to supply calories because it is rapidly and completely metabolized. It therefore prevents carbohydrate, protein, and fat breakdown. It has also been used as a sedative and analgesic agent and can inhibit the secretion of ADH, the antidiuretic hormone.

Volume of Solution to Be Used

A total daily dose of 1000 to 2000 mL can be given.

Route of Administration

Alcohol solutions should be given only intravenously.

Rate of Administration

An adult can metabolize approximately 10 mL of pure alcohol per hour. This is equivalent to 200 mL of a 5% alcohol solution. Therefore, 200 to 300 mL of a 5% alcohol solution per hour can be given without causing symptoms of intoxication.

Solutions Available

Alcohol is available in a 5% solution with 5% dextrose in water.

One gram of ethyl alcohol provides 7.1 kcal. Therefore, 1 liter of a 5% alcohol, 5% dextrose solution will provide 525 kcal (50 g alcohol, 355 kcal; 50 g dextrose, 170 kcal) in contrast to 170 kcal that 1 liter of 5% dextrose would provide.

Alcohol solutions are contraindicated if shock is present, in epilepsy, or if severe liver or renal disease is present. There is potentiation of ethyl alcohol by sodium pentothal, and these two should not be given together.

Amino Acid Solutions

When a patient is receiving parenteral fluids for a day or a short time, it is not necessary to provide proteins. However, if parenteral fluid therapy is maintained more than 3 to 4 days, the patient should receive protein parenterally in the form of amino acids. One liter of a solution of 3.5% amino acid contains 5.5 g of nitrogen. This is the equivalent of 35 g of protein, or 140 kcal.

Side Effects

Patients with hepatic insufficiency may develop metabolic alkalosis, prerenal azotemia, hyperammonemia, stupor, and coma. Patients with impaired renal function may develop a marked rise in BUN. However, a modest rise in BUN occurs normally. Metabolic or respiratory alkalosis may be exacerbated because of the acetate ions in the amino acid solution. Also, amino acid preparations should be used in burn patients only during the convalescent phase.

Amino acid solutions may cause the following reactions especially if given at an excessive rate: nausea, vomiting, headache, flushing, chills, or fever. Local venous thrombosis may also occur.

Solutions Available

Numerous amino acid preparations are available. The 3.5% solution (without additives) is essentially isotonic. The 5% solution (without additives) is slightly hypertonic.

Amino acid solutions can be given in conjunction with 5% or 10% dextrose solutions or with intravenous fat emulsion.

Volume of Solution to Be Used

For peripheral IV infusion, 1 to 1.5 g/kg/day of total amino acids will achieve optimum sparing of protein catabolism. If one uses a 3.5% solution, 1 liter will contain 35 g of the amino acids. Therefore, if one decides to infuse 1 g/kg/day, a 70-kg (154 pound) patient will need 70 g of the amino acids, or 2 liters of the 3.5% solution daily.

Route of Administration

All amino acid preparations should be given IV.

Rate of Administration

One should calculate the amino acid and fluid needs per 24 hours and give the amino acid solution over a 24-hour period.

Fat Emulsions

Several fat emulsions are available for IV use that contain soybean or safflower oil stabilized with egg phosphotides and made isotonic with glycerol. The 10% emulsion supplies 1.1 kcal/mL of the emulsion. The 20% emulsion supplies 2 kcal/mL.

Indications

Fat emulsion can be used as a source of calories and essential fatty acids when a patient needs parenteral nutrition for an extended period (usually for more than 5 days).

Contraindications

Fat emulsion is contraindicated if a patient has a disturbance of normal fat metabolism, such as pathological hyperlipemia, lipoid nephrosis, or if the patient has acute pancreatitis accompanied by hyperlipemia. It must also be used cautiously if a patient has severe liver damage, pulmonary disease, anemia, a disorder of blood coagulation, or when there is danger of fat embolism.

Side Effects

These may be immediate (acute) or long-term (chronic).

Immediate side effects may include allergic reactions, hyperlipemia, dyspnea, cyanosis, flushing, dizziness, headache, sleepiness, nausea, vomiting, increased temperature, sweating, chest and back pain, thrombocytopenia, hypercoagulability, and transient increases in liver enzyme values.

Long-term side effects include hepatomegaly, jaundice due to central lobular-cholestasis, splenomegaly, thrombocytopenia, leukopenia, transient increases in liver enzyme values, *overloading syndrome* (which consists of focal convulsive seizures, fever, leukocytosis, splenomegaly, and shock), and the deposition of a brown "fat" pigment in the reticuloendothelial cells of the liver (the significance of which is unknown).

Other side effects include irritation at the site of the infusion, or thrombophlebitis. This can be avoided if the infusion site is changed every 12 hours.

Dosage and Administration

The fat emulsion can be given intravenously either through a peripheral vein or through a central venous catheter. The initial rate of infusion in adults for the first 15 minutes should be 1.0 mL/min for the 10% solution, or 0.5 mL/min for the 20% solution. If no adverse reactions occur (see Side Effects above) the infusion rate can be increased to allow no more than 500 mL of the 10% solution or 250 mL of the 20% solution to be given over a period of 4 to 6 hours.

The daily dosage of the fat emulsion should not exceed 2.5 g/kg body weight. In addition, it should provide no more than 60% of the total caloric intake of the patient. (The remaining 40% of the calories should be supplied by carbohydrates and amino acids.)

The fat emulsion should be infused separately from any other intravenously administered solution, to avoid disturbing the stability of the emulsion. However, it can be infused into the same peripheral vein as a carbohydrate or amino acid solution, by means of a Y-connector located near the infusion site. The flow rate of each solution should be controlled separately by infusion pumps. A filter should *not* be used with the fat emulsion.

Periodic liver function tests should be done when fat emulsions are used for a long term.

Peripheral Parenteral Nutrition

Total parenteral nutrition, using an amino acid solution with a concentrated dextrose solution, intravenously through a central venous catheter, is available. However, a 10% or 20% lipid emulsion in combination with a 10% dextrose solution and amino acid solution can be infused through a peripheral vein, if a patient is only moderately debilitated or cachectic. This procedure is known as *peripheral parenteral nutrition.* The following is an example of solutions that can be used:

Solution	kcalories
750 mL 10% fat emulsion (1.1. kcal/mL)	825
500 mL 10% dextrose (50 g) 3.5% in water (3.4 kcal/mL)	170
1000 mL 3.5% amino acid solution in 5% dextrose solution (50 g)	
35 g protein-equivalent (4 kcal/g)	140
50 g dextrose (3.4 kcal/g)	160
Total kcalories	1290

Bibliography

AMA Drug Evaluations, 5th ed., Chicago: American Medical Association, 1983.

American Hospital Formulary Service, Drug Information 84.

Borges, HF, et al: Mannitol intoxication in patients with renal failure. Arch Intern Med 142:63, 1982.

Blackburn, GL, et al: Peripheral intravenous feeding with isotonic amino acid solutions. Am J Surg 125:447, 1973.

Decaus, G, et al: Treatment of syndrome of inappropriate secretion of antidiuretic hormone by urea. Am J Med 69:99, 1980.

Diehl, JT, et al: Clinical comparison of hetastarch and albumin in postoperative cardiac patients. Surg Forum 32:260, 1981.

Clemetson, CAB, and Moshefghi, MM: Strange effects of "dextrose 5% in water." N Engl J Med 280:332, 1969.

Cooke, RE, and Crowley, LG: Replacement of gastric and intestinal fluid losses in surgery. N Engl J Med 246:637, 1952.

Crossley, K, and Matsen, JM: The scalp-vein needle. JAMA 220:985, 1972.

Darrow, DC, et al: Disturbances of water and electrolytes in infantile diarrhea. Pediatrics 3:129, 1949.

FDA Drug Bulletin: Users reminded about adverse reactions to dextran. 13:no. 3, Nov. 1983.

Felig, P: Intravenous nutrition. Fact and fancy. N Engl J Med 294:1455, 1976.

Flatau, E, and Resnitzky, P: Fatal anaphylactoid reaction after dextran 40 administration, letter. JAMA 243:1035, 1980.

Frazer, IH, et al: Is infusion phlebitis preventable? Br Med J 2:232, 1977.

Freeman, JB, et al: The current status of protein sparing. Surg Gynecol Obstet 144:843, 1977.

Fye, WB: Sydney Ringer, calcium, and cardiac function. Circulation 69:849, 1984.

Grady, GF: Transfusions and hepatitis. Update in '78. N Engl J Med 298:1413, 1978.

Grindon, AJ: The use of packed red blood cells. JAMA 235:389, 1976.

Hanson, SM: Ringer, Hartmann, and their solutions. JAMA 204:272, 1968.

Hartmann, AF, et al: Further observations on metabolism and clinical uses of sodium lactate. J Pediatr 13:692, 1938.

Hartmann, AF, and Senn, MJE: Studies on the metabolism of sodium-r-lactate. J Clin Invest 11:327, 337, 345, 1932.

Heller, WM: Ringer. JAMA 207:2103, 1969.

Kohen, M, Mattikow, M, and Middleton, E, Jr: Study of three untoward reactions to dextran. J Allerg 46:109, 1970.

Letters to the Editor: pH of intravenous solution. N Engl J Med 280:900, 1969.

Mailloux, L, et al: Acute renal failure after administration of low molecular weight dextran. N Engl J Med 277;1113, 1967.

Makim, DG, Goldmann, DA, and Rhame, FS: Infection control in intravenous therapy. Ann Intern Med 79:867, 1973.

Mead, WB: Particles in intravenous fluids. N Engl J Med 287:1152, 1972.

Nahas, GG: Tris buffer vs sodium bicarbonate. N Engl J Med 275:1024, 1966.

Oliver, WJ, Graham, BD, and Wilson, JL: Lack of scientific validity of body surface as basis for parenteral fluid dosage. JAMA 167:1211, 1958.

Questions and Answers: Parenteral fluids by hypodermoclysis to elderly patients may be hazardous. JAMA 226:1127, 1973.

Sarma, DP: Use of blood in elective surgery. JAMA 243:1536, 1980.

Siberman, H, et al: Parenteral nutrition with lipids. JAMA 238:1380, 1977.

Talbot, NB, Crawford, JD, and Butler, AM: Medical progress; homeostatic limits to safe parenteral fluid therapy. N Engl J Med 248:1100, 1953.

Talbot, NB, et al: Medical progress; application of homeostatic principles to the practice of parenteral fluid therapy. N Engl J Med 252:856, 1955.

The Medical Letter: Parenteral water and electrolyte solutions. 12:19, 1970.

The Medical Letter: Plastic containers for intravenous solutions. 17, no. 10, May 9, 1975.

Tse, RL, and Lee, MW: pH of infusion fluids. A predisposing factor in thrombophlebitis. JAMA 215:642, 1971.

Tullis, JL: Albumin, 1. Background and use. 2. Guidelines for clinical use. JAMA 237:355, and 460, 1977.

Turco, S, and Davis, NM: Glass particles in intravenous injections. N Engl J Med 287:1204, 1972.

Vidt, DG: Use and abuse of intravenous solutions. JAMA 232:533, 1975.

Wakim, KG: "Normal" 0.9% salt solution is neither "normal" nor physiological. JAMA 214:1710, 1970.

Weisberg, HF: Osmolarity of parenteral fluids. JAMA 194:471, 1965.

Zintel, HA, Rhoads, JE, and Ravdin, IS: Use of intravenous ammonium chloride in treatment of alkalosis. Surgery 14:728, 1943.

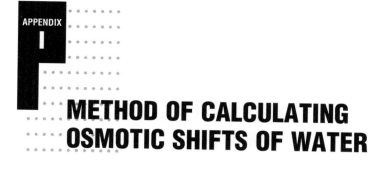

METHOD OF CALCULATING
OSMOTIC SHIFTS OF WATER

The osmotic shift of water in Figure 2–3 (page 19) can be calculated from the osmotic formula:

Osmotic concentration × volume = total osmolality

In the NaCl compartment, 14 liters of sodium chloride is present with an osmolal concentration of 290 mOsm/L, and a total osmolality of 14 × 290 = 4060 mOsm.

In the K_2HPO_4 compartment, 28 liters of potassium phosphate is present, with an osmolal concentration of 310 mOsm/L, and a total osmolality of 28 × 310 = 8680 mOsm.

The total volume of solution is therefore 14 + 28 = 42 liters, with a total osmolality of 4060 + 8680 = 12,740 mOsm.

When osmotic equilibrium occurs, the 12,740 mOsm will be equally divided among the 42 liters, giving an average osmolal concentration of 12,740/42 = 303 mOsm/L.

The 4060 mOsm will remain in the NaCl compartment but will be now contained in 4060/303 = 13.4 liters.

The 8680 mOsm will remain in the K_2HPO_4 compartment, but will now be contained in 8680/303 = 28.6 liters.

In other words, the NaCl solution has a lower osmotic pressure than the K_2HPO_4 solution. Therefore, 0.6 liter of water will flow from the NaCl solution to the K_2HPO_4 solution to equalize the osmotic pressure in this example.

APPENDIX II

CALCULATION OF THE OSMOTIC SHIFT OF WATER WHICH OCCURS AS A RESULT OF WATER LOSS

Figure A1*A* shows the normal volumes of extracellular and cellular water in a 70-kg male. (The total body water volume is 60% of the body weight: $0.6 \times 70 = 42$ liters. The extracellular water is 20% of the body weight: $0.2 \times 70 = 14$ L; $42 - 14 = 28$ L, the volume of the cellular water.)

Notice that the osmolality of both the extracellular and cellular water is the same, namely, 310 mOsm/L, and the serum sodium concentration is 142 mEq/L. The total osmolality of the extracellular water equals the osmolal concentration per liter times the volume of the extracellular water: $310 \times 14 = 4340$ mOsm. The total osmolality of the cellular water also equals the osmolal concentration per liter times the cellular water volume: $310 \times 28 = 8680$ mOsm. The body water equals $4340 + 8680 = 13,020$ mOsm.

In Figure A1*B*, 3 liters of extracellular water has been lost. Osmotic equilibrium has not yet occurred. Notice that the volume of the extracellular water has decreased to 11 liters, and its osmolal concentration has increased to 394 mOsm/L. (The reason for this is that only water [but no electrolytes] has been lost.) Therefore, 4340 mOsm is now contained in 11 liters. This gives a concentration of $4340/11 = 394$ mOsm/L. Notice also that the serum sodium concentration has also risen proportionately to 180 mEq/L:

$$142:X = 310:394$$

$$X = \frac{142 \times 394}{310} = 180$$

382

Notice also that the osmotic pressure of the extracellular water (394 mOsm/L) is now greater than that of the cells, which is still 310 mOsm/L.

Figure A1 C shows the volume and osmolal changes after water has flowed from the cells to the extracellular water. The new osmolal concentration in the extracellular water and in the cells can be calculated from the following osmotic formula:

Osmolal concentration $\times$ volume = total osmolality.

Because 3 liters of water has been lost, the total volume of body water is now $42 - 3 = 39$ liters. The total osmolality of the extracellular and cellular water remains the same as before the water loss, namely, 13,010 mOsm.

The formula can now be rewritten:

$$\text{Osmolal concentration} \times \text{volume} = \text{total osmolality}$$
$$X \times 39 \quad = 13{,}010$$
$$X = \frac{13{,}010}{39} = 334 \text{ mOsm/L}$$

Just as the osmolality falls from 394 to 334 mOsm/L, the serum sodium concentration also falls proportionately from 180 to 152 mEq/L ($180 : X = 394 : 334$).

The osmotic formula can now be used to calculate the volumes of extracellular and cellular water that are present after osmotic equilibrium occurs:

$$\text{Osmotic concentration} \times \text{volume } V = \text{total osmolality}$$
$$334 \times V = 4340$$
$$V = \frac{4340}{334} = 13 \text{ liters (extracellular water)}$$
$$334 \times V = 8680$$
$$V = 26 \text{ liters (cellular water)}$$

Normal

	A
14 L 310 mOsm/L 4340 mOsm ECW Serum Na 142 mEq/L	28 L 310 mOsm/L 8680 mOsm Cellular water

Water loss— 3 liters
before osmotic equilibrium

	B
11 L 394 mOsm/L 4340 mOsm Serum Na 180 mEq/L	No change

Water loss
after osmotic equilibrium

	C
13 L 334 mOsm/L 4340 mOsm Serum Na 152 mEq/L	26 L 334 mOsm/L 8680 mOsm

FIGURE A1. Diagrams showing the effect of water loss on osmotic equilibrium. See text.

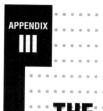

THE AMOUNT OF SODIUM CHLORIDE NEEDED TO RAISE THE SERUM SODIUM CONCENTRATION BY 10 mEq/L

To raise the serum sodium concentration by 10 mEq/L, a volume of 5% sodium chloride solution should be given that is equal (in mL) to 6 times the patient's weight in kilograms.

This rule is derived in the following way: Even though the sodium chloride is confined to the extracellular water, it causes a shift of water between the cells and the extracellular water when it is either added to, or removed from, the extracellular water. Therefore, its osmotic effect is distributed throughout the entire volume of body water.

Example: Man, weighing 70 kg. Total body water is 60% of the body weight, or 42 liters. The extracellular water volume is 20% of the body weight, or 14 liters; the cellular water is 40% of the body weight, or 28 liters.

If the serum sodium concentration is 132 mEq/L, this represents a deficiency of 10 mEq/L (142, normal − 132). This is equivalent to a deficit of 20 mOsm/L (because sodium chloride ionizes into sodium and chloride ions). Since the normal osmolal concentration is 310 mOsm/L, the present osmolal concentration must be 290 mOsm/L. Furthermore, since the extracellular water volume is 14 liters, there is a deficit of 20 × 14 = 280 mOsm/L in the extracellular water.

When sodium chloride is added, it will increase the osmolality of the extracellular water above that of the cells. As a result, pure water will flow from the cells into the extracellular water. Therefore, as Welt has pointed out, enough sodium chloride must also be added to raise the osmolality of this water to 310 mOsm/L. Since the initial volume of the cell water in this patient is 28 liters, and its osmotic concentration is 290 mOsm/L, the cells have a total of 28 × 290 = 8120 mOsm. When water flows from the cells to the extracellular water, the osmotic concentration of the cells will be raised to 310 mOsm/L.

Using the osmotic formula (Appendix I), we know that:

$$\text{Osmotic concentration} \times \text{volume V} = \text{total osmolality}$$

$$310 \times V = 8120$$

$$V = \frac{8120}{310} = 26.194 \text{ liters of cell water}$$

Therefore, the volume of water that flow out of the cells is 28 − 26.194 = 1.806 liters.

Since the osmolality of these 1.806 liters must be raised from 0 to 310 mOsm/L, it will require 310 × 1.806 = 560 mOsm of sodium chloride.

The total sodium chloride requirement is therefore:

280 mOsm to raise the extracellular water osmolality from 290 to 310 mOsm/L, plus 560 mOsm of sodium chloride to raise the osmolality of the pure water that flows from the cells to the extracellular water from 0 to 310 mOsm/L.

280 + 560 = 840 mOsm of sodium chloride is needed. This is equivalent to 840/2 = 420 millimoles or milliequivalents of sodium chloride.

Notice that the value 420 mEq is identical with that obtained by multiplying the patient's weight by the factor 6.

Since 420 mEq of sodium chloride is contained in 420 mL of 5.85% sodium chloride, 420 mL of 5.85% sodium chloride solution will raise the serum sodium concentration by 10 mEq/L. (A 5.85% solution of NaCl contains 58.5 g/L. Since the molecular weight of NaCl is 58.5 [Na, 23; Cl, 35.5], each milliliter of 5.85% NaCl contains 1 mEq Na.)

It should also be pointed out that all of these calculations are merely approximations and do not represent absolute amounts or volumes of sodium chloride that must be used. In addition, the above calculations assume that 420 mEq of solid sodium chloride has been added. However, the sodium chloride is dissolved in 420 mL of water. This will also dilute the body water and cause the serum sodium concentration to rise less than 10 mEq/L.

As has been pointed out earlier, the body is not a closed system. As soon as the hypertonic sodium chloride solution is infused, the blood volume rises, aldosterone secretion stops, and the kidneys begin to excrete this excess sodium. However, the sodium is infused in a hypertonic solution, but is excreted in urine of lower sodium concentration. As a result, a large amount of water is excreted along with the sodium. This also causes the serum sodium concentration to rise.

Bibliography

Spital, A, and Sterns, RD: The paradox of sodium's volume of distribution: Why an extracellular solute appears to distribute over total body water. Commentaries. Arch Intern Med 149:1255, 1989.

Welt, LG: *Clinical Disorders of Hydration and Acid-Base Balance.* Boston: Little Brown, 1955.

Wynn, V: The osmotic behavior of the body cells in man. Lancet 2:1212, 1957.

THE EFFECT OF HYPERGLYCEMIA ON THE SERUM SODIUM CONCENTRATION

Since glucose does not penetrate cell membranes passively, it has an osmotic pressure. However, its normal concentration in the blood (100 mg/dL) is relatively low. Therefore, it does not normally exert a significant osmotic pressure. However, in a patient with severe diabetes mellitus, for example, where the blood glucose concentration may be very high, the glucose will exert a significant osmotic pressure. This will cause the osmotic pressure of the extracellular water to rise above that of the cells, and the serum osmolality will rise.

As a result, water will flow from the cells to the extracellular water, which will become diluted. This will lower the concentration, not only of glucose, but of all the electrolytes. As a result, the serum sodium concentration may appear to be low. This really represents a dilutional effect and not a true decrease or loss of sodium.

The following rule can be used to determine the effect of hyperglycemia on the serum sodium concentration:

The serum sodium concentration will decrease 1.6 mEq/L for each 100 mg/dL increase of serum glucose concentration (above the normal level of 100 mg/dL).

Proof of this is as follows (Katz): When the serum glucose concentration rises, it increases the osmolality of the blood and extracellular water above that of the cells. Therefore, water flows from the cells into the extracellular water to equalize this difference. As the water flows from the cells, the osmolality of the extracellular water will decrease and the osmolality of the cells will increase, until a point is reached when the extra and intracellular osmolalities will be equal. This point can be calculated from the osmotic formula: osmotic concentration × volume = total osmolality.

Example: Patient's weight, 70 kg; serum sodium concentration, 140 mEq/L; blood glucose concentration, 100 mg/dL. (5.5 mOsm/L): *plasma (and cell) osmolality, 285 mOsm/L.

If 1000 mOsm glucose are now added to the blood and extracellular water (assuming that the water in which the glucose is dissolved has negligible volume), the osmolality of the blood and extracellular water will rise as follows:

Since the extracellular water is 20% of body weight, a 70-kg person has $70 \times 0.2 = 14$ liters of extracellular water (and a total of $285 \times 14 = 3990$ mOsm).

Since the cell water is 40% of body weight, this person has $70 \times 0.4 = 28$ liters of cell water (and a total of $285 \times 28 = 7980$ mOsm).

The total body water is therefore $14 + 28 = 42$ liters (and a total of $3990 + 7980 = 11,970$ mOsm).

When the 1000 mOsm glucose are added, the total body water osmolality increases to 12,970 mOsm. However, this is still contained in 42 liters of body water. Therefore, each liter of body water now contains $12,970/42 = 308.8$ mOsm/L.

The cell water that originally contained 7980 mOsm in 28 liters now has $7980/308.8 = 25.8$ liters — a loss of 2.2 liters, which have moved to the extracellular water. The extracellular water volume now is therefore $14 + 2.2 = 16.2$ liters.

The final serum glucose concentration is therefore

$$\frac{1000 + (5.5 \times 14)}{16.2} = 66.48 \text{ mOsm/L, or } 1197 \text{ mg/dL}$$

The final serum sodium concentration is $(140 \times 14)/16.2 = 121$ mEq/L.

When these results are repeated for different amounts of added glucose, the results indicate that the serum sodium concentration decreases 1.6 mEq/L for each 100 mg/dL rise in serum glucose concentration (above a normal level of 100 mg/dL).

Bibliography

Crandall, ED: Serum sodium response to hyperglycemia. N Engl J Med 290:465, 1974.

Jenkins, PG, and Larmore, C: Hyperglycemia-induced hyponatremia. N Engl J Med 290:573, 1974.

Katz, MA: Hyperglycemia-induced hyponatremia. Calculation of expected serum sodium depression. N Engl J Med 289:843, 1973.

Robin, AP, Ing, TS, et al: Hyperglycemia-induced hyponatremia. A fresh look. Clin Chem 125:496, 1979.

---

*The molecular weight of glucose is 180. Therefore, 1 mOsm equals 180 mg, and a concentration of 5.5 mOsm/L is equivalent to a concentration of 100 mg/dL.

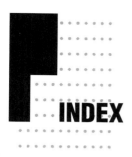

INDEX

A "t" or an "f" following a page number indicates a table or a figure, respectively.

DATE DUE

GAYLORD   PRINTED IN U.S.A.